T0323380

BRAIN–MIND

Brain–Mind

FROM NEURONS TO CONSCIOUSNESS AND CREATIVITY

Paul Thagard

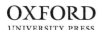

OXFORD
UNIVERSITY PRESS

Oxford University Press is a department of the University of Oxford. It furthers
the University's objective of excellence in research, scholarship, and education
by publishing worldwide. Oxford is a registered trade mark of Oxford University
Press in the UK and certain other countries.

Published in the United States of America by Oxford University Press
198 Madison Avenue, New York, NY 10016, United States of America.

Library of Congress Cataloging-in-Publication Data
Names: Thagard, Paul, author.
Title: Brain–mind : from neurons to consciousness and creativity / Paul Thagard.
Description: New York, NY : Oxford University Press, [2019] |
Includes bibliographical references and index.
Identifiers: LCCN 2018033233 | ISBN 9780190678715
Subjects: LCSH: Cognitive neuroscience. | Mind and body.
Classification: LCC QP360.5 T43 2019 | DDC 612.8/233—dc23
LC record available at https://lccn.loc.gov/2018033233

9 8 7 6 5 4 3 2 1

Printed by Sheridan Books, Inc., United States of America

To Chris, for pointing to the best semantics.

Contents

List of Illustrations

Foreword

Frank E. Ritter

THREE DECADES AGO, Newell, Anderson, and Simon shared a desire for a unified theory of how cognition arises and what a mechanistic explanation would look like. Today, much still remains to be done to pursue that desire, but much has been accomplished.

Allen Newell talked about narrow and deep theories, and broad and shallow theories, and that theories could differ in these ways. Many psychology theories are deep, explaining a few phenomena in great detail but not explaining many phenomena nor how they interact and mutually constrain each other.

In the trio of books making up his treatise, Paul Thagard creates a much broader and more accessible explanation than we have seen before of what a mechanistic explanation of mind and human behavior would look like. These books explain the cognitive science approach to cognition, learning, thinking, emotion, and social interaction—much of what it means to be human—and what this means for a wide variety of sciences and philosophy. His treatise provides a good overview of cognitive science and its implications. Different readers will be drawn to the treatise in different ways. It does not matter where they start. In this book, *Brain–Mind*, Thagard explains how the semantic pointer architecture (SPA) by Chris Eliasmith, Thagard's colleague at the University of Waterloo, can be used to explain the mind, cognition, and related concepts. The SPA architecture is a very useful dynamic theory that can do multiple tasks in the same model, and it is explained in journal articles and by Eliasmith's (2013) book in the Oxford Series on Cognitive Models and Architectures. Most of the implications based on SPA are also supported by and have lessons for other computational models of cognition, so these books can be useful to users of other cognitive architectures.

In his book, _Mind–Society,_ Thagard examines what this approach means for social science and related professional fields, and the mechanisms account for successes and failures of major professional activities. In his book, _Natural Philosophy,_ he examines what this approach means for philosophy, including important topics of philosophy of mind and of beauty. This book provides a useful and engaging overview of philosophy, particularly for those interested in cognitive science or working in cognitive science.

These books introduce several useful theories and methods about how to do science as well. Beyond allowing and using explanations via multilevel mechanisms, particularly helpful are Thagard's introduction and use of three-analysis for definitions and coherence. The three-analysis definitions are a way to explain concepts without using simple definitions. They define a concept using _exemplars, typical features,_ and _explanations._ This approach resolves several problems with simple dictionary definitions.

Also valuable is the development of coherence as a concept for reasoning. Coherence is used in this book as a way to describe the quality of theories—that theories are not just good when they predict a single result, but how they cohere with multiple sources of data and with other theories. Coherence is hard to quantify itself, but it is clearly useful. But the use of coherence is not just normative—we should use it—it is also descriptive in that scientists and laypersons appear to already use it, at least implicitly. Making the use of coherence explicit will help us to apply, teach, and improve the process.

Not only will these books be helpful to cognitive scientists and those interested in cognitive science, they will also appeal to those who simply want to learn more about the world and cognition—they offer one of the best and broadest explanations we have for cognition. Thus, humanists and social scientists interested in knowing how cognitive science works will find some answers here.

These books contain powerful ideas by one of the most highly cited living philosophers. They can change the way you think about the world, including brains and mind, and how you might think that the mind works and interacts with the world. Thagard calls these trio of books a treatise, and I found them so compelling that I've decided to use them in a course this next semester.

REFERENCE

Eliasmith, C. (2013). _How to build a brain: A neural architecture for biological cognition._ New York, NY: Oxford University Press.

Preface

THIS BOOK BELONGS to a trio (Treatise on Mind and Society) that can be read independently:

Brain–Mind: From Neurons to Consciousness and Creativity
Mind–Society: From Brains to Social Sciences and Professions
Natural Philosophy: From Social Brains to Knowledge, Reality, Morality, and Beauty.

Brain–Mind presents a unified, brain-based theory of cognition and emotion with applications to the most complex kinds of thinking, right up to consciousness and creativity. Unification comes from systematic application of Chris Eliasmith's powerful Semantic Pointer Architecture, a highly original synthesis of neural network and symbolic ideas about how the mind works. I show the relevance of semantic pointers to a full range of important kinds of mental representations, from sensations and imagery to concepts, rules, analogies, and emotions. Neural mechanisms can then be used to explain many phenomena concerning consciousness, action, intention, language, creativity, and the self.

Because of their broad importance, I have tried to make Chris's ideas accessible to a broad audience with no special background in neuroscience or mathematics. For readability, I have omitted references from the main text, but extensive citations are in the Notes section at the end of each chapter. These references also point to papers that provide the mathematical and computational details too technical for general presentation. Most of my papers can be found via paulthagard. com, which also contains live links for the URLs in this book.

The value of a unified theory of thinking goes well beyond psychology, neuroscience, and the other cognitive sciences. *Mind–Society* melds the mental mechanisms in this book with complementary social mechanisms to explain a wide range of social phenomena. The result is an integrated account of six social sciences (social psychology, sociology, politics, economics, anthropology, and history) and five professions (medicine, law, education, engineering, and business). *Natural Philosophy* considers the implications for the humanities of the resulting account of mind, brain, and society. The main topic is philosophy, with a systematic treatment of fundamental questions about knowledge, reality, morality, and meaning. But the book also shows the relevance of neural-social explanations to the arts, especially painting and music.

The goal of this trio of books is to harmonize the cognitive sciences, social sciences, professions, and humanities as a coherent system of thought, not to reduce one to the other. I call my general approach *social cognitivism*, because it combines cognitive neuroscience (including a heavy emphasis on emotions) with social processes of communication. Social cognitivism is not a new field but rather an integrated theoretical approach to thought, society, and values.

Brain–Mind has a distant ancestor in my textbook *Mind: Introduction to Cognitive Science* (first edition, 1996; second edition, 2005). That book covered some of the same ground by considering different kinds of cognitive theories (e.g., rules and neural networks) and several challenges to the whole enterprise of cognitive science (e.g., consciousness and embodiment). The last decade has brought major advances that make it now possible to unify what were once disparate theoretical approaches and to provide plausible answers to all of the challenges.

Acknowledgments

MOST OF THIS book was newly written in 2014–2018, but I have incorporated some extracts from other works, as indicated in the notes and in the figure and table captions. I have also used some paragraphs from my *Psychology Today* blog, *Hot Thought*, for which I hold the copyright.

I have benefitted enormously from the ideas of numerous collaborators, especially Chris Eliasmith, Tobias Schröder, and Terry Stewart. I am grateful for 23 years of grant support from the Natural Sciences and Engineering Research Council of Canada. My students in PHIL 371 furnished valuable corrections to an earlier draft, especially Lucas Connors and Louise Upton. For helpful suggestions, I am grateful to William Bechtel, Richard Carlson, Shawn Clark, Christopher Dancy, William Kennedy, Laurette Larocque, Marcin Milkowski, Jonathan Morgan, Steve Read, Frank Ritter, Jose Soto, and anonymous reviewers. I thank Joan Bossert for editorial advice, Phil Velinov and Shanmuga Priya for organizing production, Alisa Larson for skilled copyediting, and Kevin Broccoli for professional indexing. CBC Radio 2 and Apple Music provided the accompaniment.

1

What Are Minds?

Marvin Minsky wrote: "What magical trick makes us intelligent? The trick is that there is no trick. The power of intelligence stems from our vast diversity, not from any single, perfect principle." This book will argue that the diversity of mind that makes people intelligent comes from different kinds of mental structures such as images, concepts, rules, analogies, and emotions. But this diversity has an underlying unity, because all of these structures come from the same basic set of brain processes. Intelligence—the capacity to solve problems, learn, understand, reason, act, and manage other mental functions—requires neural mechanisms for representation, transformation, and competition. All these mechanisms employ special neural entities that Chris Eliasmith calls *semantic pointers*, whose operation will be explained in chapter 2.

Why should you care about how the mind works? The answer is easy if you are interested in topics like these: good decisions, personal relationships, mental health, language, emotions, consciousness, free will, creativity, politics, economics, history, literature, music, religion, artificial intelligence, robots, or human–machine interaction. Engaging in these concerns requires a mind that enables you to think about what you are doing when you pursue them on your own or through interactions with other people. Knowing how the mind works, and why it sometimes fails to work well, should help you to understand the successes and failures of people in the full range of human pursuits.

Perhaps you think you already know how minds work, just from having experience with your own thoughts and ability to speak about mental ideas such as *belief, desire*, and *feeling*. That assumption would make you as naïve as people who think they can understand the world without any knowledge of physics, chemistry, and biology. Introspection and ordinary language are as limited in what they can tell us about mental operations as they are about topics such as gravity, chemical bonds, and natural selection. Fortunately, great progress has been made in the interdisciplinary field of cognitive science that provides insights into how minds work and sometimes fail. This book describes basic neural mechanisms that can explain the full range of human thinking, from problem solving to emotions and consciousness.

WHAT ARE MINDS?

Dictionary definitions of the word "mind" are not very informative, making vague reference to whatever makes people capable of thinking, perceiving, willing, feeling, and so on. As chapter 4 argues, we usually do not understand concepts by giving them strict definitions but rather by identifying exemplars (standard examples), typical features, and explanations. What I call "three-analysis" is the method of characterizing a concept by specifying these three aspects rather than by giving a definition using necessary and sufficient conditions. Let us now apply three-analysis to the concept of mind by examining its exemplars, features, and explanations. Table 1.1 provides a concise summary.

Exemplars for minds are easy to find. Just consider yourself and all the people you know, ignoring the philosopher who responded to the question, "Are there other minds?" by saying, "Not many." You and your friends are all examples of having a mind. For now, we should not ignore the possibility that nonhuman

TABLE 1.1

Three-Analysis of *Mind*	
Exemplars	People including you and everyone you know, and advanced nonhuman animals such as chimps
Typical features	Sensing, perceiving, learning, thinking, deciding, feeling, acting, problem solving, communicating
Explanations	Explains: behaviors, experiences
	Explained by: neural mechanisms?

animals such as chimpanzees and dogs also have minds, and we should not rule out the possibility that computers and space aliens might also turn out to have minds. But it is better first to focus on the many good examples of minds in people we know, including you, your mother, and even Justin Bieber.

Typical features of these minds include capacities for

1. sensing the external world by seeing, smelling, touching, tasting, and hearing.
2. sensing internal bodily states such as pain, hunger, balance, and heat.
3. perceiving recognizable objects in the world.
4. thinking to solve problems, make decisions, and reason.
5. feeling emotions.
6. having conscious experiences.
7. having intentions and performing actions.

These capabilities should not be taken as definitional, for there may be simple minds that lack some of them, but a majority belong to most exemplars of minds. Capacities are dispositions to behave in various ways in various circumstances, as the result of underlying causal mechanisms.

We frequently use concepts to explain important observations, and we also look for explanations of the phenomena described using the concept. The six features just listed enable minds to figure prominently in explanations of why people behave the ways they do, because their behavior is caused by their sensations, thoughts, emotions, and intentions. For example, we can explain why two people got married by supposing that they love each other, where love is an emotional mental state.

To take these explanations beyond the superficial ones used in everyday life, we need a theory that tells us what minds are and how they work. For example, the concept of love becomes much richer if we can explain what makes two people fall in love. Here are some historically important claims about the nature of mind.

1. Minds are souls. This theory is assumed by religions such as Christianity, Islam, and Hinduism that presuppose that minds survive death, which requires that minds be separable from mortal bodies.
2. Minds are fictions. Behaviorism, which dominated psychology from the 1920s through the 1950s, claimed that science requires avoiding postulating nonobservable entities like mental states and processes and should only study how behavior is shaped by physical environments.

3. Minds are computers. The development of computational ideas in the 1940s and 1950s provided a new way of understanding how minds work by analogy to computer programs. On this view, thinking is not just analogous to computing—it *is* computing.

4. Minds are brains. Rapidly increasing knowledge about how brains operate using billions of neurons has encouraged the identification of mental operations with neural processes.

5. Minds are dynamical systems. A dynamical system is a collection of interacting objects and states whose changes are describable by mathematical equations. Minds are embodied systems capable of perception and action.

6. Minds are social constructions. Thinking should not be understood as a capability of isolated individuals but rather as the result of interactions among people who are part of a society.

Depending on your background, you may view one of these theories as obviously true and the others as ridiculous.

We shall see that these views are not as incompatible as they might seem. The first theory does conflict with a scientific approach to the mind, because it places mind beyond the standard scientific tools of experiment and theorizing. In contrast, the other five ways have affinities. My main emphasis in this book will be on the fourth theory—that minds are brains—but we will also see the relevance of ideas about behavior, computation, dynamical systems, and social interactions. The theory that minds are brains can be greatly enriched by understanding how neural operations employ representations and computations to help us interact dynamically with the world and other people.

COGNITIVE SCIENCE

Cognitive science is the interdisciplinary investigation of mind and intelligence, combining insights from psychology, neuroscience, linguistics, philosophy, anthropology, and computer modeling. It began intellectually in the 1950s when visionaries such as Herbert Simon, Marvin Minsky, and George Miller realized that understanding the mind could not be accomplished using the ideas and methods from any single field. This realization was institutionalized in the 1970s when the term "cognitive science" was coined and the Cognitive Science Society was formed. Today, cognitive science is a thriving interdisciplinary enterprise with multiple journals, annual conferences, and programs at many universities worldwide.

The first key assumption of cognitive science is that the mind can be studied scientifically by combining experimental studies and theoretical explanations of the results of those studies. This assumption rules out the claim that minds are supernatural entities like the souls assumed by many religions and also the claim that the mind is just too complicated to be subject to scientific explanation. The second key assumption of cognitive science is that no one field such as psychology, neuroscience, or philosophy has a monopoly on the ideas and methods needed to gain a full understanding of mind. Rather, cognitive science requires embracing and synthesizing ideas and methods from many fields.

This book will treat cognitive science as the integration of disciplinary insights, not just the sum of what various disciplines have learned about the mind. A third key assumption of cognitive science, shared by the theories that minds are computers and that minds are brains, is that mental operations can be understood in terms of representations and processes that operate on them. The next section will describe how these explain mental activities.

First, I want to provide a brief introduction to the main fields that currently constitute cognitive science. The most ancient is *philosophy*, which has been concerned with the nature of mind since the ancient Greek thinkers, Plato and Aristotle. Like many later philosophers, Plato tried to understand the mind by abstract reasoning alone, using thought experiments to determine how the mind *must* work. Aristotle's approach to mind was more biological, and many subsequent philosophers, from Locke and Hume to many current ones, have tried to tie the understanding of mind to scientific findings. From a cognitive science perspective, the most valuable contributions of philosophers have been their concerns with generality, dealing with broad questions about the nature of mind that cross many disciplines, and with normativity, dealing with how minds should work better as well as with the descriptive question of how they do work. On this view, the best method for philosophers is to integrate and reflect on scientific advances, rather than to delude themselves that thought experiments alone can provide information about the mind.

Psychology emerged as an experimental field distinct from philosophy in the 1870s. Led by pioneers such as Wilhelm Wundt and William James, psychology shared philosophy's concern with mental states but adopted a different method of systematic observations and careful experimentation, with theories aimed at explaining these findings. During the first half of the twentieth century, psychology became dominated by behaviorism, the doctrine that a scientific approach to mind should avoid theorizing about mental states and processes and stick to understanding how environmental stimuli produce behavioral responses. One of the spurs to the cognitive revolution that hit psychology in the 1950s was growing realization that even the behavior of rats could not be explained without considering mental processes. Today, psychologists still conduct behavioral experiments but often combine them with neural measurements and computational theorizing.

Modern *neuroscience* began in the 1880s with the realization by Santiago Ramón y Cajal that brain functioning is due to cells that were later called neurons. Neural explanations of thinking were thin, however, until the 1980s when two major developments occurred that produced the rise of a new subfield, cognitive neuroscience. The first experimental development was the introduction of new techniques for neuroimaging, including positron emission tomography and functional magnetic resonance imagery (fMRI). The second theoretical development was the creation of new mathematical techniques for studying neural networks and modeling how groups of neurons can carry out complex cognitive functions. The next chapter will describe in more detail how basic ideas from cognitive neuroscience explain mental processes.

The scientific study of language is called *linguistics*, which has a big place in cognitive science because of the importance of language in human thought and communication. At the same time as psychologists were beginning to throw off the shackles of behaviorism, Noam Chomsky attacked behaviorist accounts of human language and began to develop alternative theories that explained human linguistic capabilities in terms of mental representations of syntactic structure. Subsequently, linguists have moved beyond syntax (grammatical structure) to also consider semantics (meaning) and pragmatics (purpose and context). The brain is a marvelous engine for integrating syntax, semantics, and pragmatics in the generation and comprehension of language. Linguists use various methods including the collection of grammatical intuitions of speakers of one language and the cross-cultural investigation of differences in the thousands of languages spoken worldwide.

The social aspects of language are also part of anthropology, which studies the origins, distribution, social relations, and culture of human beings. Culture is the way of life of a society, including its beliefs and behaviors. Whereas philosophy, psychology, neuroscience, and linguistics have largely been concerned with thinking in individuals, anthropology recognizes that cognition also has many important social dimensions. Along with sociology, economics, and political science, anthropology helps to expand the study of cognition to encompass social mechanisms that enable people to function in groups and to accomplish tasks that would be beyond the capabilities of any individual. Anthropology thus overlaps with social psychology, which has become increasingly concerned with cultural matters.

The final major field contributing to cognitive science is *computer modeling*. The introduction of computational ideas in the 1940s and 1950s provided new theoretical ideas for understanding mental processes, and computers also contributed a new method. Building and testing theories about the mind is difficult because mental operations are not easily captured by a few mathematical equations. Instead, researchers can write computer programs that incorporate theoretical claims about thinking and then run the programs to see whether they produce results similar to what people do. A crucial part of the rise of cognitive science in the 1950s was the creation of the new field of artificial intelligence, which tries to get computers to perform tasks that require intelligence when people do them. There has been a regular flow of ideas among computer modeling, psychology, and neuroscience that has contributed to all three. Computational ideas from artificial intelligence have stimulated theorizing in psychology and neuroscience, while attention to how minds and brains work has suggested new computational approaches. Computer modeling is also now contributing to the understanding of social processes because computers can simulate the interaction of multiple intelligent agents.

Later chapters will provide much more information about the ideas, methods, and interactions of these six fields that contribute to cognitive science. We will see how the investigation of all kinds of thinking, from perception to high-level reasoning, can benefit from integrated multidisciplinary insights. The six disciplines just mentioned are the main contributors to the theories and methods of cognitive science, but many other fields are relevant, from professional areas such as education and law to humanistic areas such as literature and music.

REPRESENTATIONS AND PROCESSES

To understand how minds work from a cognitive science perspective, you need to grasp two central ideas: representation and process. A representation is something that stands for something, and the most familiar kinds of representations are words. I follow the convention of using quotes to indicate linguistic entities such as words and sentences, and italics to indicate mental representations such as concepts. For example, the word "tree" stands for trees in the world, which your mind understands using the concept *tree*. Verbal representations can be combined into sentences, as when someone says that "A tree grows in the forest," which is a representation that stands for a state of affairs in the world. It is a mistake, however, to suppose that all representations are verbal. A picture of a tree is also a representation of it, as is a heard sound that reproduces the rustling of leaves. In a computer, a representation might just be a string of zeros and ones that also stands for trees. Many kinds of visual representations are in everyday use, such as maps, diagrams, and clocks.

To explain thinking, we need to consider representations that operate inside people's heads when they use a mental state or process to stand for something else. Here are some examples of mental representations that you can easily acquire: the look of the Eiffel Tower, the smell of grass, the taste of wine, the touch of sandpaper, the sound of a guitar, the sadness of losing a friend, the joy of winning a contest, the feeling of pain, and the urgency of a full bladder. Like words, these representations can be combined, as when you imagine yourself drinking wine on the lawn in front of the Eiffel Tower after winning a race with sore feet. Behaviorists rejected the existence of mental representations because they cannot be directly observed, but science often proposes nonobservable entities such as electrons and black holes that are accepted because they provide good explanations of observed facts. Similarly, cognitive science proposes various kinds of mental representations, including sensory images and verbal concepts, to explain many kinds of thinking.

Representations by themselves do not explain thinking, however, because on their own they do not do anything. Hence, we need to add the second central idea of cognitive science: mental process. A process in the world is a series of operations or changes that bring about a result. For example, the process of digesting food requires operations that include chewing, swallowing, dissolving, absorbing, and excretion. Similarly, a mental process occurs when your mind carries out a series of operations that together accomplish a result. For example, if you need to decide what clothes to wear, you can imagine yourself wearing various outfits and weigh their relative attractiveness. I have already mentioned one important kind of mental process—combination—that serves to build the sentence "A tree grows in the forest" out of the words "tree" and "grows" and to build the scenario of you at the Eiffel Tower out of sensory images of different kinds. Another important kind of mental process is inference—for example, when you use the beliefs that there is a tree in the forest and that trees have roots to conclude that there are roots in the forest. A mental process takes one or more mental representations and transforms them into other representations. Inference is different from reasoning, which is an explicit verbal process, whereas inference can be unconscious and nonverbal.

Mental representations and processes are not directly observable by our senses, so it helps to understand them by analogy with more familiar things. Consider, for example, a food recipe, which consists of a list of ingredients and a set of instructions for what needs to be done to the ingredients. To make macaroni and cheese, you need to boil the noodles and mix them together with cheese and other ingredients. Boiling and mixing are processes that are applied to macaroni and cheese to produce the desired result, something to eat. Similarly, mental processes such as combination and inference apply to sensory and verbal representations to produce desired results such as solving problems.

A more technical analogy will make sense to readers who have some familiarity with computers. A computer program consists of data structures such as numbers, strings, lists, and arrays that can be manipulated by precisely defined algorithms that perform tasks such as addition, sorting, and searching. Before the development of computers, theorizing about the mind was hindered by weak analogies to currently available mechanical analogies, such as clockworks, vibrating strings, and telephone switchboards.

The advent of computational ideas provided a more appropriate analogy, suggesting that mental representations and processes are like the data structures and algorithms that are familiar in computer programming. These computational analogies were remarkably fertile in the beginnings of cognitive science but have since been challenged by very different ideas about representation and processes derived from neuroscience. The next chapter will describe how processes operating on groups of neurons can produce representations and perform operations on them. We will see that these representations and processes are still computational but differ from the operations of most current computers. For example, processes in brains do not proceed step by step but rather require the simultaneous, parallel action of billions of neurons.

The ambition of cognitive science is to show that the full range of human thinking—including perception, problem solving, learning, language, emotions, and consciousness—can be explained by interacting representations and processes. Fulfilling this ambition has major implications for a vast range of important applications including the social sciences, but understanding the social dimensions of human thought requires attention to mechanisms that go beyond mental representations and processes.

MECHANISMS

Around 2,700 years ago, the ancient Greek philosopher Thales initiated scientific explanation in terms of natural processes such as water waves. Before then, the dominant form of explanation of events was theological: What happens is the result of the actions and will of the gods. In contrast, natural explanations are often mechanistic, explaining observations as the result of systems of parts whose interactions produce regular changes. For example, a mobile phone is a mechanism with many parts, such as the screen, computer chip, and antennae, which interact in ways that enable people to make calls and carry out Internet tasks. Cognitive explanations in terms of representations and processes are also mechanistic, with representational parts that interact by virtue of mental processes to produce changes in representation that lead to actions. Table 1.2 provides a three-analysis of the concept of mechanism that is more informative than a simple definition of a mechanism as a combination of connected parts whose interactions produce regular changes.

People often react negatively to the suggestion that thinking is mechanistic. Does that mean you are just a robot with no will or imagination? Well, you are obviously much more complicated than any current robots, whose abilities are restricted to limited tasks. You certainly have imagination, because you can combine representations together to produce ones that are novel, such as thinking what you would look like with a hawk perched on your head. Assessing whether you have free will requires a neural theory of intention and action like the one presented in chapter 9. Putting prejudice aside, I hope that you can at least entertain the hypothesis that thinking is mechanistic, a hypothesis that gains credibility from the increasing availability of neural explanations of thinking. Such explanations are clearly mechanistic, because brain changes result from interactions of billions of neurons.

Part of the resistance to mechanistic explanations of mind is that familiar mechanisms like bicycles and can openers seem too simple to account for anything as complex as thinking. In contrast, today there are mechanisms like smart phones and robots that can carry out much more complicated tasks. We will see in chapter 2 how complex mechanisms like neural networks can have emergent

TABLE 1.2

Three-Analysis of *Mechanism*

Exemplars	Machines such as bicycles, physical systems such as the solar system, organisms such as bacteria, organs such as the brain, groups such as political parties and markets
Typical features	Wholes, parts, connections, interactions, regular changes
Explanations	Explains: changes in parts and wholes
	Explained by: underlying mechanisms inside parts

properties that are different from the sum of their parts. An emergent property belongs to a whole but not to any of its parts and is not the aggregate of the property of the parts because it results from the interactions of the parts. For example, water is liquid at room temperature, even though the hydrogen and oxygen that make it up are gases. To take a social example, a group of adolescents may engage in a risky social behavior such as stealing a car that no individual would do alone. Even machines can have emergent properties, for example, a bicycle that can carry people through the interactions of its parts such as wheels and handlebars, none of which can carry people.

Emergence is an important result of social mechanisms such as communication and emotional contagion, a process in which emotions spread through a population. Mental mechanisms consist of interacting representations, but social mechanisms consist of interacting people. It may seem demeaning to think of people as parts in a mechanism, but doing so provides a helpful way of understanding how societies operate. Each person has properties and relations, including mental representations and processes. People interact by various forms of communication that transfer verbal and other kinds of information including emotional reactions. Chapter 12 will provide a much more detailed account of a variety of social mechanisms that are important for understanding the self.

Table 1.3 summarizes four levels of mechanisms relevant to explaining human thinking. The aim of this book is not to reduce one level to another—the social to the mental, the mental to the neural, or the neural to the molecular. Rather, it will show the usefulness of considering mechanisms at all of these levels, taking into account their interactions rather than trying to identify one level as fundamental. For example, in explaining people's shopping behavior, it helps to go down to the

TABLE 1.3

Four Levels of Mechanisms Relevant to How the Mind Works

Level	Parts	Interactions	Changes	Results
Social	People	Communication	Group behavior	Social practices
Mental	Mental representations	Processes such as inference	Shifts in representations	Thought, action
Neural	Neurons	Electric/chemical transmission	Neural firing patterns	Representations, inferences
Molecular	Genes, proteins, neurotransmitters	Chemical reactions	Neural properties	Neural firing

neural and molecular levels to understand how their brains are making decisions but also up to the social level to understand how people's decisions are influenced by social interactions such as the opinions of friends and the manipulations of advertising. The term "mental" is a bit misleading, because it will turn out that mental mechanisms include neural and molecular ones. But I use it concisely to stand for what goes on at the level of individual psychology based on inferences using mental representations.

My emphasis in this book will be on the mental and neural levels, with occasional allusions to molecular processes; social mechanisms are saved for chapter 12 and *Mind–Society*. The four levels of mechanisms are not independent, because they interact in two ways. First, changes in one level can influence another. For example, circulating alcohol in the brains of people changes their social interactions, and interacting with people at a bar increases the consumption of alcohol. Second, the molecular–neural–psychological connections are even more direct, because mental representations are patterns of neural firing that result from chemical interactions among neurons.

In popular accounts, neuroscience is often associated with brain scans, particularly ones using fMRI. These machines can be used to produce vivid pictures that seem to indicate what parts of the brain are used for particular mental processes, but there is much more to neuroscience. First, there are methodological problems associated with fMRI, for example, that they are expensive and therefore often used in experiments with small numbers of participants. The result is that statistically significant neural firing is found in fewer brain areas than are actually operating. Fortunately, databases are being compiled from thousands of studies that provide a much broader view of brain processing than can be gained from individual fMRI studies.

Second, fMRI is only one of many experimental methods that can be used to study brains. For example, single-cell recording can directly measure firing activity in small numbers of neurons, and transcranial magnetic stimulation can interfere with the operation of accessible brain regions, changing rather than measuring what they are normally doing. Diffusion tensor imaging can be used to track the movement of water along axons that connect different areas, and much current research concerns the connections between brain areas rather than local activity.

Third, the vast amount of neuroscience data accumulated by experimental methods can be organized and explained through the development of theories that use mathematics and computer models to describe the mechanisms responsible for neural phenomena. This increasingly fruitful procedure operates by identifying an important mental phenomenon such as pain. Then, what is known about brain operations can be used to form conjectures about the kinds of representations and processes that might produce the phenomena. Next, theorists can spell out these conjectures with sufficient rigor that they can be implemented in computer simulations and then determine whether the computer simulations match the behavior of people in psychological experiments. If the mechanisms specified provide the best available explanation of the mental phenomena, this justifies the tentative identification of a familiar mental process with a novel neural process.

Like all theoretical claims in science, the proposed identification is fallible and may be found wanting, either because there are important phenomena for which it cannot account or because better theories come along. The procedure for identifying mental processes with neural processes is like many cases in the history of science, where everyday notions become understood scientifically through their identification with newly proposed mechanisms; for example, fire is rapid oxidation and lightning is the flow of electrons.

LOOKING AHEAD

The rest of this book will describe mechanisms that are responsible for all mental operations. Chapter 2 provides an outline of how brains work, focusing on several main kinds of neural mechanisms. First, we need an account of how brains can represent both the external world and internal operations of the body. I will describe neural representations that are patterns of firing in groups of neurons. Second, neural firing by itself is insufficient, for we also need to be able to consider how representations can be transformed and combined into more complicated ones. Combination requires a description of the mechanisms of binding, which joins representations into more powerful ones. Binding is crucial for understanding both basic functions like perception and advanced processes like language and creativity. Chris Eliasmith's semantic pointers are rich neural representations that result from repeated bindings. A third mechanism, competition among semantic pointers, is important for inference performed by satisfying constraints in parallel and for the role of attention in consciousness explained in chapter 8. Additional mechanisms are needed for memory and learning.

These neural mechanisms provide the basis for explaining more advanced mental processes, including the uses of imagery, concepts, beliefs, rules, and analogies, discussed in chapters 3 to 6. In chapters 7 and 8, I provide semantic pointer theories of emotions and consciousness that smoothly integrate them with other cognitive mechanisms. The justification for considering just these kinds of mental representation is that they suffice for explaining the full range of human thinking.

To understand human behavior, we need to consider how actions result from intentions. Chapter 9 describes the mechanisms by which intentions sometimes lead to action but also sometimes fail. This theory of intention has strong implications for the traditional problem of free will.

The integrated account of language in chapter 10 provides new perspectives on syntax, metaphor, conceptual blending, and meaning. The semantic pointer hypothesis provides a bridge between basic neural processes found in all animals and the sophisticated linguistic inferences made by people. A recurring theme, found in discussions of concepts, rules, and analogies as well as language, is the importance of an integrated account of syntax, semantics, and pragmatics. Researchers in philosophy, linguistics, and artificial intelligence are often beguiled by the syntactic dream that intelligence can be explained by formal operations on abstract symbols. In contrast, semantic pointers show how neural representations can deal with meaning and purpose at the same time as formal structure, without putting syntax first.

The best human activities are creative in that they do not simply repeat previous ideas and practices but introduce ones that are new, valuable, and surprising. I show in chapter 11 how neural processes can explain creativity. Finally, chapter 12 considers the self as emerging from social and molecular mechanisms as well as neural and mental ones. Social and mental explanations are complementary rather than competitive. I see no battle between the cognitive and social sciences but rather a promising partnership that looks at ways in which cognitive and social mechanisms interpenetrate.

In particular, the social mechanisms of communication among people are intimately tied with the kinds of mental mechanisms that operate in people's heads, so that having a rich account of mental mechanisms makes possible a much deeper understanding of how social mechanisms work. Communication needs to be understood not just as a matter of verbal presentation in which people pass word-like representations to each other but a matter of how emotions and values spread through society as well. The sketch of neural-social mechanisms in the discussion of the self sets the stage for a much more detailed consideration of social sciences and professions in the second book of this treatise, *Mind–Society*. The third book, *Natural Philosophy*, applies the full range of mechanisms to answer important questions in the humanities concerning the value for human lives of philosophy, painting, and music.

Like any scientific hypothesis, my claims concerning the relevance of neural theories to this huge range of applications might be false. They would be false if dualism is true and minds require the operations of some kind of nonphysical, spiritual soul. They would be false if behaviorism is correct and we can explain human operations just in terms of the causal effects of environments. They would be false if everything is socially constructed so that mental processes are irrelevant to human behaviors. There are good reasons, however, to conclude that dualism, behaviorism, and social constructionism are inadequate for understanding human activity. Another purported alternative to brain-based cognitive science is one that emphasizes embodiment and dynamic systems, but I will show that its insights, stripped of rhetorical exaggerations, can be absorbed within a sufficiently rich account of mind and brain. As with all scientific theories, acceptance and rejection of theories of mind should be the result of an inference to the best explanation of the full range of relevant evidence.

SUMMARY AND DISCUSSION

Minds enable people to perceive, understand, learn, speak, reason, and be emotional and conscious. Competing explanations of how the mind works have been proposed, identifying it as soul, computer, brain, dynamical system, or social construction. This book will explain minds in terms of interacting mechanisms operating at multiple levels, including the social, mental, neural, and molecular. Mechanisms consist of parts that interact to produce regular changes. At the mental level, we can explain much of human behavior in terms of mental representations and processes that operate on the representations. Chapters 3 to 7 will present the most important kinds of representations and processes, covering sensations, images, concepts, rules, analogies, and emotions.

At the complementary neural level, the operations of brains can be explained by the interactions of billions of neurons whose molecular interactions are accomplished by neurotransmitters. Chapter 2 will contend that mental representations and processes result from these neural mechanisms: patterns of firing, transformations of these patterns, binding of representations into semantic pointers, and competition among them.

Because humans are inherently social, social mechanisms such as communication between individuals are also highly relevant to explaining human thought. Cognitive science combines empirical and theoretical insights from many fields, especially psychology, neuroscience, linguistics, anthropology, philosophy, and computer modeling. This combination of insights has dramatic implications for other fields, including all of the social sciences, professions, and humanities.

The trick quote is from Minsky 1986, p. 308.

General introductions to cognitive science as an interdisciplinary field include Bermudez 2014, Friedenberg and Silverman 2011 and Thagard 2005b. The best history of cognitive science is Boden 2006, but see also Gardner 1985. Good introductions to cognitive psychology are Smith and Kosslyn 2007, Anderson 2010, and Holyoak and Morrison 2012. An introduction to artificial intelligence is Russell and Norvig 2009. On neuroscience, see Kandel, Schwartz, Jessell, Siegelbaum, and Hudspeth 2012, Banich and Compton 2018, and Finger 1994. On cultural psychology, see Heine 2011. For an introduction to linguistics, see Akmajian, Demers, Farmer, and Harnish 2010. Schutt, Seidman, and Keshavan 2015 discuss social neuroscience.

On philosophy of mind, see Mandik 2013 and Churchland 2002, 2011. On philosophical method compatible with science, see Thagard 2009, 2010, 2012d, 2014d and http://www.psychologytoday.com/blog/hot-thought/201212/eleven-dogmas-analytic-philosophy. *Natural Philosophy* connects philosophy of mind with epistemology, metaphysics, ethics, and aesthetics.

See chapter 4 for references on exemplar, prototype, and explanation views of concepts. Sets of typical features are sometimes called prototypes or stereotypes. The justification for using the method of three-analysis is the semantic pointer theory of concepts in Blouw, Solodkin, Thagard, and Eliasmith 2016.

Here are some databases for summarizing results of neural experiments:

Neurosynth: http://www.talyarkoni.org/blog/tag/neurosynth/
Cognitive Atlas: http://www.cognitiveatlas.org
Human Connectome Project: http://www.humanconnectomeproject.org
Human Brain Project: https://www.humanbrainproject.eu
Neuroimaging methods: http://psychcentral.com/lib/types-of-brain-imaging-techniques/0001057. Other methods include optogenetics which uses light to control genetically modified neurons.

Work in the philosophy of science on mechanistic explanations includes Bechtel 2008, Bunge 2003, Craver and Darden 2013, and Findlay and Thagard 2012. I write of parts and interactions, whereas others discuss components and operations, or entities and activities. These are just terminological variations, except that Craver and Darden assume that mechanisms have start and finish conditions, which does not fit well with brains whose neural mechanisms operate for decades. For more on mechanisms and emergence, see chapter 2 of *Mind–Society* and chapter 5 of *Natural Philosophy*.

My account of emergence adapts Wimsatt 2007 and Bunge 2003. Emergence occurs in complex systems because of features such as feedback loops, chaos, nonlinearity, multiple attractors, and tipping points, all of which occur in brain networks. Chapter 12 describes the self as an example of multilevel emergence from interacting mechanisms that are molecular, neural, psychological, and social.

Like the mechanistic philosophers and McCauley 2007, my account of levels is based on size, organization, scope, and age of the systems. Very different is Marr's 1982 view of computational, algorithmic, and physical levels of analysis, which does not reflect the practice of theoretical neuroscience described in chapter 2: Neurophysiology and computational analyses are tightly interconnected.

For a fuller account of the methodology of computer simulation, see Thagard 2012d. Analysis of many historical cases of explanatory identities can be found in Thagard 2014b.

On inference to the best explanation, see Thagard 1988, 1992 and Lipton 2004. The term "abduction" or "abductive inference" covers both inference to the best explanation and the initial generation of explanatory hypotheses; see Magnani 2009.

PROJECT

Perform a three-analysis (exemplars, typical features, explanations) of some rich mental concept that interests you, such as *perception, intelligence, action, causality, emotion,* or *consciousness.*

2

How Brains Make Minds

In one of my favorite poems, Emily Dickinson wrote:

> The brain is wider than the sky,
> For, put them side by side,
> The one the other will include
> With ease, and you beside.

This stanza notices the enormous power of the human brain that enables it to represent the universe and even the person who does the representing. The aim of this chapter is to provide a gentle introduction to how brains are capable of mental representations and processes such as problem solving and learning.

The hypothesis that the mind is the brain, that all mental processes are neural processes, is revolutionary. It potentially overturns thousands of years of philosophical and religious assumptions that the mind is something spiritual rather than material and mechanistic. If true, mind–brain identity has enormous consequences, not only for philosophy and psychology but also for the social sciences, professions, and humanities. I do not directly defend the identity hypothesis but set the stage by describing key mechanisms that can explain the full range of mental phenomena discussed in later chapters, including emotions, consciousness, action, language, and creativity. My overall aim is to show that mind = brain provides a better explanation of these phenomena than available alternatives, including the seductive hypothesis that mind = soul.

THINKING WITH CELLS

Your mind is a bunch of cells. That suggestion sounds ridiculous, given that your mind is capable of wonderful activities such as feeling happy when spring arrives, whereas cells are just tiny collections of proteins and other molecules. Cells were not even discovered until 1665, when Robert Hooke used a microscope to examine the structure of cork. The modern theory that all living things consist of cells was only proposed in the 1830s, and the role of brain cells in mental functions only started to become evident in the 1890s. How could mental processes such as thoughts, emotions, and consciousness result from the activity of cells?

The first clue to how cells can contribute to thinking comes from noticing that brains contain a special kind of cells, neurons, that can function to represent the world and make inferences about it. The second clue comes from seeing how neurons interact to perform their representational tasks by working in groups. The third clue comes from appreciating how neural groups can further combine to provide more complex representations that go well beyond simple sensory representations. Thinking in the brain comes about through the escalating capacities for representation and processing found in single neurons, neural groups, and interactions of neural groups operating across multiple brain areas.

Compare how music is produced by your favorite band. One key on a piano cannot produce a song, but when keys are played together they can make a tune, which gets even better when the piano is combined with other sounds like guitars and singing. The resulting music comes about because of a collective effort produced by processes in groups of instruments. Similarly, your thoughts result from the collective activity of many groups of neurons. This chapter introduces basic neural mechanisms, and later chapters will show how these can contribute to more complex processes from imagery to creativity.

NEURONS

Your body has trillions of cells, but most of them, like the cells in your skin and bones, are not capable of helping you to think about the world. Neurons have special properties that make them capable of contributing to representation.

Figure 2.1 shows the structure of a typical neuron that allows it to receive and transmit information. The chemical reactions inside each cell body enable it to accumulate electrical charge, which it can discharge in a process called firing or spiking. Each neuron has an axon, a fiber that connects it to other neurons by means of extensions (dendrites) that have junctions (synapses) with the axon.

When a neuron fires, an electrical signal travels along the axon toward other neurons whose dendrites are connected to the axon of the neuron sending the signal. Transfer of the signal is usually not just an electrical process, however, as most neurons use a chemical process to transfer a signal from one neuron to another. The electrical signal in the axon causes it to release neurotransmitters, which are molecules that travel across the synapse between two neurons to stimulate receptors on the dendrites of the second neuron. These receptors initiate

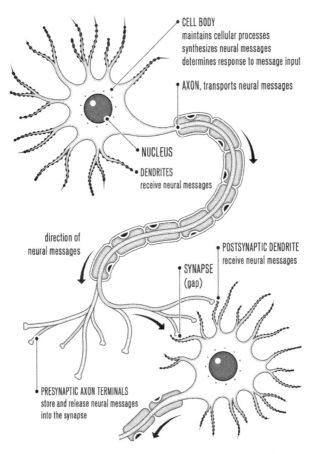

FIGURE 2.1 Two connected neurons. Reprinted from Thagard (2010) with permission of Princeton University Press.

chemical processes in the second cell that change its electrical charge to increase its ability to fire.

Figure 2.1 shows how one neuron can send a message to another, but how does a neuron represent anything in the world, for example, when your brain represents the coldness of an ice cube? Your skin contains receptors for heat and cold that can initiate signaling through chains of neurons that go from your fingers through your spinal cord to the brain. Processing in the brain requires the interaction of many neurons, but let us focus on just one simplified neuron that receives signals that originated with the ice cube. That neuron receives signals from thousands of other neurons whose axons connect to its dendrites, and the chemical activity in its dendrites produce its firing. The neuron can represent cold by changing its rate and pattern of firing.

Rate just means how fast the neuron is firing. A typical neuron might be capable of firing 100 times per second, so we might think of its representation of cold as being carried by how fast it fires. For example, firing five times per second might mean NOT COLD, whereas firing 90 times per second might mean VERY COLD. This method is the simplest way in which neurons can represent things in the world, when a specific neuron has a firing rate that tracks presence or absence. Most neural representation in the brain is far more complicated than this method, but there actually seem to be specific neurons in some people's brains that respond to pictures of famous movie stars and characters like Jennifer Aniston and Luke Skywalker!

The first complication in this simple picture is that neurons can represent things by means of firing patterns as well as firing rates. The patterns are not visual like the ones in a plaid shirt, but rather temporal like the beat of a song. Here are two patterns of firing that have the same rate but different orders of firing:

1. FIRE REST FIRE REST FIRE
2. FIRE FIRE FIRE REST REST

In both these cases, a neuron is firing 60% of the time, say 60 times a second, but the first pattern of alternating firing and not firing is different from the second pattern of firing three times and then resting two. Using firing patterns rather than just rates greatly increases the representational power of a neuron. Whereas a neuron using a rate strategy might be able to signal the presence or absence of Jennifer Aniston, a more complicated neuron could use one firing pattern to signal Jennifer Aniston and another to signal Luke Skywalker.

A second complication in the simple picture of a single neuron using its rate of firing is that most representations require a lot of neurons. Psychologists rightfully disparage the idea of a "grandmother neuron" that fires just in the presence of your grandmother. That idea presumes a one-to-one relationship between what is represented and a neuron that represents it, each thing getting its own special neuron. Most representations in the brain, however, are many-to-many, with each thing in the world represented in the brain by the firing patterns (not just rates) of many neurons and each neuron contributing to the representation of many things. To understand how this works, we need to consider neural groups.

NEURAL GROUPS

People form organizations such as companies and governments to accomplish tasks that one person could not do alone. Similarly, there is not much that one neuron can do by itself, but groups of neurons working together have amazing abilities to represent and process information. Neural groups, also called populations, assemblies, or ensembles, consist of neurons that are connected to each other by the axons, dendrites, and synapses shown in Figure 2.1.

A group consisting of 10 neurons is shown in Figure 2.2, with the connections divided into links that are excitatory or inhibitory. Information flows into this group from the left in the form of electrochemical signals passed to the first column of neurons, which pass signals on to the other neurons. The function of an *excitatory* link from a neuron A to a neuron B is to ensure that the more A is firing, the more B will be firing. So, if A is part of the representation of the concept *tree* and B is part of the representation of *green*, then the firing of A will lead to the firing of B, corresponding to the linguistic inference that trees are generally green.

If there were only excitatory links in neural groups, then firing would just spread throughout the neural network, rendering it incapable of useful discriminations.

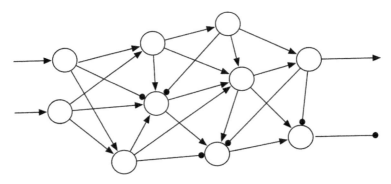

FIGURE 2.2 Neural group with excitatory and inhibitory connections. Arrows indicate excitatory links, and circles indicate inhibitory links.

For example, firing would spread from neural groups for *green* to *bush*, leading the network to conclude that something is both a tree and a bush. To make more selective distinctions, neural networks also need inhibitory links. The function of an inhibitory link from a neuron A to a neuron C is to ensure that the more A is firing, the *less* C will be firing. So if A is part of the representation of *tree* and C is part of the representation of *bush*, then the firing of A will suppress the firing of C, corresponding to the linguistic inference that trees are not bushes.

A neural group like the one shown in Figure 2.2 can take sensory inputs (from the left), develop new patterns of firing among the whole collection of neurons shown in the middle, and send output signals on to other neural groups via the connections shown on the right. Approximately 20% of the links between neurons are inhibitory, with the rest excitatory.

Where do the connections between neurons—the excitatory and inhibitory links—come from? Some are innate, formed in the brains of fetuses by genetics. A newborn baby does not need experience to figure out that mother's milk tastes good, thanks to innate connections between neural groups that detect sweetness and fat, which in turn are connected with neural groups that produce experiences of pleasure. A newborn baby actually has more synaptic connections than a two-year old, because learning often consists of connections being dropped rather than added, in line with the saying "use it or lose it." A toddler knows a lot more than a newborn—for example, that chocolate tastes good—the result of excitatory and inhibitory links that have been established by learning.

The simplest kind of neural learning is called "Hebbian," after the psychologist Donald Hebb. When two neurons are connected by a synapse and they both fire at the same time, then chemical changes take place that make it more likely that they will continue to fire together. The slogan for this is: Whatever fires together, wires together. Some wiring in the brain by excitatory and inhibitory connections is innate—you are born with it—but most wiring occurs as the result of the adjustment of synaptic connections.

Hebbian learning is unsupervised—it does not require an external reward to train a neural group to perform in ways that accomplish an animal's goals. But other kinds of learning do respond to rewards and punishments provided by physical and social environments that reinforce successful behaviors. Supervised reinforcement learning revises excitatory and inhibitory links to help the animal acquire representations that support its goals such as finding food and mates. For example, if an animal tries a new food and finds it sweet and fatty, it will get a reward that rewires its neural connections to shape its behavior toward eating more of that food in the future. Hebbian and reinforcement learning usually require many experiences to revise the connections between neurons, but humans can also learn from single examples, as when you eat a nasty new food and decide never to try it again.

Neural groups provide much richer representations and processing than is possible with individual neurons. Brains represent the world by having groups of neurons that collectively encode inputs from the world through the excitatory and inhibitory links between neurons. These connections produce a form of representation different from the words, pictures, and other images that are familiar in everyday experience. In neural groups, the representation of something is *distributed* across all the neurons by virtue of their interconnections that produce patterns of firing. What matters is not just the pattern or rate of firing of each individual neuron but rather the pattern of firing across all the neurons in the group. The resulting patterns are both temporal and collective, like the performance of a band that requires the coordinated activity of many musicians and their instruments.

Representations in brains are not things or properties but rather processes consisting of patterns of firing that result from the synaptic connections among neurons. These learned or innate connections enable neural groups to produce useful patterns of firing in response to inputs from the environment or other neural groups. Such production licenses a secondary sense of representation as the collection of synaptic connections that disposes a group of neurons to produce patterns of firing in response to inputs.

Neural groups are tiny, occupying less than a cubic millimeter of space in the brain, so there is room for many millions of them. The brain's organization is usually described in terms of large regions like those shown in Figure 2.3, including the cortex (responsible for most cognitive functions), cerebellum (important for motor control), and brain stem (needed for sensory transmission, control of breathing, and other functions). In turn, these regions divide into many more specific anatomical areas, such as the 52 Brodmann areas in the cortex. There is a rough correspondence between brain areas and cognitive functions, for example, with area 17 playing an important role in vision.

When brain imaging took off in the 1990s, researchers expected to find a close correspondence between brain areas and functions. This expectation made sense from the perspective of familiar mechanisms like a car, which has a simple mapping between parts and functions: the wheels, steering column, and engine parts each play their respective roles. But thousands of studies have revealed that brain functions are usually spread out over many brain areas, and the current emphasis is on tracking the *connectome*, the map of the interconnections among all the areas of the brain. For example, pain is not just a pattern of firing of neural groups in one area of the brain but rather a pattern that is distributed across groups in many areas and regions. Hence, representations and processes in the brain are

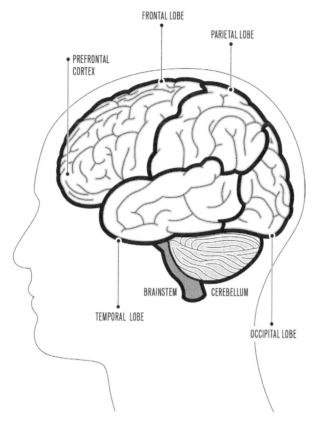

FIGURE 2.3 Sketch of some major regions of the brain. Reprinted from Thagard (2010) with permission of Princeton University Press.

doubly distributed, first across multiple neurons in each neural group and second across multiple areas. Representation in brains is therefore an emergent process resulting from the interactions of many neurons, not just the sum of the limited representational capability of each neuron.

COMBINING NEURAL REPRESENTATIONS

An organism with representations consisting of neural groups can do a lot. For example, the tiny worm *Caenorhabditis. elegans* has only 302 neurons, but these suffice for behavioral functions such as eating and mating. Such functions use patterns of recognition and action, with some neural groups detecting something worth eating or mating with and other neural groups directing motor actions to accomplish these tasks. But thinking in humans and other animals is capable of much more complicated kinds of representation and inference than are found in recognize-and-act structures. Such complexity requires the transformation of neural representations into different ones that need not be tied so closely to sensory inputs. A single pattern of firing can be transformed by changing the pattern, as a band might do by playing a song faster or louder. But powerful transformations can result from combining representations.

Recognizing objects requires combinations of features, for example, when a monkey identifies a banana. Different neural groups may serve to encode different features of bananas, such as yellow, long, and round. However, when you recognize an object as a banana, you do not see it as a completely disjointed set of features. Rather, you see yellow, long, and round as being bound together into a single object. Similarly, when you recognize a friend's face, you do not see it as an unconnected, disorganized group of features that include eyes, nose, and mouth. Rather, you see these features as bound together into a unified face.

Binding is also important for constructing complex representations in other modalities, such as hearing and taste. When you hear your favorite band play, you do not separately hear the different instruments but rather appreciate ways in which they are integrated into a common sound. Similarly, when you taste a cheese sandwich, the separate tastes of bread, cheese, and tomato get combined into something that tastes like a whole sandwich, not just like the sum of the parts. We will see that binding is also important for higher-level cognitive operations, including emotions, language, consciousness, and creativity.

How does the brain bind simple neural representations into more complex ones? There are two currently available theories about brain mechanisms that can accomplish binding. The most popular one is neural synchrony, the idea that neural representations get bound together because they become temporally coordinated. To understand this process, the musical band metaphor is again useful. A band does not perform well if each of the instruments is played at its own pace. Rather, the band needs to get coordinated so that everyone is playing at the same beat. In a symphony orchestra, the synchronization is arranged by the conductor, and in some popular bands, a similar role is played by the drummer. In more informal bands, everyone manages to coordinate with each other.

Analogously, even though different neurons have independent firing patterns, they can become coordinated. For example, there are conditions under which the brain displays brain waves of approximately 40 Hertz, which means that the neurons are firing in temporally organized fashion around 40 times per second.

The neural synchrony hypothesis is that binding takes place because the representations that need to be bound together are firing in the same temporal patterns. For example, when you see a banana, the group of neurons representing *yellow* start firing in a pattern that is temporally similar to the pattern for *long* and the pattern for *round*. Then, the perception of a banana as yellow, round, and long comes about because of the temporal coordination of these individual representations.

However, there are reasons to doubt whether synchrony really is the main mechanism of binding. First, it is not clear that binding by synchrony can produce representations that play all the cognitive roles that even perceptual representations of objects are required to do. For example, you can make inferences about bananas. Once you have identified something as a banana, you can infer that is sweet and that it will taste good. How does binding by neural synchrony make possible additional inferences such as that the banana will be sweet?

Second, no one has explained how binding by neural synchrony can allow for manipulations of the resulting bound object. You can easily imagine a banana that is being eaten by a monkey, which requires you to be able to manipulate the representation of the banana to see it in the hands of a monkey, watch the monkey peel it, and see the monkey bring it into its mouth. Neural synchrony may seem to tie together the perceptions of yellow, long, and round, but it does not explain how you can deal with the representation thereby produced, either verbally or by some kind of imagistic manipulation. Third, neural firing in real brains is noisy in the sense of containing much random fluctuation, making exact synchronization difficult to achieve. The synchrony observed in brain waves may just be a side effect of neural operations rather than a mechanism for binding.

An alternative explanation of how binding works in the brain is the proposal of convolution by Chris Eliasmith, building on ideas of Tony Plate. Suppose that each feature of a banana is represented by a pattern of firing in a group of neurons. Neural processes can produce a new pattern of firing in a group of neurons that may overlap with the existing groups. The new group accomplishes the binding of all the previous representations using a mathematical procedure called "circular convolution." The idea is that the previous representations are twisted together in a way that preserves much of the original representations so that they can subsequently be taken apart.

A simple metaphor for convolution is braiding hair. Hair can be braided together when separate strands are woven into a single strand, and then it is also possible to take the strands apart to regain their original form. Similarly, neurons can compute a mathematical function, convolution, that takes representations and weaves them together to produce new patterns of firing that are capable of being decomposed into the contributing representations.

Most important, the result of this binding can be representations that can then serve for additional manipulations and inference, as in my examples of the inference that the banana is sweet and the image of the monkey eating the banana.

Sufficiently complicated binding by convolution can produce the important kind of representation described in the next section on semantic pointers.

There are currently no experimental methods that can tell whether the brain accomplishes binding by means of neural synchrony or by means of convolution. It is possible that the brain uses both mechanisms and maybe others that no one has thought of yet. It is not unusual for biological systems to find multiple ways to accomplish the same ends. The good news is that we have at least two ways of understanding how the brain builds up complicated patterns of neural firing.

With enough neurons and processing time, a human brain can do much more than produce patterns of firing from sensory inputs. Brains not only perform bindings but also bindings of bindings and even bindings of bindings of bindings. Visualizing a monkey eating a banana requires binding representations of the monkey, the banana, and the activity of eating. Such complex combination is required whether the representation is produced by visual imagery or by language. Highly sophisticated brains, like those of humans, can make it even more complicated by producing whole stories that introduce additional complex relations. For example, I can tell a verbal story or produce a mental image of a situation where a monkey eating a banana causes a child to laugh, introducing the higher-level relation of causality. Binding is recursive, repeatedly feeding back on itself to generate structures that can then be further bound. In language, this can produce sentences as complicated as the cartoon where a man says to a woman: "Of course I care about how you imagined I thought you perceived I wanted you to feel."

Later discussions of imagery, conceptual combination, language, and creativity will describe the intelligent behaviors that result from recursive bindings, that is, bindings of bindings of bindings. Even with more than 80 billion neurons operating in our brains, people have limited capacity for bindings that produce more complicated representations, because both the representations and the binding operations require a lot of neurons. Nevertheless, the neural capacity for recursive binding provides the basis for the most creative intellectual achievements, discussed in chapter 11.

SEMANTIC POINTERS

The peak of repeated binding is construction of powerful neural representations that Chris Eliasmith calls "semantic pointers." Chris began his education in engineering at the University of Waterloo, did an MA in philosophy there, and completed his PhD at the Philosophy, Neuroscience, and Psychology program at Washington University in St. Louis. There, he melded philosophical studies on meaning with extensive work on neuroscience, collaborating with Charles Anderson on a new framework for computational neuroscience that became their book *Neural Engineering*. Now he has appointments at the University of Waterloo in three departments (Philosophy, Systems Design Engineering, and Computer Science) and directs the Centre for Theoretical Neuroscience. His unusual background in philosophy, neuroscience, and computation makes him uniquely qualified to help solve the daunting problem of how neural processes can be meaningful.

Semantic pointers combine the flexible capabilities of neural representations understood as firing patterns with the symbolic capacity that enables people to accomplish language and reasoning. Semantic pointers result from binding multiple representations together by means of convolution. Neural synchrony is not adequate to generate semantic pointers because it does not produce new representations that can function as symbols. To understand how semantic pointers work, we need to appreciate how they are formed, how they can be taken apart, and how they can be used to perform mental functions. These operations can be characterized mathematically using vector algebra, as in the appendix to this chapter, but here I resort to diagrams.

Formation

Figure 2.4 pictures how binding takes multiple neural representations and combines them into a semantic pointer. The circles do not stand for individual

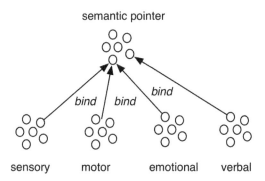

FIGURE 2.4 Semantic pointers are neural representations (patterns of firing) formed by binding sensory, motor, emotional, and/or verbal representations, which are also patterns of firing in neural groups. The circles indicate representations accomplished by thousands or millions of neurons. Here "verbal" does not mean having the full capabilities of language but just patterns of firing for particular words. Reprinted by permission of Elsevier from Thagard and Stewart 2014.

neurons but rather for groups of thousands of neurons. These groups encode different kinds of information, including the sensory and motor inputs described in chapter 3, the emotional reactions described in chapter 7, and the verbal symbols discussed in chapter 10. Binding is not a physical operation like tying things together with a cord but rather a functional operation that transforms the firing patterns of the contributing neural groups into a new firing pattern in a different neural group that may have some overlap with the contributing ones.

For example, the concept of a cat can be viewed as a semantic pointer that binds sensory features such as what cats look and sound like, motor features such as how it feels to pick up a cat, emotional features such as how much you like cats, and verbal features such as that cats are a kind of mammal. Binding does not simply duplicate the neural patterns of the bound representations but rather packs the information in the patterns into a compressed form, just as computers can compress music and picture files into smaller files that retain most of the functionality of the originals. Extending the unpacking metaphor, you can think of a semantic pointer as like a big suitcase full of suitcases: The big one makes it easy to carry around the small ones, but it can always be unpacked to yield the smaller ones, which can be unpacked further.

Figure 2.5 pictures the functioning of semantic pointers as symbols and their unpacking into the lower-level representations from which they were formed by binding. The compression of different representations can be approximately reversed by operations that unpack or decompress the semantic pointer, just as compressed computer files can be used to generate useful pictures and sounds. For example, from the semantic pointer for *cat*, it is possible to extract much of

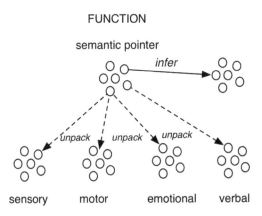

FIGURE 2.5 Semantic pointers function to provide inferences by virtue of relations to other semantic pointers and can also unpack (decompress) into the sensory, motor, emotional, and/or verbal representations whose bindings formed the semantic pointer. Reprinted by permission of Elsevier from Thagard and Stewart 2014.

the sensory, motor, emotional, or verbal information out of which the pointer can be constructed. However, some of the information is lost during compression, so that decompression provides only an approximation of the original inputs, in the same way that MP3 music files and JPEG picture files are only approximations.

Semantic pointers have the unique capability of *modal retention:* They retain in partial, compressed form the information resulting from the particular sensory or motor modality that produced them. Moreover, this information can be partially regenerated through decompression, when semantic pointers are unpacked to produce some approximation to the sensory inputs that went into them. Chapter 3 shows how visual, auditory, and other kinds of imagery can be understood as operations on semantic pointers in ways that depend on modal retention, as do sensory–motor aspects of causality. Moreover, concepts, rules and analogies discussed in chapters 4 to 6 have embodied aspects that modal retention accommodates but which are otherwise mysterious. Chapter 7 argues that emotion is best explained as a combination by neural binding that includes bodily inputs as well as cognitive appraisals, where representation of physiology retains some of the character of internal sensing.

Modal retention is also crucial for explaining why there are different qualitative feelings associated with different states of consciousness (chapter 8). Chapter 11 highlights the role of multimodal concepts and rules in creativity, which again work much better with modal retention than with translation of physiological inputs into abstract symbols.

Function

Despite being performed by neural networks, constructed semantic pointers can function in symbolic inferences, for example, enabling the deduction from "Fluffy is a cat" to "Fluffy is a mammal." Semantic pointers can also function in nonverbal inferences such as ones resulting from imagining a monkey eating a banana because semantic pointers can be produced by combining images of a monkey, a banana, and eating.

Semantic pointers are semantic in that they carry with them two kinds of meaning, from (a) sensory inputs that provide a causal connection with things in the world and (b) connections among symbols. For example, the meaning of *cat* comes from its connections to sensory processes such as vision and hearing and also from its inferential connections to other concepts such as *mammal* and *pet*. Semantic pointers are pointers in that they unpack into the various kinds of neural representations out of which they were compressed. Unlike neural representations produced by learning from examples, semantic pointers are produced by binding small numbers of existing neural representations rather than by training from numerous inputs and can be further bound into more complicated semantic pointers. This capability is crucial for many kinds of creative processes discussed in later chapters, including image manipulation, conceptual combination, rule generation, and language production.

Another function of semantic pointers is competition. Deciding whether an object is a banana or a pear requires a neural process of competition between the semantic pointers for the two kinds of fruit. Semantic pointers can compete with each other even when they are represented by the same neurons, as shown in Figure 2.6. That is, since a group of neurons forms a distributed representation of a concept (i.e., each concept is some pattern of firing across all these neurons), those same neurons can represent a combination of semantic pointers via a firing pattern that is a convolution of the two firing patterns for the two concepts. To make them compete, we add recurrent (looping back) connections between the neurons that ensure that the firing pattern for one semantic pointer such as *banana* will discourage the firing pattern for alternatives such as *pear*, using inhibitory connections between relevant neurons.

As with the binding mechanisms of neural synchrony and convolution, there is currently no way to determine whether brains really do function using semantic pointers. The various ways of investigating brains mentioned in chapter 1 are not sensitive enough to establish whether groups of neurons are producing semantic

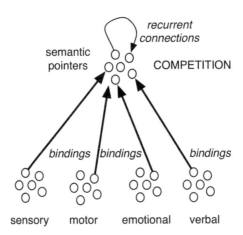

FIGURE 2.6 Competition between semantic pointers. Two or more semantic pointers are produced in the same neural group by bindings of multimodal representations, shown by dark arrows to indicate that more than one semantic pointers are produced. Recurrent connections among the neurons in a group that jointly encodes the semantic pointers generates competition among them by looping backward with inhibitory links.

pointers and applying them to cognitive tasks. Nevertheless, the idea of semantic pointers is theoretically valuable, because we can use it to explain many aspects of thinking, as future chapters will show. Theoretical entities in science such as electrons, genes, and viruses have proven valuable even when it was not possible to observe them directly. Similarly, the hypothesis that brains operate with semantic pointers is legitimate in the current state of neuroscience if it provides ways of explaining mental phenomena that are beyond the reach of other kinds of representation.

Analogies for Semantic Pointers

Because of their explanatory power across the social sciences and humanities, semantic pointers should be of interest to many people who lack backgrounds in biology and computation. Accordingly, I present a suite of analogies designed to explain semantic pointers to a broader audience.

The brain's production of semantic pointers is roughly like a cook baking a cake or making a stew. A cake is not just an agglomeration of ingredients such as flour, butter, sugar, and eggs but rather a binding of them into something new with properties such as taste and texture not found in any of the ingredients. Similarly, semantic pointers take a variety of sensory and motor representations and bind them into something new. Moreover, a cake can then repetitively be used through other operations, such as adding icing or berries, just as semantic pointers can be repeatedly bound into more complex semantic pointers. In a cake, the binding occurs through the application of heat to ingredients such as eggs, whereas binding in semantic pointers results from convolution.

Another analogy for convolution is the formation of new strands of rope by winding together smaller strands. This analogy is better than the baking one for understanding convolution, because ropes can be taken apart, just as semantic pointers can be decomposed approximately into their original sensory–motor components. For cooking, a stew is a better analogy for semantic pointers with respect to decomposition, because items in the stew such as pieces of meat and potato can be picked out afterwards.

The major limitation of these cooking and braiding analogies is that they suggest that semantic pointers are things rather than dynamic processes, unlike patterns of firing in groups of neurons. A more dynamic analogy is with musical bands, where several musicians play together to produce a better sound than they could do individually. For example, a drummer, guitarist, and singer perform together by coordination that include synchronization and mutual attention, roughly as neural firings can be bound into new ones by convolution.

Further coordination is required for combination with another unit such as a horn section, analogous to the recursive binding of semantic pointers into more complex ones.

Finally, the term "pointer" in "semantic pointer" was inspired by the use in some computer programming languages such as C of objects that refer (point) to values stored elsewhere in memory. This analogy is limited because in semantic pointers both the pointing and what is pointed to are dynamic processes of neural firing, not just objects and values. A more dynamic comparison would be to the processes when a nod from one musician serves as a pointer to another musician's playing. The appendix to this chapter provides comparisons of semantic pointers with more familiar ideas about mental representation.

THE SEMANTIC POINTER ARCHITECTURE

A cognitive architecture is a general proposal about the representations and processes that produce intelligent thought. The architecture of a building concerns not just its physical structures such as beams and windows but also its many functions such as human purposes, plumbing, and heating. Similarly, an architecture for the human mind needs to describe its most important structures, which are various kinds of mental representations, and also the most important processes that enable it to accomplish important functions such as perception and inference.

Cognitive architectures have primarily been used to explain important aspects of human thinking such as problem solving, memory, and learning. But they can also be used as blueprints for designing computers and robots that possess some of the cognitive abilities of humans. The most influential cognitive architectures that have been developed are either rule-based, using if–then rules and procedures that operate on them to explain thinking, or connectionist, using artificial neural networks.

Eliasmith's Semantic Pointer Architecture provides a synthesis of connectionist and rule-based approaches, because it shows how neural networks can perform if–then reasoning. In this architecture, the most important representations are semantic pointers, and the most important processes include compression, transformation, and action selection. Semantic pointers have already been useful for explaining many psychological phenomena, including recognizing patterns, serial memory, controlling motor actions, learning, and inference.

Structures and Processes

Figure 2.7 depicts the overall structure and processing of Spaun, a computational implementation of the Semantic Pointer Architecture, with millions of spiking neurons. The brain gets inputs from the visual system through signals from the eyes that go to visual areas of the brain such as V1. Other senses such as hearing and pain also provide inputs. This information gets encoded and transformed by areas in the brain's prefrontal cortex and elsewhere to make it useful for decisions about what cognitive and motor actions to select. These actions are selected and carried out by interactions among areas such as the basal ganglia and temporal cortex. Information about action selection is passed to areas for motor processing such as the primary motor cortex, leading to motor outputs as various forms of bodily movement. All of these components interact with working memory, which operates in the frontal, parietal, and temporal cortex to keep active those neural representations most relevant to the task at hand.

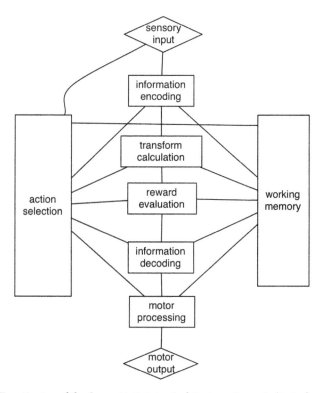

FIGURE 2.7 Functioning of the Semantic Pointer Architecture. Boxes indicate functions carried out by identified brain areas. Lines indicate flows of influence carried out by neural interactions.

Communication between the components of the model efficiently uses semantic pointers. These compressed representations are performed by spiking
neurons that transform the complexity of sensory inputs into features that guide
action selection and motor performance. Many other cognitive architectures have
been proposed to explain mental processes such as problem solving and learning.
The appendix to this chapter contrasts the Semantic Pointer Architecture with
these alternatives.

Constraint Satisfaction

Sufficiently complex neural representations can carry out mental tasks that are
much more complicated than simply recognizing objects. I have already mentioned how semantic pointers can be used for making inferences and constructing
imaginary situations. Consider also decision-making. Suppose you need to decide
whether to eat a banana now or to save it for later. Such inferences require the incorporation of multiple constraints. Perhaps you are on a diet and do not want to
eat the banana until later to not exceed your calorie quota for the day. Or perhaps
you are currently eating something else, such as a cheese sandwich that you think
does not go well with a banana. Making a decision requires you to balance multiple
constraints, not just applying a simple rule such as *do not eat a banana until it is
time for dessert.*

Neural networks provide a computationally efficient way of figuring out how to
satisfy multiple constraints. Whereas formal logic and most computer programs
operate serially, one step at a time, neural networks operate in parallel, with many
neurons firing at once. A simple neural network can represent your different options by individual neurons for eat-banana-now and eat-banana-later. We can see
that there is a constraint between eating the banana now and saving it for later
because you cannot do both.

These constraints can naturally be captured in a neural network by having inhibitory links between the neurons that represent the two options, in this case
between the neurons for eat-banana-now and eat-banana-later, as in Figure 2.8.
Excitatory links also play a role because you can make connections between the
neurons for eat-banana-now and eat-banana-later to the goals that would be accomplished. For example, you could have a neuron representing eat-banana-now
connected to another neuron representing a goal of satisfying hunger. The competing neuron for eat-banana-later can be connected to a different neuron representing a different goal of avoiding calories. Solving this problem need not be a
matter of making a series of logical inferences but rather a matter of satisfying
constraints in parallel.

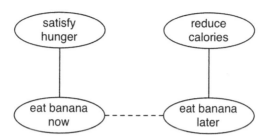

FIGURE 2.8 Simple constraint network for deciding whether to eat a banana now or later. The solid lines indicate excitatory links, and the dotted line indicates an inhibitory link.

Of course, no brain has a single neuron for eat-banana-now with an inhibitory link to eat-banana-later. The actions of eating a banana now or later need to be represented by semantic pointers that use thousands or millions of neurons, many of which are also employed in similar representations. Competition cannot be accomplished merely by having inhibitory links but requires the recurrent (looping backward) connections shown in Figure 2.6. Then, highly distributed neural networks like those in the Semantic Pointer Architecture can carry out parallel constraint satisfaction. This process is important for explaining many phenomena described in later chapters such as perception in chapter 3, concept application in chapter 4, rule selection in chapter 5, analogical mapping in chapter 6, emotional appraisal in chapter 7, and consciousness in chapter 8. Cognitive processes involving high-level inference and language require an assessment of coherence that can be accomplished by parallel constraint satisfaction and hence by semantic pointer competition.

The Semantic Pointer Architecture does not require any central processor or blackboard for computation, which is accomplished by interacting neurons organized into groups. Some of these groups, or groups of groups, provide hubs for communication among different parts of the brain that are variously called "neural hubs," "convergence zones" or "association areas." Hence, the brain is very different from modern computers that have at most a small number of processors through which information flows.

Another major way in which brains differ from computers is that memory does not work by storing exact digital encodings but rather by transforming sensory experiences into neural connections that are only approximations to the experiences. To store memories of episodes such as what you are doing right now, the brain's hippocampus produces a summary of what is happening, represented by a pattern of neural firing. This activity causes changes in synaptic connections between neurons that allow the memory to be retrieved by reactivating the neural pattern in response to relevant inputs from the senses or other thoughts.

Semantic pointers integrate semantics and syntax because they accommodate sensory–motor and inferential meanings into structures that can be bound into sentences. Later chapters describe how this integration allows semantic pointers to supplant the syntactic dream that has misdirected studies of inference and language. Moreover, the Semantic Pointer Architecture can handle pragmatics, the need for thinking to be sensitive to context and to practical goals such as actions that respond to environments, because it has powerful ways of controlling attention and action described in later chapters.

Semantic pointers can be both embodied and transbodied (i.e., going beyond bodily senses). Embodiment comes by virtue of bindings of sensory, motor, and emotional information. Transbodiment comes from bindings that enable human thought to surpass sensory experience, for example, in the novel concepts of *infinite banana* and *altruistic cat*. Embodiment is important for keeping human thought tied to the world, but transbodiment allows thought to soar into the higher reaches of science, philosophy, and poetry. Even transbodied thought is not some mysterious spiritual activity that is fully disembodied but rather a neural process with remote connections with the senses and the world. Human creativity abounds because recursive binding gives us the capacity to break the fetters of bodily perceptions. Many semantic pointers are learned from sense experience, but others powerfully transcend the senses through recursive binding.

INNATENESS VERSUS LEARNING

Various kinds of structures and processes can be innate, including concepts, rules, and procedures for carrying out different kinds of tasks such as learning language. The alternative hypothesis to innateness is learning. Which representations and procedures are learned from experience, and which are built into our brains by evolution?

Although many philosophers and psychologists have emphasized learning over innateness, at least some procedures must be innate. Consider the mechanisms described earlier in this chapter. Representation by patterns of firing in neural groups is clearly innate. Genes shared by all animals make proteins that produce fetuses whose neurons have connections and firing patterns. No animal has to learn how to get its neurons to fire. As we saw, learning consists of the formation of synaptic connections between neurons, but some of these synaptic connections can be formed by genetic instructions, prior to learning. The difficult question is how much is wired into human brains by evolution and how much is the result of learning from experience, which begins before birth. The question is complicated by the fact that some evolved capacities like walking do not appear immediately but require physical maturation.

Like neural representation, the mechanisms of binding and competition are built into the operations of the brain. Also built-in are basic mechanisms of learning such as Hebbian and reinforcement learning. Binding operations make possible kinds of learning that are not directly tied to environments. You can bind together two experience-based concepts to generate a new concept that goes beyond anyone's experience. For example, you can take the concept of horse and the concept of horn and form an image of a unicorn, thereby generating the concept about previously unobserved unicorns. Similar binding operations can generate hypotheses built out of concepts, for example, the hypothesis that some strange noises are caused by unicorns. Hence, innate learning mechanisms such as neural representation and binding can produce knowledge that goes far beyond what is innate and what can be observed by perception.

It is possible that some specific kinds of representations are built into the brain, for example, ones that can lead to the expectation that the world consists of objects that are connected by causal relations. It is often difficult to tell, however, whether the knowledge that appears in babies early on is there as a result of its having been wired into brains by evolution or whether there is simply a tendency to acquire the appropriate sorts of information by learning.

My own inclination is to hypothesize innate mechanisms just when they are the best explanation of the capacity for humans and other animals to develop representations and behaviors. For particular representations such as concepts, rules, and emotions, I recommend asking the following questions. Are they culturally universal or only found in some societies? Are there specific brain areas where they are found? Are there precursors in animals from which humans evolved? Is there evidence that they were adaptive during the period when the organisms evolved? Are they mere side effects of other features that are innate because of natural selection? Are they better explained by cultural innovation and learning rather than innateness? Answers to these questions do not provide necessary and sufficient conditions of innateness, but they do identify typical features that can serve as criteria.

Often, human mental operations depend on both innate procedures and learned information. For example, chapter 7 describes how emotions have a large innate component that is common to all humans, along with culturally specific aspects that are acquired by learning in a social environment. It would be ridiculous to insist that nothing is innate or that everything is; the better procedure is to figure out case by case what proportions are supported by the evidence. The issue of innateness will be discussed in more detail in later chapters with respect to images, concepts, rules, analogies, language, emotions, and consciousness.

Evidence is mounting for the claim that mental operations can be explained via neural mechanisms that include the following. First, mental representations work by patterns of firing in neural groups. Second, more complicated representations that go beyond sensory experience can be formed by binding representations together, combining patterns of firing into new ones. In particular, binding can produce semantic pointers that coalesce and compress different kinds of information, including sensory, motor, emotional, and verbal information. Semantic pointers retain connections to sensory and motor experience while also acquiring the autonomy that is usually attributed to symbols. Eliasmith's semantic pointer hypothesis shows how neural cells can interact to produce high-level thinking.

Third, different representations compete with each other to provide accounts of what is going on in the world through a parallel process of satisfaction of multiple constraints. Fourth, neural networks can learn by changing the synaptic connections between neurons. There are various methods of learning, including: Hebbian learning, which does not require a supervisor; supervised learning such as reinforcement by rewards and punishments where the supervisor can be the environment; and higher-level kinds of learning resulting from the generation of new representations by means of binding. Learning and inference allow the brain to change as the result of new information that comes from the senses as well as from transformations of stored mental representations into new ones.

Emergence of properties of wholes that are not properties of their parts occurs in many ways. Groups of neurons represent aspects of the world that no single neuron can. Semantic pointers are symbol-like neural representations that result from the compression and recursive binding of perceptual, motor, verbal, and emotional information. Semantic pointers have capacities for meaning and inference not found in any of the simpler representations that they bind together. Recursive binding of semantic pointers can produce radically new and valuable images and sentences that are the quintessence of creativity.

Neuroscience is both an experimental field and a theoretical field. The experimental side of neuroscience has exploded in recent decades because of the development of scanning techniques such as functional magnetic resonance imagery. But no science aspires only to collect data, as researchers want to make sense of their data by developing new theories that provide causal mechanisms from which the experimental phenomena result. Because of the complexity of neural operations and their interactions, the typical way of building neural theories is to postulate mechanisms that can be simulated using computer models. The success of the models in approximating the results of experiments provides evidence that theoretical progress is being made.

Theoretical neuroscience has been identifying mechanisms for explaining thinking, just as biology has been identifying mechanisms for explaining life. In the nineteenth century, some biologists and philosophers argued that life was so unlike other physical processes that it could only be explained by the operations of a special vital force. But this idea turned out be superfluous as life increasingly became explained by mechanisms such as cell division, digestion, respiration, and reproduction. Analogously, more and more aspects of thinking are being explained by neural mechanisms of representation, binding, competition, and learning. Evidence for this claim is presented in the chapters to come. Images, concepts, beliefs, and emotions are all kinds of semantic pointers that carry out their cognitive functions by means of bindings of neural representations.

APPENDIX: DETAILS AND COMPARISONS

For readers with more background in cognitive science, this section provides some technical details about semantic pointers and comparisons with related ideas.

Mathematics and Computation

A typical neuron has a firing rate of around 100 times per second, which gives it 100 possible firing rates but 2^{100} possible firing patterns over a second, which is more than 1 followed by 30 zeros. Ten neurons working together with each firing 100 times per second can have $10^{(2^{100})}$ firing patterns over a second, which is more than the number of atoms in the universe. Hence, the representational capacity of groups of neurons firing in coordination with each other is enormous.

Learning changes the connectivity of groups of neurons by adjusting the strengths of the synaptic links between them in response to inputs from the environment, disposing the neurons to fire in appropriate patterns when similar inputs are received. But patterns of firing should be able to respond not only to simple features but also to combinations of features, so that concepts like *cat* and *pet* can substantially increase an organism's ability to understand the world.

Mathematically, patterns of firing in neural groups are conveniently represented by vectors, which are strings of numbers that represent a collection of dimensions. For example, the speed and direction of a car can be represented by the two-dimensional vector (20, 90), where 20 indicates that the car is going 20 kilometers per hour and 90 indicates an angle of direction. Speed and location could be represented by a three-dimensional vector that includes map coordinates, for example, where (20, 10, 20) indicates 20 kilometers per hour and map indicators of 10 units across and 20 up.

The firing rates of a group of neurons are naturally captured by vectors with the dimension of the number of neurons, for example when (0.2, 0.4, 0.6, 0.8) represents the rates of four neurons firing with increasing frequencies expressed as a maximum of their capacity. Here 0.8 means that the neuron is firing at 80% of its firing capacity, which would be 80 times per second in a neuron capable of firing 100 times per second. Using vectors to represent firing patterns rather than rates requires many more dimensions, up to 1,024 in the Semantic Pointer Architecture.

Once the firing pattern of a group of neurons is represented by a vector, we can define convolution of patterns as a mathematical operation on vectors. The addition of vectors is simple, for example, when adding (0.2, 0.4, 0.6, 0.8) and (0.1, 0.1, 0.1 0.1) yields (0.3, 0.5, 0.7, 0.9). But vector addition and multiplication of vectors cannot perform convolution, because they obliterate the information in the input, which cannot be reconstructed even approximately. The vector (0.3, 0.5, 0.6, 0.9) could have resulted from the addition of many other pairs of vectors.

Convolution solves this problem by using a more complex function that wraps the dimensional values of two vectors around each other (using multiplication and modular arithmetic) to produce a vector that is not similar to the original vectors but can nevertheless be decomposed into an approximation of the originals. For details, see Eliasmith (2013, p. 406) and Crawford, Gingerich, and Eliasmith (2016, p. 788). In the Semantic Pointer Architecture, the convolution of vectors is computed by feed-forward neural networks, thereby implementing binding by convolution in spiking neurons.

Semantic pointers formed by convolution are a key component of a general account of neural computation called the Semantic Pointer Architecture, which produces motor outputs in response to visual inputs and numerous other processes including working memory and action selection. This architecture is implemented in a specific computational model called Spaun, which has been used to simulate many cognitive processes and even to control robots. For a diagram and more detail, see http://compneuro.uwaterloo.ca/research/spa/semantic-pointer-architecture.html.

Semantic pointers can be further characterized by contrasting them with more familiar theoretical ideas in cognitive science, including mental representation, distributed representations, rules, schemas, modality-specific simulations, Bayesian inference, and somatic markers.

Mental Representation

A mental representation is a structure in the mind that stands for something. A semantic pointer is a neurocomputational process that explains how mental representations might operate in the brain. To make this conjecture plausible, it needs to be shown how each kind of empirically supported mental representation (e.g., concepts and rules) can be implemented as semantic pointers.

Distributed Representations

In connectionist architectures such as the influential parallel distributed processing (PDP) account, concepts are not represented by single word-like nodes but rather by groups of neurons working together: The representation is distributed across multiple neurons as occurs in the brain (Rumelhart & McClelland, 1986; Rogers & McClelland, 2004). Semantic pointers are a kind of distributed representation, but they differ from standard accounts in two ways. First, the neurons employed in the Semantic Pointer Architecture are spiking neurons, capable of firing with many different patterns that affect the firing activity of other neurons. In contrast, PDP models use rate neurons, whose activity is determined by how fast they fire, not their particular patterns. Second, whereas PDP connections are formed by training using algorithms such as backpropagation, semantic pointers are formed by convolution of other neural patterns, including ones formed by learning. This formation enables semantic pointers to be subject to further convolutions into sentence-like representations, functioning as symbols.

Rules

In rule-based architectures such as ACT-R, rules are IF–THEN structures where the IF and THEN parts are groups of word-like symbols (Anderson, 1983, 2007). Semantic pointers are not rules, but they can be used to model rule-like problem solving, for example, in the Tower of Hanoi problem (Eliasmith, 2013, chapter 5). The IF and THEN parts in the Semantic Pointer Architecture are not traditional symbols but are represented by vectors created in part by convolution in ways that can be encoded as patterns of neural firing.

Schemas

In psychology, a schema is a mental representation of a class of objects, events, or practices. Semantic pointers provide a mechanistic explanation of what schemas are and how they work in the brain. For example, the restaurant schema is a combination of a concept and expectations for what to do in restaurants. Concepts can be explained as semantic pointers (Blouw, Solodkin, Thagard, & Eliasmith, 2016), and expectations can be modeled as rules of the sort just described. Hence, schemas in the brain are one kind of semantic pointer, but there are other kinds of semantic pointers such as representations of individuals.

Modality-Specific Simulations

Barsalou (2016) has emphasized that concepts are grounded in particular modalities such as vision rather than being amodal, language-like representations. Such concepts can be used in simulations, for example, when visual images associated with a restaurant allow people to imagine themselves being seated and fed. Semantic pointers provide neural explanations of how concepts can combine different modalities and can serve in simulations using nonverbal rules. Hence, Barsalou's psychological theories are mechanistically explained by the Semantic Pointer Architecture.

Bayesian Inference

Bayesian cognitive architectures explain human thought using network structures that make inferences using probability theory. The Semantic Pointer Architecture does not explicitly use probabilities, but semantic pointer vectors can be interpreted as probability distributions, and Bayesian inference is approximately implemented by neural computations (Eliasmith, 2013, p. 281). Bayesian networks translate sensory inputs into values of variables rather than performing modal retention.

Somatic Markers

According to Damasio (1994), cognitive processes such as decision-making are heavily influenced by neural responses to bodily changes. These somatic markers enable the brain rapidly to evaluate and anticipate different actions and outcomes. Somatic markers are naturally understood as semantic pointers if they involve bindings of inputs from various internal physiological sensors and signals concerned with situations. Hence, somatic markers are part (but not all) of the semantic pointer theory of emotion presented in chapter 7.

Summary

In sum, semantic pointers are processes in groups of spiking neurons that provide representations by repeatedly binding sensory, motor, and verbal patterns of firing. Such processes provide neurocomputational explanations for many psychological ideas such as schemas and emotions.

Comparisons with Other Cognitive Architectures

Dozens of other cognitive architectures have been proposed, but it would be tedious to provide detailed comparisons of the Semantic Pointer Architecture with each of them. Fortunately, John Laird, Christian Lebiere, and Paul Rosenbloom propose a standard model of the mind that encompasses what they see as the common core of current cognitive architectures, so it is useful to compare the Semantic Pointer Architecture with this model.

The Standard Model assumes the physical symbol system hypothesis, according to which the manipulation of symbols in physical systems such as brains and computers is both necessary and sufficient for intelligence. It is open both to the traditional computational understanding of symbols as uninterpreted labels and to more recent understanding of symbols as statistical patterns such as those in neural networks. The Standard Model views these symbols as interacting via five components: perception, motor, working memory, declarative long-term memory, and procedural memory. Long-term memory is permanent, high-capacity storage of representations, in contrast to working memory, which holds information temporarily to keep it available for processing. Declarative memory concerns facts or events, whereas procedural memory is unconscious storage of skills and how to do things.

The heart of the Standard Model is the cognitive cycle in which interactions among the various kinds of memory lead to the selection of a deliberate act roughly every 50 milliseconds. Problem solving occurs by sequences of such deliberate acts, sometimes leading to motor actions. Perception converts sensory inputs into symbolic structures, which motor control can convert into external actions. Learning consists of changes to long-term memory content, both declarative and procedural.

At first glance, the Semantic Pointer Architecture seems like an instantiation of the Standard Model, because it also has perceptual inputs, motor control, and working memory. Long-term declarative and procedural memory are not explicitly shown in Figure 2.7 but are consistent with the standard assumption that neural networks store memories through synaptic connections between neurons. Action selection using semantic pointers is analogous to the deliberate act cycle of the Standard Model.

Careful inspection, however, reveals that the Semantic Pointer Architecture diverges from the Standard Model in at least four respects. First, the Semantic Pointer Architecture is explicitly tied to the structure of the brain, as is ACT-R, whereas the Standard Model assumes that cognitive systems can be implemented by a diversity of physical devices such as various kinds of computers. Simulations of the Semantic Pointer Architecture are commonly run on regular digital computers, but they work much better on recent versions of neuromorphic chips that mimic the operations of biological neurons by having millions of artificial neurons that operate in parallel. The Semantic Pointer Architecture recognizes that brains have large advantages over digital computers in energy efficiency, consuming only about 40 watts of power while accomplishing tasks such as pattern recognition and inference with effectiveness only now being approximated by banks of computers. Hardware matters for both energy efficiency and for carrying out required tasks in real time, as biologically required for survival and reproduction.

Second, the Semantic Pointer Architecture complies with the massive parallelism of the brain, which has billions of neurons capable of firing at the same time with no central coordination. The Standard Model allows for parallel processing across its five components (e.g., with perception and memory operating independently), but it has only limited parallelism within components for processes such as matching and firing rules. In the Semantic Pointer Architecture as in the brain, neurons operate asynchronously; that is, they fire independently in their own time patterns determined by thousands of inputs coming from other neurons. In principle, such parallelism can be simulated by serial processes, but the brain gets its practical effectiveness for real-time performance by much greater parallelism than the Standard Model requires.

Third, the Semantic Pointer Architecture differs from the Standard Model in how it deals with perceptual and motor information. The Standard Model assumes that perception converts external signals into symbols but does not require that the resulting symbols retain any connection with the sensory input. In contrast, many semantic pointers result from compressing and binding sensory signals that are transformed but not completely lost. Standard computer systems translate sensory information into nonsensory values of variables, a process that might be called "amodal transduction": Inputs from some sensory modality are transduced (translated) into modality-free representations, abandoning the sensory character of the information.

In contrast, semantic pointers accomplish modal retention, preserving in compressed form the information resulting from the particular sensory or motor modality that produced them. Modal retention is crucial for the ability of the

Semantic Pointer Architecture to explain many important psychological phenomena that are not currently within the scope of the Standard Model, including imagery, emotions, and consciousness (chapters 3–8). The Standard Model does not forbid modal retention, but the cognitive architectures on which it is based (Soar, ACT-R, Sigma) do not have mechanisms for preserving sensory information in internal representations.

The fourth divergence of the Semantic Pointer Architecture from the Standard Model concerns the contentious question of the meaning of symbols. A standard objection against traditional artificial intelligence is that the physical symbols it employs have syntax but no semantics. But symbols acquired in the Semantic Pointer Architecture via sensory inputs do have physical grounding because of the causal processes that connect senses with the world. The connection between symbols and the world through semantic pointers is much tighter than the connection for symbols that arise from sensory inputs to a Standard Model–type system, because of modal retention.

As chapter 10 on language clarifies, the meaning of symbols comes from both connections to the world and from connections to other symbols. Without modal retention, cognitive architectures have abundant symbol–symbol connections but are limited in symbol–world connections. Semantic pointers also have abundant symbol–symbol connections because their compression enables them to function with some independence from sensory experience. Moreover, new semantic pointers can be formed by binding other semantic pointers, allowing the Semantic Pointer Architecture to account for transbodiment (going beyond bodily senses) as well as embodiment.

NOTES

Books on theoretical neuroscience include Dayan and Abbot 2001; Eliasmith and Anderson 2003; Hebb 1949; O'Reilly and Munakata 2000; O'Reilly, Munakata, Frank, Hazy, and Contributors 2012; and Shallice and Cooper 2011. Poldrack and Yarkoni 2016 discuss the use of brain scans in cognitive neuroscience.

For a philosophical discussion of mind–brain identity, see *Natural Philosophy*, chapter 2. Rather than the simple identity theory that mind = brain, that book defends multilevel materialism which incorporates social mechanisms, including semantic pointer communication described in *Mind–Society*, chapter 3.

I cannot define "pattern," but a three-analysis can provide exemplars (e.g., visual, musical, tactile), typical features (e.g., regular, recurring, static or temporal), and explanations (e.g., patterns explain sensory reactions and are

explained by underlying mechanisms such as designers, natural selection, and social cooperation).

On semantic pointers, see Eliasmith 2013 and Eliasmith et al. 2012. Eliasmith
(2013, p. 83) characterizes semantic pointers in three different but corresponding
ways: physically as occurrent activity in biological networks (which is equivalent to
my description of patterns of firing), functionally as compressed representations
that point to fuller semantic content, and mathematically as vectors in a high-
dimensional space (see this chapter's appendix). Construction of semantic pointers
uses addition of vectors as well as binding by convolution. Chris's last name,
Eliasmith, is a compressed binding of his last name before marriage (Elias) and his
wife Jennifer's maiden name (Smith). For a video of Chris explaining the Semantic
Pointer Architecture, see https://www.youtube.com/watch?v=-bBqWHenYNA.

Specific neurons for movie stars are reported by Quiroga Reddy, Kreiman, Koch,
and Fried 2005.

On binding by convolution and related methods, see Eliasmith 2013, Eliasmith
and Thagard 2001, Stewart and Eliasmith 2011, Plate 2003, and Smolensky 1990.
For another approach to binding by indirection, see Kriete, Noelle, Cohen, and
O'Reilly 2013. Newly hatched chicks can do visual binding: Wood, 2014.

Proponents of binding by neural synchrony include Engel Fries, König, Brecht,
and Singer 1999; Hummel and Holyoak 2003; and Shastri and Ajjanagaddi 1993.
Wang and Fan 2007 present a neural network model of attention based on
competition.

In this chapter, I use the term "symbol" in the sense employed in logic, computer science, and linguistics to mean any verbal representation. In anthropology,
"symbol" has a richer sense discussed in *Mind–Society* (Thagard, 2019a).

Figure 2.7 is based on Eliasmith et al. 2012, which describes simulations using
the program Spaun (Semantic Pointer Architecture Unified Network). See that
paper's Figure 1 for more detailed depiction of functions and brain areas, as well as
Eliasmith (2013, Table 7.2).

On parallel constraint satisfaction, see Rumelhart and McClelland 1986; Read,
Vanman, and Miller 1997; and Thagard 2000.

For a review of cognitive architectures, see Thagard 2012a. For a list of cognitive
architectures, see https://en.wikipedia.org/wiki/Cognitive_architecture.

On moderate embodiment compatible with mental representations, see Barsalou
2009 and Gibbs 2005. On the radical and implausible view that embodiment eliminates representation, see Chemero 2009. Antirepresentationalists tout dynamic
systems as alternatives to representation and procedures. The brain is undoubtedly
a dynamic system, but it is a special kind that uses representations: Eliasmith 1996.

On memory and retrieval in neural networks, see Eliasmith 2013 and O'Reilly et al. 2012. Deep learning, currently popular in artificial intelligence, is a kind of supervised learning in multi-layered neural networks: Mnih et al. 2015.

Discussions of innateness and learning include Carey 2009 and Elman et al. 1996.

Brown 1991 provides a list and analysis of human universals.

On the Standard Model for cognitive architectures, see Laird, Lebiere, and Rosenbloom 2017. It is a generalization of three well-established cognitive architectures (Soar, ACT-R, and Sigma), all of which have a distant ancestor in the General Problem Solver of Newell and Simon 1972. Chapter 5 contains more on rule-based architectures. Neural network architectures such as Leabra (O'Reilly et al., 2012) and Clarion (Sun, 2014) are more like the brain but lack the Semantic Pointer Architecture's neural realism and modal retention. Eliasmith (2013, chapter 9) compares the Semantic Pointer Architecture with six other cognitive architectures.

PROJECT

To demonstrate that parallel constraint satisfaction can generally be modeled as semantic pointer competition, implement classic tasks such as concept application, visual interpretation, semantic ambiguity, analogical mapping, and explanatory coherence in the Semantic Pointer Architecture.

3

Perception and Imagery

Albert Einstein wrote about his discoveries:

> The words or the language, as they are written or spoken, do not seem to play any role in my mechanism of thought. The psychical entities which seem to serve as elements in thought are certain signs and more or less clear images which can be "voluntarily" reproduced and combined.

This comment is surprising, because Einstein is rightly regarded as one of the great minds of the twentieth century, but people usually associate intelligence with verbal operations of speaking and writing. In contrast, Einstein claimed to get his major insights from pictorial images. That puts him in the company of animals like chimpanzees, crows, and octopuses, which lack language and therefore must rely on images or associations for their impressive problem solving.

According to empiricist philosophers like John Locke and David Hume, the source of all knowledge is experience from the senses such as seeing and hearing. Later chapters on concepts, rules, and analogies will show that this claim is an exaggeration, but much of human knowledge does derive from our senses. You know the colors of apples, as well as their tastes, textures, smells, and the sounds they make when you drop them on the floor. You also know how it feels when eating too many apples gives you a stomach ache or diarrhea, relying on internal bodily senses as well as external ones such as vision. This chapter shows how perception and imagery can be understood using neural mechanisms of representation, binding, competition, learning, and memory.

Humans can easily go beyond sensory stimulation to create images of things they have never directly experienced. You can imagine a purple apple, or one eaten with spicy mustard, or one that smells like a rose, or one with a scratchy skin, or one that makes a strange sound when thrown against a metal gong. These imaginings require neural mechanisms for transforming representations into new ones. Imagery also operates on internal senses, as when you think of having an intense pain in your left earlobe. People are also capable of emotional imagery, for example, when you imagine how you would feel if you won the lottery or if your best friend died. All forms of imagery support basic transformations such as intensification, combination, and juxtaposition, but some transformations such as rotating a visual object are specific to particular kinds of sensing.

Later chapters will show the relevance of perception and imagery to other cognitive processes including concept application, inferences based on rules and analogies, planning, metaphoric language, and empathic understanding of other people. Perception and imagery are also relevant to social applications such as political ideologies and religious rituals. Political and religious practices include visual images like pictures of candidates and martyrs, auditory images like campaign songs and hymns, and even olfactory images like incense. Treatments of cognition often emphasize the verbal communication that is such an important part of human interactions, but more basic are the sensory mechanisms that people share with other animals.

FROM SENSATION TO PERCEPTION TO IMAGERY

Sensation is the stimulation of bodily receptors, for example, when photons of light hit cells in the retina to excite neurons in the optic nerve that connect the retina with the brain. Perception is the brain's interpretation of these signals, for example, when you see a rabbit rather than a squirrel. Imagery occurs when perceptions are stored and later reactivated, for example, when you remember that the rabbit you saw yesterday was limping.

Even bacteria have simple sensors such as ones for detecting chemicals like glucose that indicate food sources, but they lack brains to interpret those sensors. Plants can sense and react to light, moisture, gravity, temperature, sound, touch, and other stimuli, but they are limited in their capacity to interpret these inputs because they lack neurons that evolved in simple animals such as jellyfish and worms. The roundworm *C. elegans* has only around 7,500 synapses that suffice for finding food and mates. More complicated animals have multiple ways of sensing the external world and also have ways of sensing what is going on inside their bodies.

Both external and internal sensation operate by means of five capacities. First, an animal needs to have sensors that can send signals to the brain. Second, the animal needs to have ways of converting the signals into patterns of neural firing that can represent aspects of the world, turning sensations into perceptions. Third, the animal needs to be able to convert what it has learned from the signals into courses of action that can accomplish its goals, which in all organisms include surviving and reproducing. Fourth, the animal needs to be able to learn from experience, that is, to change the connections among its neurons so that it can be better at accomplishing its goals in the future. Fifth, for more complicated kinds of representation and action, an animal benefits from being able to combine its sensations into organized images by means of neural binding.

This chapter considers the familiar external senses: vision, hearing, touch, taste, and smell. But the human body also is capable of many different internal senses, such as pain, heat, balance, hunger, thirst, acceleration, time, stomach distension, kinesthesia (muscle movement sense), proprioception (sense of spatial location), and the need to urinate or defecate. All of these kinds of sensation operate with neural codes based on patterns of firing in groups of neurons.

Primitive organisms like worms are only capable of firing patterns that represent simple stimuli. But humans are able to go beyond external and internal inputs and generate them by imagination. A mental image is a representation that resembles the representations that the senses have produced, but people can transcend the senses by combining images. Imagery enables humans to go far beyond anything that they have ever experienced, for example, when you form the mental picture of something that has never been seen before by anybody, such as a galloping unicorn ridden by a basketball player.

Most research on imagery in cognitive science has been done on vision, but other kinds of imagery are also important. For example, you can imagine the sound of your favorite singer executing a song such as "Happy Birthday." This image can combine multiple modalities, when you make a visual picture of the singer at the same time as you imagine the song being sung. You might even be able to integrate this visual–auditory image with the other external senses, such as smell, touch, and taste. Imagery can also operate on the internal senses, for example, when you imagine having a severe pain in your left hand.

EXTERNAL SENSES

Each of the senses that animals use to gain information about the external world has its own sense organs and its own brain areas where representations are primarily formed. For example, vision uses the eyes and the brain's occipital lobe. Nevertheless, the senses are similar in using sensors, neural signals, and neural representations. The senses in other animals are not the same as in humans. Dogs have a more powerful sense of smell than humans with the ability to bind smells to specific locations in their environment. Birds can sense ultraviolet light. Bats are capable of echolocation, using sound waves to navigate. Some fish are able to sense electromagnetic fields, and some birds do long-distance migration by virtue of their ability to sense magnetic fields of the earth. The human sensory apparatus is just one way of forming representations of the world that are useful for operating in it.

In humans, as in our monkey ancestors, the most powerful form of sensation is vision. Plato thought that vision works by the eyes sending out rays that are reflected back into the eye, a view still held by many people (Winer, Cottrell, Gregg, Fournier, & Bica, 2002). We now know that no such rays are needed, because light from any source reflects off objects in the world into the eye. At the back of the eye are millions of cells in the retina that are capable of detecting light. These cells initiate neural signals that send information to the visual cortex in the occipital lobe at the back of the brain, where signals must be processed before inferences can lead to object recognition.

To develop visual representations, the brain needs to be able to detect edges, notice lines, and build these into recognition of various kinds of shapes such as circles and rectangles. These shapes can be three dimensional, for example, spheres and cubes rather than circles and squares. Moreover, the shapes can have important associated characteristics such as texture and color. Processing such information is not straightforward, for there are always multiple possible interpretations that can be made of different shapes, textures, and colors. The result of choosing among interpretations is always a pattern of firing in a group of neurons.

Hearing also depends on neural transformations. When sound waves enter our ears, they produce a chain of events that affects different internal parts such as the ear drum and cochlea. The result is a rapid series of neural firings that travel by nerves into a part of the temporal lobe called the auditory cortex. As with vision, the information carried by the signals encodes multiple features, including loudness, pitch, and timbre. In the auditory cortex, millions of neurons combine these pieces of information into a unified sound, for example, Paul McCartney singing the song "Yesterday." Further processing is required for the brain to recognize a sound using familiar sounds stored in memory.

Touch sensors are found all over the body in skin cells. When an object impinges on those cells, a signal is sent via neurons to the somatosensory cortex in the parietal lobe. The brain integrates the information that comes from many different cells, for example, ones at the tips of all of your fingers. As with vision and sound, the causal pattern runs from sensor cells to neural signal to patterns of firing operating in the brain that represent what is being sensed, for example, a pen that you are holding in your hand. There are many kinds of skin sensors such as for temperature, air flow, and air pressure.

Taste and smell often work together even though they operate with different kinds of sensors and neural pathways. Your tongue has detectors for a small number of characteristics, including sweet, sour, salty, bitter, and umami, the sensation of glutamate in such foods as soy sauce and parmesan cheese. Smell has a much larger range of detectors, because your nose is able to detect thousands of different kinds of molecules that stimulate sensors in your nose. You are able to smell more different kinds of things than you can taste, although not as many as a dog can. When we eat or drink, our overall sensation is the result of the combination of taste and smells, all of which result in neural firing patterns in brain areas such as the olfactory bulb. As with vision, hearing, and touch, the neural response to external sensors is not confined to one brain area but can be affected by many others, ranging from the amygdala to the prefrontal cortex. Chapter 8 explains how such patterns of neural firing give rise to conscious experiences.

Combination of sensations can sometimes have surprising results, for example, in synesthesia, which affects approximately 5% of the human population. Synesthetes combine aspects of sensation that for most people are separate, for example, seeing the shape of the number 9 associated with particular colors such as yellow, or a particular sound such as that of a trumpet, or even a particular taste. Synesthesia can also be induced in people who do not normally have it by means of drugs such as LSD that disrupt neural processing.

Many people naively assume that they perceive the world as it really is. This assumption requires a simple causal relation between the world and the perceptions produced by the senses. There is substantial evidence, however, that visual perception is shaped by prior assumptions, context, and even motivations: people are prone to "wishful seeing," for example, seeing desirable objects as closer than they really are and categorizing visual information in ways that suit their goals.

The crucial role that inference plays in perception is illustrated by the ambiguity in Figure 3.1. The picture can be seen as either of two different cubes depending

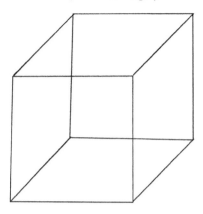

FIGURE 3.1 Ambiguous pictures that can be perceived in different ways depending on context and focus. To make it flip, attend to different corners of the cube.

on which corners you focus on. The capability of the brain to perceive whole forms is called the gestalt effect, and the switch between forms is a gestalt shift. Gestalt shifts are prime examples of emergence: The perception of the whole is other than the sum of the parts because it results from interactions among the neurons that represent the parts. Small changes in sensory inputs, resulting from shifts in attention between different aspects of the figure, can cause a critical transition (tipping point) from one perceptual whole to another. Perceptual inferences are performed by neural groups using parallel constraint satisfaction, which can integrate top–down expectations with bottom–up sensory inputs.

INTERNAL SENSES

Just as important for human functioning are the internal senses that tell us what is going on in our bodies. Our skin contains sensors not only for touch and temperature but also for pain. Nociceptors found in the internal organs as well as the skin detect potentially damaging changes and send signals through the spinal cord to multiple brain areas, including the parieto-insular cortex, with interconnections to the amygdala and other areas related to emotions.

The brain also has neural patterns capable of detecting and representing other kinds of internal operations, including heart rate, respiration, and levels of the stress hormone cortisol. Chapter 7 describes how representing these physiological changes is important for generation of emotions. Other internal sensors that support human functioning include the sense of fullness when one has eaten enough and the genital engorgement that accompanies sexual arousal. The human gut is rich in sensors and neural processing, with around 100,000 neurons, as many as are found in the brain of a fruit fly or lobster. The neural patterns generated in the human gut are important for regulating digestion but can also have effects on emotions and therefore on high-level cognition.

For walking, dancing, and sports, a sense of balance is very important. People need to be able to detect when they are falling or tilted, and there are organs such as the eyes, ears, and muscular system that send signals to the brain, for example, from the vestibular system in the inner ear to the brain's cerebellum. Another important internal sense is kinesthesia, which is produced by signals sent from the muscle to the cerebellum to produce an overall representation of the location and motion of muscles. Kinesthetic representations are important for many actions such as picking up objects, throwing a ball, or opening a door.

An organism does not need to have a complicated brain to have sensation. Even jellyfish have simple sensors that detect aspects of their environment and prompt them to act in ways that promote their survival. But an organism with multiple sensors can pick up different aspects of the environment, using this information to generate actions that will be far more effective for survival and reproduction than mere reflexes. Combinations of sensations can support multimodal object recognition, for example, when humans are able to identify something as a dog by virtue of its shape, color, feel, and smell. Combinations of sensory information requires binding sensations into integrated representations which can then support imagery.

IMAGERY

The empiricist philosophers Locke and Hume assumed that sensation was the most fundamental form of thinking and that ideas are merely copies of sensation. Many contemporary philosophers err in the opposite direction, supposing that thinking is essentially a matter of language, with sensation merely generating information that needs to be transformed into linguistic format before thinking gets underway. Even cognitive psychologists sometimes write as if the most obvious form of thinking is with language, with imagery providing a supplementary code on top of linguistic processing. From an evolutionary point of view, this emphasis on language is peculiar, given that animals other than humans do not have anything like our linguistic capacity.

During the 1970s and 1980s, a strong case was made from experimental work in both psychology and neuroscience that human thought employs visual imagery. This section will review the experimental evidence that supports the existence of imagery, making it plausible that most people use visual and other kinds of imagery to solve problems and perform other varieties of thinking.

A visual image is a mental representation that has approximately the same spatial structure as what it represents. Since the 1970s, psychologists have produced many clever experiments that support the view that visual imagery is an important part of human thinking. Some kinds of visual thinking seem to involve rotation, for example, when you imagine what the Eiffel Tower would look like if it were turned upside down, as in Figure 3.2. Psychologists got the idea of trying to determine experimentally whether mental rotation is what it seems. If you really are rotating the Eiffel Tower, then it should take longer to rotate it 180° until it is fully upside down than it takes to rotate it 90°, which puts it on its side. Experiments

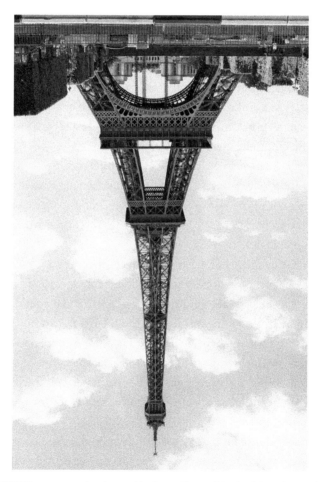

FIGURE 3.2 Eiffel Tower rotated to be upside down. Try making it right side up. Photo from public domain.

showed that mental rotation has just the expected temporal properties: People are slower to answer questions that require longer rotations then shorter ones.

Other psychological experiments that provide evidence that people are using visual imagery include the finding that it takes longer for people to answer a question when they have to scan a long way across a map than merely a short way. For example, it takes longer to scan a mental map from New York to California than it does to scan from New York to Chicago. These experiments do not conclusively prove that people are capable of using visual representations in their thinking when they answer questions, because there might be some kind of weird verbal inference that produces the same results for rotation and scanning.

In the 1980s, however, new experimental evidence became available that has convinced most psychologists that visual imagery is a special form of representation operating in human brains. With brain scans, one can detect the flow of blood to regions that may require visual imagery when people are given tasks such as rotation and scanning. The important finding is that when people do these tasks neurons fire in parts of the brain that are typically involved in visual processing. There is also activation in motor areas, as if mentally rotating the Eiffel Tower uses your muscles to physically move the tower. For these reasons, most cognitive psychologists support the conclusion that thought operates with visual imagery as well as linguistic representations.

Visual imagery can be very useful for solving problems. How can you find a key that has fallen under your sofa? To answer this question, you can imagine yourself pushing the sofa out of the way or, alternatively, sliding a ruler under the sofa to push the key within reach of your hand. Both these solutions involve a combination of visual and kinesthetic imagery.

Whereas visual imagery has been extensively investigated by psychologists, much less research has been done on other kinds of imagery that are also important. For example, you can take your memory of a particular sound, say a musical note, and imagine it played higher, lower, or louder. You can imagine a favorite food such as lasagna with a slightly different taste, for example, saltier or spicier. When I was asked by nurses after a hip operation to report my degree of pain on a scale of 1 to 10, I recalled the worst pain I have ever experienced, a burst ear drum. I labeled that pain as number 9 and then used it as a mark to compare the pain I was feeling in my hip.

The anecdotal evidence for many other kinds of imagery seems convincing: You should have no problem imagining a caress, dizziness, or urgently full bladder. Does this mean that the brain has many codes besides the dual code that has been taken to operate by combining linguistic and visual representations? Chapter 2 offered a much simpler way of thinking about how the mind works, namely, with a common underlying code that comes from patterns of firing in groups of neurons. Nevertheless, because there are different pathways by which sensory inputs lead to neural firing in different brain areas, it is not surprising that various sensations feel different consciously, as discussed in chapter 8.

Auditory imagery has been studied with respect to features of sounds, including pitch, timbre, loudness, musical melody, harmony, tempo, and speech. Sound imagery preserves many structural and temporal properties of auditory stimuli, including pitch distance, loudness distance, timbre, and melody. Just as the time to identify a rotated visual image is proportional to the degree of rotation, the time to compare two pitches is proportional to the auditory difference between them. Just as generation of visual imagery involves activation of brain areas involved in perception of visual stimuli, generation of auditory imagery involves activation of many brain areas involved in perception of sounds. There are therefore good reasons to believe that visual and auditory imagery are legitimate mental representations that require neural explanation.

MENTAL MECHANISMS FOR IMAGERY

A general theory of imagery needs to specify the mental and neural mechanisms responsible for the construction, transformation, and comparison of images. It should apply to all modalities, covering external senses such as vision, internal senses such as pain, and emotions that integrate internal senses with cognitive appraisals (chapter 7). It should be compatible with theories of perception that combine sensory inputs with cognitive elements such as expectations. It should apply both to simple transformations such as intensifying the color or loudness of an image and to more complex ones that require combining multiple images. A unified theory of imagery needs to show that the same neural mechanisms accomplish imagery across all modalities.

Other kinds of imagery use operations like those for visual imagery. I have already described some of the ways in which visual images can be manipulated, for example, by rotating and scanning them. Another important operation for visual imagery is zooming, for example, when you start with an image of the Eiffel Tower in the distance and then imagine myself getting closer to it until you can focus on the metal structure in more detail.

Zooming and focusing have analogues that operate in other kinds of imagery as well. For example, in tasting lasagna, you can try to focus in on one aspect of it such as the flavor of the cheese or the degree of saltiness. In thinking about the sound of the song "Happy Birthday," you can zoom in or focus on the sound of the notes as the phrase "to you" is sung. You can also zoom in on a pain in a particular part of your foot rather than pain in the whole foot.

Another useful kind of imagery operation is juxtaposition. You can imagine the Eiffel Tower with a gorilla climbing on top of it, thereby placing the image of the ape beside the image of the Eiffel Tower or possibly on top of it, which is superposition. Juxtaposition also works with other modalities. You can imagine "Happy Birthday" being sung but then add that the singing is accompanied by a trombone, producing a combined auditory image of "Happy Birthday" being sung with a trombone accompaniment. Juxtaposition and superposition also work with taste and smell, for example, in imagining the taste of lasagna accompanied by mushroom sauce. These operations are important for constructing new images and therefore for creativity discussed in chapter 11.

Table 3.1 is a rough attempt to characterize the operations in mental imagery. I will show in the next section how these changes can be accomplished by the neural mechanisms of representation, binding, and competition described in chapter 2. Table 3.1 considers imagery based on two kinds of external sensation— sight and hearing—and two kinds of internal sensation—pain and movement. The table provides examples of five classes of operations in all four kinds of imagery. There are many other kinds of internal and external imagery, and there may be other operations besides the ones discussed here.

Intensification occurs when you take a characteristic of an image and make it stronger, for example, imagining making a color brighter, a sound louder, a pain worse, or an arm move faster. Weakening of the characteristics of an image is just the reverse of intensification, for example, making a sound quieter. Imagery intensification applies to all external senses, as it is easy to imagine a saltier taste, a

TABLE 3.1

Five Operations on Four Kinds of Imagery

	Intensify	Focus	Combine	Juxtapose	Decompose
See	Color, size	Zoom, scan	Features	Objects, movies	Look at parts
Hear	Loudness, pitch	Concentrate, scan	Sounds (e.g., chords)	Melody	Examine parts
Pain	Hurt	Concentrate	Location	Sequence	Separate
Movement	Speed	Concentrate	Complex action	Series of actions	Break down into steps

fouler smell, or a firmer touch. Similarly, internal sensations can be transformed into intensified images such as greater hunger, thirst, nausea, dizziness, imbalance, and fullness. The qualitative character of experiences varies across the wide range of internal and external senses, but intensification operates across the range.

Focusing also applies to all kinds of imagery, although it is most familiar in vision. Think of the face of your favorite movie star, and now focus in on the eyes to see if you can identify their color. Scanning a visual image such as a map is sequentially focusing on various aspects like the placement of countries. Music provides a good domain for auditory images, and you can run a favorite song in your head and focus on one of the salient features, such as a particular set of notes or an instrumental part such as the violin. You can also scan through a remembered song to focus on a solo. With pain, you can concentrate on a particular aspect of it such as its intensity or location. Focusing on motor actions can involve concentrating on one aspect of a motion, for example, how you are moving your wrists when you swing a tennis racket.

Combination occurs when you take two or more characteristics of sensations and locate them in the same entity, such as an apple that you imagine to be both round and red. In music, multiple notes can combine into a chord, and a sophisticated musician can also think of how different instruments will sound together. Beethoven was deaf when he composed his *Ninth Symphony* with the rousing "Ode to Joy," but he was able to imagine complex combinations of notes and sounds. Pain involves the combination of a hurt and a location, which can be transformed by changing the combined location, for example, imagining that pain is in a different toe.

Complex motor actions require simultaneous combinations of motions in different body parts, as when shooting a basketball requires combination of wrist, elbow, and shoulder movements. These examples of visual, auditory, pain, and motor imagery each involve a single kind of sensation, but imagery can also operate across modalities. For example, you can imagine a red apple that tastes sweet, a rock guitarist who is painfully loud, or a football kick that has both a feel and a look.

Juxtaposition is more complex than combination because it requires changes in spatial or temporal organization involving separate images, not just integration of features into a single image. Imagining a purple giraffe requires only a combination of the giraffe and the color in the same object, but imagining a giraffe eating an apple requires placing two separate objects in the same spatial location. Visual imagery can also require temporal juxtaposition, as when you mentally picture a giraffe grabbing an apple off a tree and then eating it. Spatial and temporal juxtaposition enable you to run a kind of movie in your head, as when you think of yourself crossing the finish line of a race, which might also involve motor, pain, and auditory imagery as the crowd cheers.

Auditory juxtaposition is usually temporal rather than spatial, as in imagining a sequence of notes that form a melody. Some composers can hear a new melody in their heads as a temporal juxtaposition of notes and then write them down or play them on an instrument. Temporal juxtaposition can occur if you imagine yourself in a dental procedure feeling the jab of an anesthetizing needle, the numbness of a frozen jaw, and the dull pain when the anesthetic wears off. Motor juxtaposition can be both spatial and temporal, as when you imagine taking a violin in one hand and a bow in the other and then working them together to produce a song. This complex image also involves motor imagery (holding and moving the instrument) auditory imagery (the sounds produced), and possibly pain imagery if the violinist is incompetent.

Spatial and temporal juxtaposition can produce rich images. The operation of rotation for visual imagery requires both spatial and temporal changes as an image such as a tower is turned around. Imagining difficult motor tasks such as driving a car, shooting a basketball, typing, and cooking require temporal sequences of actions across multiple locations. Superposition is a special kind of juxtaposition where one image is put on top of each another, for example, imagining someone donning a mask.

The final main class of imagistic transformation is decomposition, in which a complex image is taken apart. In contrast to focusing, the result of decomposition is not just a particular part but an image of all the parts. For example, you can make a mental picture of a bicycle taken apart with the wheels, pedals, and frame all lying on the ground. Similarly, sounds and motor behaviors can be taken apart into their components by reversing the combination and juxtaposition operations that produced them. The key question now is how these mental operations are performed by the brain. How does the brain manage intensification, focusing, combination, juxtaposition, and decomposition?

NEURAL MECHANISMS FOR IMAGERY

All imagery requires the neural mechanisms of representation, binding, competition, storage, retrieval, and transformation. Simple perceptions such as seeing red, smelling beer, or hearing a bang only require basic neural representations accomplished by firing patterns, the first of the mechanisms discussed in chapter 2. Perceptions can be stored by translating neural firing patterns into synaptic connections, and retrieval occurs by reactivating neural patterns. More compli-cated mental operations require more powerful operations such as binding into semantic pointers, which are firing patterns in groups of spiking neurons that provide representations by binding sensory, motor, and verbal patterns.

Chapter 2 described how binding is crucial for object recognition because of the need to put multiple features together to tell the difference between a dog and a cat or between the sound of a trumpet and the sound of a saxophone. Object recognition also requires competition among semantic pointers to select among candidate interpretations of sensory inputs.

Compressed representations like semantic pointers are needed to support the operations that can be carried out in different kinds of imagery. To answer the question of what the Eiffel Tower would look like upside down, you need to be able to treat the representation of the tower as a whole separated from the sensations that produced it. Like linguistic symbols, images can be manipulated, although the forms of manipulation are different. Words are combined into sentences and sen-tences into stories, whereas sensory images are subject to operations like juxtapo-sition that put images beside each other in space or time. Only when images have manageable representations can they contribute substantially to problem solving and learning.

Imagery requires neural mechanisms for memory that can store and retrieve per-ceptions and images. A perception is stored by the memory mechanism described in chapter 2: forming of new synaptic connections between neurons. For example, you see a BMW car, and the experience is stored initially as neural connections in the hippocampus that can become more permanent in the cortex. A perception is retrieved from memory when external stimuli or internal neural processing lead to the reactivation of the pattern of neural firing that originated with the initial visual experience of the BMW. For the pattern to be useful in image manipula-tion, the pattern of firing must be maintained by recurrent (looping) connections among the neurons. Not all maintained patterns are adequate for imagery, which requires both the sensory aspects of the various modalities and the symbol-like susceptibility to manipulations. Semantic pointers combine manipulability with sensory connections because of their production by binding and compression.

The major remaining question is how neural transformations can perform all the mental operations that are applied to imagery. A pattern of firing must be changed in various ways to generate images different from the retrieved sensory representation retrieved. For example, you can make the image of the BMW larger or smaller or combine it with another image such as adding Taylor Swift as the driver.

Intensification is the transformation most easily explained in terms of neurons. Start with the assumption that neural representations of features such as color, size, loudness, pitch, painfulness, and motor movement are all patterns of firing in groups of neurons. The easiest way to produce greater intensity of experience would be to increase the rapidity of firing of the relevant neurons. If the sensation of red results from neural firing, then brighter red might just be the result of more spikes per second in the relevant group. Similarly, all it would take to produce a louder song, stronger pain, or faster arm movement would be faster firing in the corresponding group of neurons. However, the neural process for intensification might use more than rapid firing, with different neurons recruited to handle greater quantities of stimulation or with different firing patterns used to capture qualitative differences in intensity.

How does focusing work in the brain? In zooming and scanning of visual images, and also in changes of concentration in auditory and kinesthetic imagery, there is a shift of attention from general aspects of an image to a particular feature of it. For example, if you are asked to report the color of the door to your house or apartment building, you can form an image of the building and then zoom in on the door. As chapter 8 shows, attention is well described by the mechanism of competition among semantic pointers. Your neural representation of the building you inhabit has numerous features such as windows, walls, and a roof. The question about the color of the door initiates a competition among these different features, with the door winning out. Similarly, a question or other stimulus can lead you to focus on a particular sound in an auditory image, with attention shifting to that sound as the result of competition among neural representations.

Combination of features, for example, imagining an orange that is both round and sweet, is easily explained by the neural mechanism of binding. Neural representations for the orange object, its round shape, and its sweet taste can be bound together into a joint representation by the neural transformation of convolution. Convolution also allows musical notes to be transformed into chords and pains to be identified with particular body parts.

Juxtaposition—placing things close together in space or time—is much more complicated than combination for several reasons. First, it requires combination of more complex representations rather than just features, for example, a whole giraffe and an apple. Second, the juxtaposition requires a background representation of relations in space and/or time to capture relations such as that an apple is inside a giraffe's mouth or that a guitar plays while a person sings. Third, juxtaposition sometimes requires repetitions in space and time, for example, when a picture undergoes rotation or when a whole song is imagined in a different key. Each of these complications requires neural mechanisms that go beyond binding.

To manage juxtaposition of whole objects rather than mere combination of features, the neural representations must function as semantic pointers and not just as retrieved perceptions. The great advantage of semantic pointers is that they can be manipulated like symbols, even though they result from binding of sensory representations. Mental operations in space and time depend on neural representations that are only starting to become understood. Rats, birds, and other animals have special neurons that encode places and times. Juxtaposing in space and time requires there to be a binding of place and time representations with representations of entities such as animals and chords. Repetitive operations such as rotation and melody require iterating and modifying the spatial and temporal bindings. Figure 3.3 provides a simplified illustration of how a more complex image can be formed by juxtaposing other images. The semantic pointers that feed into the result are perceptual, not verbal. The resulting visual image of a giraffe with an apple in its mouth is an emergent result of recursive binding of semantic pointers.

The last imagery transformation in need of neural explanation is decomposition, which reverses the operations of combination and juxtaposition. Chapter 2 described how binding by convolution is reversible: Representations bound together can be unpacked (decompressed). Unbinding representations in this way should produce decomposition. For example, you can produce a novel image by binding representations to produce a visual image of Taylor Swift hugging Justin Bieber, but unpacking can extract her from the picture into a stand-alone image.

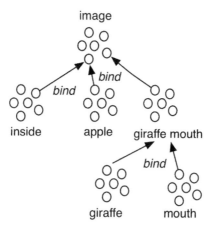

FIGURE 3.3 Generation of the visual image of a giraffe with an apple in its mouth by recursive binding of other images. The verbal labels such as "inside" are only for clarification, because the input neural groups are semantic pointers that are primarily perceptual.

USES OF IMAGERY

To illustrate the role of images in problem solving, try the following experiment. Imagine a capital letter B and then turn it on its back. Now imagine a capital letter V and place it directly below the B and connecting with it. Now, take away the back of the B. What do you see? People usually report seeing a heart, although a few see a double-scoop ice cream cone. This example illustrates all the neural mechanisms discussed in the last section. First, you need to have stored a letter B as a semantic pointer encompassing both sensory aspects (what it looks like) and verbal aspects (it is a letter). The sensory aspects combine the straight line at the back of the B with two round bumps on the front. Second, you need to retrieve the B by generating a pattern of neural firing. Third, you need to rotate the B backwards by spatial alteration. Fourth, juxtaposition with the retrieved image for V produces a new image. Fifth, removal of the back of the B—at the bottom of it after rotation—requires decomposition, taking the B apart so that the line at its back can be deleted. Sixth, the resulting image needs to be compared with other images stored in memory, yielding the match with a heart or ice cream cone to produce conscious recognition. Production and recognition of the heart requires more than the sum of the parts because it needs to be identified as a whole. Images display emergence when their parts are combined to produce unexpected features that enable detection of new relations such as the shape of a heart. Imagery is only one kind of imagination because you can also use verbal inferences to project what might happen or what might have happened.

Imagery can be an important part of planning. Like many Canadians, I face the annual problem of dealing with our long and severe winters. One solution is to get a break with a visit to someplace warm, but arranging a trip to Florida, California, or the Caribbean requires considerable planning. Imagery helps to think about whether I should go to a beach in the Caribbean or to a lively city such as Miami. My representation of these places can combine different sensory modalities, ranging from visual and tactile ones with sun, sand, and water to auditory ones such as the noise of a city and the silence of a deserted beach. Just as important are the emotional images that come with experiencing the exciting bustle of the city versus the serene calm of a beach. I can also imagine the pain that would come if I spent too much time on the beach and got a bad sunburn. When I decide what destination to make plans for, I need to be able to integrate all the different imagined sensory experiences with verbal information concerning the cost of the trip.

Imagery can also contribute to explanation. If you see a scratch on the side of your car, you can visually imagine how it might have come about, for example, by someone scraping the car with a key or by a shopping cart that rolled into the car.

Thus, imagery can contribute to abductive inference, the generation and evaluation of explanatory hypotheses. People use image-based abductive inference when they visualize an earthquake resulting from the slippage of a geological fault, a heart attack resulting from a blocked artery, or a car crash resulting from someone running a red light.

Most explanations are causal: Fault slippage causes earthquakes, blocked arteries cause heart attacks, and cars running red lights can cause crashes. But what is causality? It is common to think of it as a relation that be expressed verbally as a generalization (whenever A happens, B happens) or mathematically as a probability (B given A is more probable than B without A). But infants just a few months old have some grasp of causality, long before they have achieved linguistic let alone mathematical sophistication. For them, the most basic understanding of causality more plausibly comes from a sensory–motor–sensory schema with the structure: perception of situation + motor behavior → new perception of situation. This linguistic description, however, is misleading for infants who lack language, so a better notation is to use brackets to indicate that multimodal neural representations—semantic pointers—express the schema as <perception> <motor> → <perception>. Chapter 5 describes other multimodal rules.

Later, people's understanding of causality can become more sophisticated when they acquire concepts like probability, correlation, and common cause. But these all depend on previous, nonverbal understanding based on sensory and motor images. A three-analysis of a more sophisticated concept of causality with exemplars, typical features, and explanations is given in chapter 5.

Current evidence does not reveal whether the sensory–motor–sensory schema for causality is learned or innate. It may be that infants are born with the schema, or perhaps they are equipped to learn it quickly from combinations of sensory and motor experiences. Images are almost always learned because they result from postnatal perceptions, but it is possible that evolution encodes some images genetically because of their survival value. Perhaps people are born with images of dangerous things like snakes and spiders, but evidence suggests that evolution provides visual biases for the perception of threats rather than specific images. People may be predisposed to learn about scary things without knowing in advance what things are scary. Similarly, people may have a genetic bias to learn sensory–motor–sensory patterns without having an innate image schema for causality.

Even after language develops, people continue to use imagery in connection with language by means of gestures, the hand movements that occur with speech. Susan Goldin-Meadow describes how gestures convey information through visual imagery, for example, when a moving arm with wriggling fingers conveys a running spider. Gestures can simultaneously present information that speech has to break up into parts. Hand gestures can function as analogies to generate mental images of real things, such as a spider moving in ways that systematically resemble the wriggling hand.

As a final illustration of the usefulness of mental images, consider the theoretically powerful idea of mental models, which have been used to explain many aspects of thinking from deductive inference to human-machine interaction. Mental models correspond in structure to the situations that they represent. Suppose you are told that Adam is taller than Dan and Dan is taller than Emma. Is Adam taller than Emma? It is possible that you answer this question by logical inference using transitivity: For all x, y, and z, if x is taller than y, and y is taller than z, then x is taller than z. Most people, however, report a different experience with a mental picture of Adam, Dan, and Emma standing next to each other. Then, to determine that Emma is shorter than Adam, you only need to consult the mental image. Inference employs a mental model rather than linguistic rules. A mental model can combine multiple images with additional representations such as concepts and rules. For example, you can form a dynamic model of how lungs extract oxygen from the air that is absorbed by blood pumped by the heart throughout the body with an attendant sound of the heart beating.

The power of mental models comes from their use of images and all of their operations such as scanning, moving, and juxtaposing. The effectiveness of mental imagery is increased when it is combined with rules, as in the multimodal rules discussed in chapter 4. These arise when the parts of rules are represented by sensory images. I can have the rule, for example, that if I stub my toe, then it will hurt a lot. This rule becomes part of a mental model when the representation of stubbing includes the visual perception of the toe, the motor representation of having my toe collide with something, and the resulting pain image of my toe hurting. Hence, we can flesh out how mental models have the same structure as what they represent by virtue of the special properties of visual and other sensory images, sometimes connected via rules. Semantic pointers provide plausible explanations of mental models because of the way in which they integrate sensory, motor, and dynamic information.

SUMMARY AND DISCUSSION

This chapter provides a general account of imagery that applies to both external senses such as vision and internal senses such as pain. It identifies five mental operations that occur in all kinds of imagery: intensification, focusing, combination, juxtaposition, and decomposition. Each of these operations results from neural mechanisms that are part of the Semantic Pointer Architecture, including storage, retrieval, neural representation, binding, competition, and transformation. The special character of different kinds of imagery is respected thanks to the capability of semantic pointers for modal retention: maintaining compressed information resulting from the sensory or motor modality that produced them.

This account of imagery has competitors, ranging from the behaviorist view that there are no mental images at all to the narrowly computational view that the brain translates sensory inputs into verbal symbols and does all its inferential work by manipulating those symbols. But there is abundant psychological and neural evidence that imagery is real and that the brain's computations employ special patterns of neural representation that develop from sensory inputs. This development requires binding into semantic pointers that are susceptible to symbol-like manipulation exploiting the different sensory characters of visual, auditory, and other sorts of representation. Mental models package images into larger representations that can support many kinds of creativity, from painting to scientific discovery (chapter 11).

Imagery can foster many kinds of mental change, through generation, alteration, and replacement. Generating a new image, such as Edison's first mental picture of a light bulb, can lead to transformations in how people view the world. Altering existing images by tinkering with their parts can improve the image, for example, when you update your image of a politician by adding gray hair. The most radical kind of imagery change is replacement, when old images are supplanted with new ones that carry different emotional values. For example, many American sports teams still have names such as Redskins, associated with derogatory caricatures of indigenous people, where the names and images warrant replacement.

The ideas developed in this chapter about sensory and motor representations amplify chapter 2's remarks on embodiment. Images are profoundly embodied, because they depend on specific kinds of sensing produced by special purpose sensors that feed into dedicated brain circuitry. People would have different images if they had the sonar sensors of bats, the magnetic sensors of some fish and birds, or the laser sensors of some robots. But the power of images, for people and at least some animals, resides in our capacity to step beyond what we sense and use images to generate novel representations with emergent properties. The operations of combination and juxtaposition are especially powerful for transcending the senses and producing novel images and systems of them that form mental models. The result would be mischaracterized as disembodiment, since the body is still much involved in the emergent images. Rather, what chapter 2 called

transbodiment builds on and surpasses perceptual representations to enable creative problem solving and planning that contribute much to the intelligence of
humans.

Later chapters will display the usefulness of imagery in many cognitive processes. Chapter 4 describes how concepts are not purely verbal representations but
can also have important aspects tied to sensation and imagery. Chapter 5 presents
nonverbal rules that have a structure like *IF there is an image of one kind, THEN
there is an image of another kind.* Chapter 6 describes how analogical inference can
operate with visual, auditory, and other kinds of images, not just verbal representations. Chapter 7 on emotions portrays the role of emotional imagery in empathy.
Chapter 10 on language recounts the role that images play in metaphorical understanding. Chapter 11 on creativity illustrates the role of images in creativity. These
examples will further show that imagery is not just peripheral to human thinking
but rather permeates mental functions.

This permeation is important for understanding social phenomena such as
political ideologies and religious symbols discussed in *Mind–Society*. Moreover,
Natural Philosophy shows that mental imagery is important for dealing with deep
questions about knowledge and beauty. Hence images, understood as semantic
pointers, play an important role in explaining mind and society.

NOTES

The Einstein quote on images is from Einstein 1954, p. 25.

In defense of direct perception, see Gibson 1979. Critiques include Ullman 1980
and Fodor and Pylyshyn 1981. Gregory 1970 illustrates the inferential nature of
perception. Direct perception is made implausible by neural evidence—the large
amount of processing in brain areas V1 to V5 required to produce a perception—
and by psychological evidence, for example, ambiguous gestalt figures like the
ones in Figure 3.1 and more than 100 optical illusions: http://www.michaelbach.
de/ot/. For a full account of vision science, see Palmer 1999.

Dunning and Balcetis 2013 review evidence for wishful seeing. Vuilleumier and
Huang 2009 describe emotional bias in perception. Firestone and Scholl 2016
argue that there is no good evidence that cognition and emotion affect perception,
but numerous commentators disagree.

For a review of studies of imagery across modalities, see McNorgan 2012.
Evidence for mental imagery is reviewed by Kosslyn, Thompson, and Ganis
2006. Hubbard 2010 reviews auditory imagery. Schlegel et al. 2013 use functional

magnetic resonance imaging to identify a brain network that performs manipulations on mental images.

On place cells, see Moser, Kroppf, and Moser 2008. On time cells, see Eichenbaum 2014.

Emergence in images is discussed by Finke, Ward, and Smith 1992 (p. 50). Tversky 2011 analyzes visual thinking. Abraham 2016 reviews imagination and imagery.

For more on causality, see chapter 5; Table 5.1 provides a three-analysis of *cause*. The sensory–motor view of causality is in Thagard 2012d and *Natural Philosophy*, chapter 5. Baillergeon, Kotovsky, and Needham 1995 provide evidence for infants' appreciation of causality.

On visual explanations yielding abductive inferences, see Shelley 1996.

LoBue, Rakison, and DeLoache 2010 discuss threat perception.

Goldin-Meadow 2003 describes the communicative roles of gestures.

Semantic pointers provide a neural implementation of image schemas discussed in cognitive linguistics, for example, by Johnson 1987.

PROJECT

Use the Semantic Pointer Architecture to model operations on images, including intensification, focusing, combination, juxtaposition, and decomposition.

4

Concepts

According to Wikiquote, the novelist John Steinbeck said in an interview that ideas are like rabbits—you get a couple and learn how to handle them, and pretty soon you have a dozen. Having many dozens of ideas enables people to write novels, generate scientific theories, invent technologies, and philosophize. The term "idea" is ambiguous because it sometimes means images or beliefs, but often it means concepts, which are mental representations that roughly correspond to words.

Understanding how minds work and how minds build societies requires an appreciation of concepts. Our everyday thinking uses many physical concepts like *dog, flower,* and *butter*. Our social interactions require many relational concepts like *child, leader,* and *debt*. This chapter argues that concepts operate in our minds because they are neural structures and processes, similar to but also different from the perceptions and images discussed in chapter 3.

Concepts enable minds to accomplish many important functions for individuals and for social groups. We use concepts to recognize things in the natural world, such as rocks and squirrels, and we also use them in our social interactions when we identify someone as aggressive, friendly, or weird. Our ability to classify things depends on having the concept in the first place, for example, acquiring concepts like *squirrel* and *chipmunk* that allow us to distinguish one from the other. Concepts also serve to provide explanations, as when we say that a squirrel is gathering nuts because it likes to eat them.

An account of concepts as neural mechanisms needs to be able to explain not only how concepts function in the minds of individuals for classification and explanation but also how they contribute to social communication. Spoken and written communication use words, but behind the words are mental processes. The correspondence between concepts and words is not precise because people can have concepts that have not yet been turned into words, for example, different kinds of squirrels that are recognized as such without being labeled. Moreover, people may have words that are nonsensical and don't correspond to any mental representation, for example, the words that Lewis Carroll introduced in Jabberwocky with the lines "Twas brillig and the slithy toves, did gyre and gimble in the wabe." Educated humans have more than 10,000 words in their vocabularies, so we can suppose that they have at least 10,000 concepts.

I argue that concepts are neural processes, specifically semantic pointers that result from representation, binding, and transformation. This hypothesis contrasts sharply with traditional theories, for example, that concepts are just words or that they are abstract ideas like Plato's forms. The advantage of understanding concepts as neural processes is that we can then generate robust, scientific explanations of all the uses that people make of concepts.

THEORIES OF CONCEPTS

What are concepts? The first possibility to consider is that they are not anything at all. There are several intellectual traditions that deny the reality of concepts as a kind of mental representation. The radical behaviorist approach that dominated psychology from the 1920s to the 1950s dismissed the idea of mental representation as unscientific, since no one can directly observe the mind or its contents. From this perspective, there are no concepts, only words, which are directly observable as marks on paper or as sounds that people make. A more recent tradition, radical embodied cognitive science, is also suspicious of mental representations and therefore insists that there are no concepts. A third skeptical approach allows the idea of mental representations but maintains that concepts do not exist in a way that provides a unified explanation of their many functions of classification and inference.

Traditional philosophical views of such distinguished philosophers as Plato and Kant treat concepts as abstract entities, divorced from mundane examples that can be described using words. For example, squirrels and friends exist in the world, but there are also abstractions that are independent of things and of representations in people's minds. From a scientific perspective, however, there are no grounds for supposing the existence of things that have no causal interactions with the physical world. These abstract theories of concepts gain their only plausibility from the difficulties in understanding how processes like meaning, learning, categorization, and explanation can work biologically.

Ever since cognitive theories became prominent in the 1960s, psychologists have taken concepts seriously as a form of mental representation, but they have had trouble reaching agreement about their nature. The common-sense view of concepts is that they should be subject to strict definitions of the sort that occur in mathematics. For example, we can define a triangle as a shape that has exactly three sides and three angles. There are still many people who think that we cannot discuss complicated ideas like intelligence and consciousness without giving strict definitions that state necessary and sufficient conditions: For example, people are intelligent if and only if they satisfy conditions X, Y, and Z. However, there are many reasons for thinking that the attempt to understand concepts as definable is hopeless.

The first reason goes all the way back to Plato. In numerous dialogues, Plato has speakers attempt to give definitions of important social and ethical concepts such as virtue and justice, but the definitions are exposed by Socrates as utterly inadequate. The implication that Plato wanted the reader to draw from this failure is that concepts need to be understood as abstract entities existing independent of any natural reality. Two thousand years later, the philosopher Wittgenstein emphasized the failure by describing the difficulty of giving a strict definition of important concepts like *game*. He argued instead that we should think of the concept of game as a kind of family resemblance, not susceptible to strict definition. As an exercise, take any nonmathematical concept that interests you and see how well you can do in providing a definition that does not succumb to exceptions.

The second kind of evidence against definable concepts is experimental. In the 1970s and 1980s, the psychological experiments of Eleanor Rosch and others were used to support the claim that the structure of concepts is not given by definitions but rather by prototypes, which are sets of typical features. On this view, we do not need to define a squirrel as having necessary and sufficient features but merely say that some features are typical. Similar aspects of concepts were also emphasized by the philosopher Hilary Putnam and the artificial intelligence researcher Marvin Minsky. For a while, it seemed that the prototype view of concepts would replace the definition view, but prototypes turned out to have empirical problems, and many psychologists have pursued alternative approaches, such as thinking of concepts as sets of examples and concentrating on the role that concepts can play in explanations. The exemplar view of concepts says that they are just stored sets of examples—all the squirrels you have ever perceived. The explanation view of concepts says they are ways of explaining observations such as holes in roofs.

A third line of evidence that undercuts the definitional view of concepts, and also causes problems for all overly linguistic views, concerns the sensory and embodied aspects of concepts that have been emphasized by researchers such as Lawrence Barsalou. Behavioral and brain scanning experiments support the view that people's representations of concepts such as *squirrel* are not purely verbal but also incorporate sensory aspects such as the furry, long-tailed visual appearance of squirrels and possibly also their sound, feel, smell, and taste (for people who have eaten squirrel stew). These aspects are compatible with the exemplar views of concepts if the examples are themselves stored using sensory processes such as vision and taste. But concepts differ from sensations and images in that they are more general: The concept *squirrel* applies to all squirrels, whereas a sensation or an image is of a particular squirrel.

The difficulty of determining what concepts are may lead to the despairing conclusion that the idea of concepts is not theoretically useful. Operating only with mental mechanisms makes it hard to figure out how to have a unified theory of concepts. However, neural mechanisms, in particular the theory of semantic pointers, provide deep and useful explanations of all the relevant phenomena.

NEURAL MECHANISMS FOR CONCEPTS

If concepts are not just words, or abstract ideas in Plato's heaven, or a mishmash of psychological features, then what are they? Can concepts be identified as structures and processes in the brains of humans and other animals? It would obviously be too simple to localize a concept in the operations of a particular neuron: people do not have any single neuron that can carry out all the functions of concepts like *squirrel* and *friend*. Much more plausibly, a concept might result from the operations of a whole group of thousands or millions of neurons. This population of neurons need not be confined to a single brain area, because of the extensive connections that exist among neurons across multiple brain areas. The group of neurons for a concept may involve visual representations in one part of the brain and motor representations in another part. For example, your concept of *frying pan* has both visual and motor aspects—what it looks like and what you can do with it. The general account of representation in chapter 2 suggests that a concept is a pattern of firing in a group of neurons resulting from stored synaptic connections among the neurons and from inputs to the group from other neurons. Take this as an initial characterization, not a definition, to be filled out by the three-analysis of *concept* provided in the summary at the end of this chapter.

How are concepts different from the sensations and images described in chapter 3? As already suggested, the primary way in which concepts differ from sensations and sensory images is greater generality, for example, the general concept *giraffe* as opposed to particular sensory experiences of giraffes. The concept has greater generality because it is usually learned from more than one example by mechanisms that extract what is typical of those examples. This generality of concepts facilitates their role in classification and explanation, which requires more complicated kinds of learning than the simple storage that can happen with sensations. Like all mental representations, concepts are patterns of firing in populations of neurons, but not all patterns of firing are concepts, for example, those associated with specific sensations and images. Concepts are just one kind of semantic pointer, and others discussed later include beliefs, intentions, and emotions.

As with perceptions and images, we need to distinguish between concepts as currently active and concepts as dispositions to become currently active. Currently active concepts are patterns of neural firing that result from dispositions consisting of stored synaptic connections. Similarly, a belief such as that squirrels have bushy tails can be something that you are currently thinking about that results from connections stored more permanently in memory. In neural terms, we can view a concept both as a pattern of firing now going on in your brain when you are actually thinking of a squirrel and the capability to think of squirrels that you have whether or not you are thinking of squirrels right now. This dispositional aspect of concepts, as well as beliefs and other mental representations, results from neural connections. Learning alters the synapses between neurons so that concepts get stored in the brain in the form of excitatory and inhibitory connections. If it takes a million neurons firing together to generate a pattern corresponding to squirrels, then there are more than a billion connections among those neurons that go into making up the stored, dispositional concept. When stimulated by external stimuli such as a person's seeing or hearing a squirrel, the group of neurons generates the pattern of firing that represents squirrels.

A neural account of concepts requires them to be not just any pattern of neural firing, but rather special ones that enable learning, classification, explanation, and language use. Eliasmith's semantic pointers are well-equipped to accomplish all of these functions. Recall from chapter 2 what is special about semantic pointers as a form of neural representation. First, they can result from binding together representations of different modalities, including sensory, motor, emotional, and verbal information. Second, the bindings that go into semantic pointers can be approximately decomposed, allowing all these kinds of information to be decompressed and unpacked. If you acquire the concept of squirrel by combining various sorts of sensory and verbal information, you can still take that information apart, for example, when you need to consider what a squirrel looks like, including its head, tail, and color. The combined information in the concept *squirrel* can also include your emotional reaction to squirrels, such as how much you like squirrels or find them scary. Humans can also combine verbal information such as that squirrels are a kind of rodent, which is a kind of mammal. Animals without language, such as dogs and birds, can nevertheless have a sensory concept of a squirrel that they use in classifying animals and controlling their own behavior.

Chapter 2 describes how semantic pointers also have the powerful property that they can be used in symbol-like ways to make inferences. For humans, these inferences can be linguistic, as when someone explicitly thinks of a squirrel that it must cache nuts for the winter. But inferences can also be made with nonverbal representations, allowing a squirrel, for example, to predict that a chickpea will taste good.

In sum, concepts are processes in groups of neurons with patterns of firing that result from learned or innate connections. Like semantic pointers in general, concepts can be multimodal, resulting from binding together various sensory modalities, including ones resulting from internal sensations. For example, your concept of hunger depends in part on past bodily sensations such as hunger pangs, a growling stomach, or a feeling of weakness. Concepts construed as semantic pointers can operate with modal retention, keeping some aspects of sensory–motor information.

Despite the complexity of the multiple bindings of different sorts of information—sensory, motor, emotional, verbal—that go into them, concepts can achieve sufficient unity that they can be used in symbol-like inferential processes. The claim that concepts are semantic pointers needs to be justified by showing that this supposition generates the best available explanations of the full range of phenomena to which concepts are relevant, including innateness, learning, categorization, problem solving, planning, and explanation.

USES OF CONCEPTS

The hypothesis that concepts are neural processes of a particular kind—semantic pointers—is an explanatory identity. In the history of science, explanatory identities occur when familiar things can be identified with underlying natural processes. For example, we are confident that water is H_2O, a combination of hydrogen and oxygen, because a wide variety of phenomena can be explained by this identity. Reliably, if you run a current through water, you get hydrogen gas and oxygen gas. Many other explanatory identities have marked the advance of science, such as: the discoveries that lightning is electrical discharge; that air is a mixture of hydrogen, oxygen, nitrogen, and other gases; that fire is a process of rapid combination with oxygen; and that light consists of photons with both wave and particle characteristics. Analogously, the claim that concepts are semantic pointers is justified if it provides explanations of learning, innateness, categorization, problem solving, explanation, and language use.

Innateness

A concept is innate in a species if all members of the species are born with it, as a result of inheritance of genes acquired through evolution by natural selection. For example, if the concept of a face is innate in humans, the concept results from genes for recognizing faces that all people have. If a concept is not innate, it needs to be learned by the organisms in that species. The key question is: To what extent are concepts innate rather than learned?

The most extreme positions on this issue are that all concepts are innate or that all concepts are learned. Complete innateness has been defended by prominent philosophers such as Plato and Jerry Fodor. According to Plato's theory of forms, all humans acquired concepts as abstract entities before they were born and only lost knowledge of concepts as the result of the trauma of birth. Much more recently, Fodor has claimed that all concepts must be innate, because there are no satisfactory explanations of how they can be learned.

The hypothesis of complete innateness is regarded as implausible by most psychologists for several reasons. First, there are thousands of concepts that seem to depend crucially on people's exposure to the world after they were born. Here are just a few examples of concepts that people come to well after their entry into the world: *elephant, butter, sandwich, president, reclining chair, electron,* and *television.* Second, from an evolutionary point of view, it would be wasteful to try to store in neural connections all possible concepts that species such as humans might eventually encounter. Rather what a species needs to survive and reproduce is enough genetic endowment that it can learn to function in its environment. Third, the conclusion that all concepts must be innate because no one knows how they can be learned is premature, as the next section on the learning of concepts shows.

At the other extreme from complete innateness, philosophers such as John Locke have claimed that all concepts are learned from sense experience. This claim has two major problems. First, there is experimental evidence that babies are more inclined to learn about some aspects of the world rather than others, for example, food and faces. Second, people have many concepts that go beyond sense experience, such as *cause, electron, unicorn,* and *virus.* The most reasonable conclusion, therefore, is that some important concepts are innate in humans, but most are learned, including ones that are not learned directly from sense experience.

The issue of precisely which concepts are innate is not currently settled, but here are some prime candidates. Newborn babies do not have to learn to enjoy their mother's milk, even though they lack the verbal concept of milk. Their sense organs for taste, smell, and touch give babies the ability to recognize sweet and fat, and their innate motor abilities enable them to seek a nipple and suck. Similarly, babies react specially toward faces within an hour after being born by imitating facial movements such as sticking out tongues. Within a few months after birth, babies show interest in attending to objects and causal relations in the world. The psychologist Susan Carey has presented evidence that core (innate) concepts include *objects, number, agency, face,* and *causality.* There seem to be at least a few concepts that meet the standards for innateness suggested in chapter 2: cultural universality, dedicated brain areas, animal precursors, adaptive contribution, and absence of alternative explanations.

The view that concepts are neural processes would be hard pressed to explain how all of the thousands of concepts that people have could be innate but has no problem in explaining how some core concepts like *face* and *sweet* can be built into a species. There are genetically programmed mechanisms for the formation and organization of neurons in the brain, beginning rapidly in humans around 16 weeks after conception. The organization of the brain results from genetically influenced developmental processes and does not require any learning. By the time a human baby is born, it already has in place billions of neurons organized into brain areas with trillions of synaptic connections. Although enormous changes take place in the synaptic connections when the baby is born and exposed to new stimuli, many of the connections between neurons that will determine its subsequent behavior, including its ability to learn new concepts, are already in place by the time that it is born. That is why the baby does not have to learn to like its mother's milk, because it already has the sensory ability to identify sweet and fat and to experience pleasure as a result of exposure to them. Innateness of concepts is adequately explained by the prebirth formation of synaptic connections as a result of genes established in the species by evolution.

To summarize, concepts are patterns of neural firing that result from synaptic connections between neurons. Most synaptic connections are formed by learning, initially in the womb and much more extensively after birth. But some synaptic connections can be generated by genes, in the same way that genes determine the growth of neurons and their organization into brain areas that are common to all members of a species. Just as evolution provides people with genes to make their brains develop to have a cortex, amygdala, and so on, some synaptic connections that are particularly useful for survival and reproduction can be built into brains by genes. These connections can then generate patterns of neural firing that provide newborn babies with some idea of what to expect in their world.

Semantic pointers are innate when genetically generated synaptic connections produce patterns of firing that go beyond detection of specific features in a single sensory modality. For example, a baby's innate desire for milk seems to depend on neural binding of features from taste (sweet), touch (liquid), and motor control (suck). Similarly, the innate ability to seek and recognize faces depends not just on synaptic connections that allow babies to visually recognize simple features such as a mouth but also on bindings that unify multiple features (eyes, nose, mouth) into an organized whole that can influence motor reactions such as orienting and smiling. Hence, the neural theory of concepts as semantic pointers can explain the innateness of some concepts.

Learning

Newborn babies have some concepts but no words. Judging from vocabulary growth, we can estimate that young children gain dozens of concepts per day. How does this happen? That is, how does the brain managed to acquire thousands of new concepts over a dozen or so years? Fortunately, the learning mechanisms discussed in chapter 2 provide a good basis for explaining concept learning. We saw that learning from experience occurs when new synapses are formed and strengthened or weakened as a result of experience.

Some of this experience is sensory, as a baby encounters new sights, sounds, touches, smells, and tastes. The baby is also exposed to linguistic inputs through interactions with its parents and other humans. Hence, the basic mechanism for forming new concepts in a growing child is the adjustment of neural connections as the result of exposure to sensory stimuli. Most concept learning is unsupervised, in that there is no explicit teaching required for a child to figure out how to apply different concepts, for example, to determine the difference between cats and dogs. But concept learning sometimes is supervised when parents and other people can provide corrections to mistakes the child makes, for example, in using the word "Daddy" to refer to all males.

However, the sensory tweaking of synaptic connections is not the only way in which concepts can be learned. Once a child has acquired some linguistic sophistication, new concepts can be learned by combining old ones. For example, concepts like *unicorn* can be formed by combinations of other concepts—in this case, *horse* and *horn*. The basic learning mechanism for sensory concepts is just adjustment of synaptic connections, but for concepts learned by conceptual combination, the mechanism of binding plays a much more prominent role. In binding, a concept is formed by establishing a new pattern of activation as a result of other patterns about the world that already exist.

If the new combined concept turns out to be useful, then it can be stored in permanent memory in the form of neural connections that will generate the new pattern on appropriate occasions. Conceptual combination enables imaginative children, as well as imaginative adults such as scientists, to generate concepts that go well beyond what they have experienced within their usual sensory range. Supervised and unsupervised learning by examples is important for some concepts, but viewing concepts as semantic pointers explains how other, more creative concepts can be formed by binding. Figure 4.1 illustrates the conceptual combination of unicorn resulting from binding *horse* and *horned*. The actual concept would be much more complex, incorporating exemplars such as standard pictures of unicorns, typical features such as being magical, and explanations such as having medicinal benefits.

Here are some new concepts I acquired around 2015. Watching in one sitting many parts of a television series downloaded from Netflix is *binge watching,* analogous to binge eating. Smoking an electronic cigarette is *vaping.* Taking a picture of yourself with your phone is a *selfie,* which can be enhanced using a *selfie stick* or degenerate into a *butt selfie.* To steal a movie, TV show, or song by downloading it using the protocol BitTorrent is to *torrent* it. When a word is written with internal capital letters signaling the words melded into it, as in "BitTorrent," then it is using

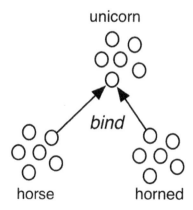

FIGURE 4.1 Concept unicorn formed by conceptual combination of *horse* and *horned*.

CamelCase, by visual analogy to the humps of a camel. People who swipe too much on the dating app Tinder can get *Tinder thumb*. When a man condescendingly explains something to a woman who knows more than he does, he is *mansplaining*. Examples may have helped me to understand some of these new concepts, such as the word "CamelCase" as an instance of the concept *CamelCase*, but the main learning mechanism for them, in both the originator and me, was combination of concepts already available, such as *binge* and *watch*.

Conceptual combination enables human thinkers to transcend sensory limitations. Empiricism is the philosophical view that all concepts derive from sense experience. It contains the grain of truth that many important concepts are based on the senses and all scientific theories need to have some empirical basis through connections to observation. But these connections can be indirect, when theories explain generalizations about experimental results that require observations. Scientific explanations routinely introduce theoretical concepts like *atom, molecule, gene,* and *virus* that go far beyond direct sensory experience but are nevertheless legitimate because they provide the best available explanations of many observable phenomena. Like radical embodiment, empiricism exaggerates the contribution of the senses to thinking.

Chapter 2 argues that imagery is capable of transbodiment by generating images of things no one has observed. Conceptual combination goes even farther beyond the senses, producing concepts of things such as quarks that no one ever could observe with human senses. Theoretical conceptual combination is a common practice, not only in science but also in religion, which is full of concepts that surpass the senses, for example, the idea of an invisible and almighty god. Transbodiment is epistemologically risky, but without it we would not have sciences such as physics, chemistry, and biology. Transbodiment by conceptual combination also produces valuable cultural ideas like *finance, ideology, social norm, war, human rights, folk rock, satire,* and *cubism*.

In sum, a sufficiently rich neural theory of concepts can explain both innateness and learning of concepts. Innateness results from genetically programmed synaptic connections, and learning results from synaptic changes. Learning of semantic pointers can come about by supervised or unsupervised exposure to examples and also by conceptual combination that binds neural representations through convolution. Hebbian learning and memory storage explain how important subsets of combined concepts end up as part of our permanent store. Some combinations of concepts such as *green tree* are too mundane and uninteresting to go into permanent storage. But other combinations are surprising and useful enough that they promote ongoing joint activity leading to Hebbian learning, ensuring that people retain concepts such as *atom* that are helpful in particular contexts. The bindings that go into semantic pointers for concepts can operate on (a) representations of sensory and motor experiences—the exemplars; (b) representations of typical features, usually other concepts; and (c) representations of rules used in explanations, as described in chapter 5. Nonneural theories of concepts, such as ones that take them to be abstract nonmaterial entities, fail to provide plausible accounts of innateness and learning.

Categorization

Once a person has acquired new concepts, they become useful for many mental processes, such as recognizing and differentiating objects. Categorization occurs when sensory stimuli prompt people to identify an object as belonging to a particular kind. For example, if you are outside and you see a small moving object, you will use your senses and stored concepts to tell you whether the object is a rabbit, squirrel, bird, or something else. A long bushy tale can help you to classify the object as a squirrel.

From the neural perspective of semantic pointers, categorization is straightforward. Sensory inputs lead to firings in neural populations for previously learned or innate concepts. When a stored pattern is reactivated, the match between the sensory pattern in the conceptual pattern warrants placing the perceived object under the category. An object is judged to be a rabbit rather than a squirrel because the neural pattern generated by the sensory inputs—including colors, shapes, and maybe sounds—approximates the neural pattern that results from the stored concept.

Frequently, there may be more than one semantic pointer that fits the sensory inputs that need to be identified. The crucial mechanism for overcoming ambiguity is competition, as described in chapter 2. Establishing the concept (semantic pointer) for rabbit as the best match for visual inputs may require it to outcompete the alternatives such as the concept for squirrel. Figure 4.2 shows how this might work, although it is important to view the ovals for *bird*, *cat*, and *squirrel* as possibly overlapping neural groups rather than as single neurons.

Categorization by competition among semantic pointers works by parallel constraint satisfaction. The positive constraints on categorization are the various ways in which the current situation or stimulus fits with the concept, including its typical sensory–motor features such as its shape. The negative constraints are mismatches between the current situation and concept, as well as the inability of more than one concept to match to the same situation. For example, we know that something cannot be equally a cat and a squirrel, producing a negative constraint

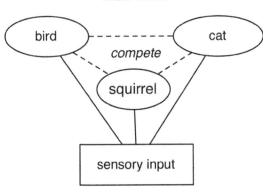

FIGURE 4.2 Neural network for competition between three concepts to determine which one best categorizes sensory input. Solid lines are excitatory links, but dotted lines are inhibitory.

to prevent us from categorizing something as both. If the concept *squirrel* outcompetes its alternatives, then the object is categorized as a squirrel.

This categorization may be of only temporary interest, or it may be significant enough to be storied as a belief. Philosophers often describe a belief as a propositional attitude, which is supposed to be a relation between a person and the meaning of a sentence. A more scientific account follows from the theory of concepts as semantic pointers. The representation of an object and the concept of squirrel are both patterns of neural firing, so that the belief that the object is a squirrel only requires binding these two representations together by convolution. The resulting belief is also a neural pattern, which can become part of permanent storage through synaptic changes. For relational concepts, binding is more complicated, because it needs to indicate the different roles played by the different objects.

For example, construction of the relational belief that a squirrel is chasing a rabbit requires binding *squirrel* to *agent* and *rabbit* to *receiver*, producing something like

$$\text{bind}\left[(\text{bind chase action})\,(\text{bind squirrel agent})\,(\text{bind squirrel receiver})\right].$$

The result, however, is not the complicated piece of syntax in the previous line but a pattern of neural firing that can be stored as a set of synaptic connections. Figure 4.3 gives some indication of how a belief can be viewed as a neural structure that results from recursive binding of semantic pointers. Simpler nonrelational beliefs about a single individual need only bind the neural representation of the individual, partly based on imagery, with the semantic pointer for the concept. For example, the belief that John is tall only requires

$$\text{bind}\left[(\text{bind object John})\,(\text{bind property tall})\right].$$

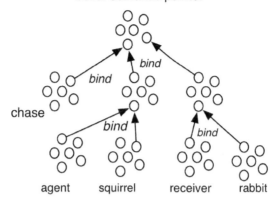

FIGURE 4.3 The belief that the squirrel chases the rabbit results from recursive binding. Not shown is the required binding of *chase* to *action*.

Problem Solving

Categorization, inference, and belief formation contribute to many kinds of problem solving, including planning, decision making, and explanation. For evolution, humans and other organisms have two fundamental goals: survival and reproduction. To survive, animals need to find food, water, and shelter and to avoid being eaten by predators. To reproduce, animals need to find at least one mate and to ensure that the resulting offspring survive. Unlike most other animals, humans are capable of generating and pursuing other more abstract goals, such as art and science.

Goals such as food, mating, and science can be expressed as concepts, but they only become goals when the semantic pointers that represent the concepts in the brain include bindings with positive emotional states such as liking, desiring, and craving. More complicated goals such as "I want to eat pizza for dinner today" require binding such states with proposition-like representations that bind the agent, object, and time. Goals can generate intentions by mechanisms described in chapter 9.

Concepts are valuable in accomplishing survival and reproduction goals. Consider the avoidance of predators, which requires recognizing another animal as a danger. If you are hiking in the woods, you need to be able to distinguish a dark shadowy object as a bear rather than a tree, because the bear could eat you. Concepts also help us to categorize objects as relevant or irrelevant to our reproduction goals through the recognition of potential mates. Once people move beyond basic goals of survival and reproduction, then many other kinds of concepts can be useful, for example, when we solve the problem of identifying a piece of music by classifying it as jazz, which requires having the concept of jazz music. The classification can use all three aspects of concepts—exemplars, typical features, and explanations—to match them against things to be identified. This process of competitive matching by parallel constraint satisfaction is fundamentally different from classification by deduction from definitions assumed by traditional views of concepts.

The simplest kind of concept-based problem solving works as follows. You have a problem to be solved, such as whether to leave a tip in a restaurant. You have various goals to be accomplished, which in this case might include not only saving money but also treating the restaurant employees fairly. Categorization can bring a solution to the problem, because if you are able to classify the restaurant as a fast-food restaurant, which you know does not normally require tipping, then you need not tip. On the other hand, if you classify the restaurant as a fancy establishment, based on features such as elegant tables with table cloths, then you can use your knowledge of that kind of restaurant to tell you that you ought to tip. In this case categorization by applying concepts such as *fast-food restaurant* or *fancy restaurant* does most of the work in solving the problem.

Much problem solving by experts can also be understood as resulting from categorization, for example, when firefighters make quick decisions by matching new fires to previously experienced prototypes. Social decisions can also be strongly affected by categorization: when you categorize people as kind, friendly, or honest, you deal with them differently from when you classify them as mean, hostile, or dishonest. Problem solving by categorization is advantageous because it does not require much inference. Chapter 5 looks at more extended problem solving using chains of if–then reasoning. For example, a trip to China from another country will require multiple steps involving buying a ticket, getting to an airport, and catching a plane.

Most problems that people solve are aimed at deciding what to do and selecting actions to be carried out as parts of plans and decisions. But people sometimes need to solve problems where the fundamental goal is understanding why something happened. For example, if you are traveling in a foreign country and you meet someone who is extraordinarily rude, you will naturally wonder why. Rightly or wrongly, people often generate explanations by using social stereotypes. Suppose you are traveling in the country Elbonia, a mythical country in Dilbert cartoons. Then you might think that the reason the person is rude is because he or she is Elbonian. Assuming you have managed to acquire a concept of an Elbonian on the basis of your previous visits or media reports, then categorization provides the explanation.

The explanation by categorization contributes to thinking in many other domains. For example, you might be able to figure out why there is a tapping noise on the side of your house by classifying a bird in the neighborhood as a woodpecker. Applying *woodpecker* provides an explanation of the noise, because your concept of woodpeckers includes the causal information that they tap on wood. Similarly, an astronomer could provide a quick explanation of some of the properties of a distant star by classifying it as a red dwarf or a black hole.

Hence concepts can be useful for solving problems that concern planning, decision making, and explanation. For all of these, the solution to the problem comes simply by recognizing the situation as being of a particular kind, which is represented by a concept. Categorization takes place by reactivation of a pattern of neural firing, a semantic pointer, that accomplishes retrieval from memory. The multimodal character of the pointers allows them to resonate to various features of the situation, including its visual, auditory, and other sensory aspects. We can recognize Elbonians by their looks, sounds, and maybe even smells. If there are alternative concepts that fit to some extent, then recognition may require competition among alternative semantic pointers in a process of parallel constraint satisfaction.

Because semantic pointers are also capable of symbolic inference, they are able to generate the actions that will accomplish planning problems and to initiate the causal reasoning that is required for explanations. The semantic pointer for Elbonian might generate actions such as avoidance if Elbonians are viewed as rude and crude. Concepts can also facilitate abductive inference, the generation of explanatory hypotheses. Chapter 3 describes how abduction can be performed using images, but concepts show how to do it nonperceptually, by applying a concept. For example, you might explain why someone is crude and has tall hair by hypothesizing that he or she is Elbonian. In science, abductive inference is often the spur for conceptual combination. For example, to explain many properties of matter, the ancient Greeks generated novel hypotheses using the novel concept of atom, which combines the concepts *particle* and *indivisible*.

Language

Concepts have numerous important functions in the generation and comprehension of language. Concepts are crucial for language because the sentences that play the central role in linguistic communication are built out of words, and concepts are the mental/neural representations that correspond to words. For example, the simple sentence "The bird landed in the tree" requires mental representations of the concepts *bird, tree*, and *landed*. Producing a meaningful sentence requires concatenating meaningful words, and words get their meaning from mental representations of concepts, best understood as semantic pointers.

People are able to generate sentences that have never been uttered before because they already have concepts that can be put into new combinations. I can produce the original sentence "Peanut butter tastes like purple socks" because I already have concepts of *peanut butter, taste, purple*, and *socks*, as well as an understanding of grammar. Going in the other direction, when someone utters a novel sentence, you are able to decode it because of the mental representations you already have: the concepts that corresponds to the words the person is using. When people struggle with unusual combination of words, as in my peanut butter example, semantic pointers provide meaning via both sensory–motor representations and internal connections with other concepts. See chapter 10 for further discussion of language and meaning.

How Concepts Change

Understanding conceptual change is crucial for many fields, including education, developmental psychology, political ideology, and history of science. The semantic pointer theory of concepts highlights many different kinds of conceptual change, including the formation, alteration, and replacement of concepts analogous to the changes mentioned for images in chapter 3. Formation involves learning from examples and by conceptual combination, generating neural patterns that integrate exemplars, typical features, and explanation. Conceptual combinations can have emergent properties, as when the mention of blind lawyers leads to further inferences about their personal characteristics, such as the grit needed to practice law without sight.

Alteration of concepts can involve changing exemplars (e.g., counting humans as animals after Darwin), typical features (e.g., shifting marriage to include same-sex), and explanations (e.g., finding new effects of genes). The method of three-analysis can be used dynamically to track changes in concepts over time.

Replacement of concepts can occur locally, as in deletion of *Negro* in favor of *African American,* or more globally, as in scientific revolutions. For example, Darwin's theory replaced accepted explanations of species in terms of religious concepts such as *divine creation* with a system of biological concepts including *evolution, variation*, and *natural selection. Mind–Society* describes the importance of understanding conceptual change for many kinds of social improvement such as better teaching and elimination of prejudice. *Natural Philosophy* identifies the substantial conceptual changes required for recognizing that minds are brains rather than souls.

SUMMARY AND DISCUSSION

Concepts are mental representations corresponding roughly to words. Construed as semantic pointers, concepts are not only capable of playing inferential roles, but they also maintain embodied connections with sensory–motor processes. Understanding concepts in this way enables us to give biologically and psychologically plausible accounts of innateness, learning, and categorization. Learning new concepts can occur not only through slow, incremental use of multiple examples but also by fast, sometimes revolutionary conceptual combinations. The process of categorization is carried out by retrieval through reactivation of neural patterns and through parallel constraint satisfaction accomplished by competition among semantic pointers. Categorization can contribute to different kinds of problem solving, including planning, decision making, and explanation.

The semantic pointer theory of concepts makes sense of the strength and weaknesses of previous theories of concepts. Concepts do not have strict definitions, but they can nevertheless be meaningful because of their relations with sensory and motor inputs and with other concepts. Concepts as semantic pointers have some of the concrete aspects found in exemplar theories, according to which a concept is just a stored set of examples, because the semantic pointers can be unpacked into sensory and motor experiences. But their inferential capacity enables concepts to go well beyond sets of exemplars and make them useful for solving problems. Concepts convey typical features, rather than definitional ones, by virtue of the sensory–motor and verbal information that is bound into the concept, and the higher-level inferential roles that the semantic pointers carry out. Concepts not only demonstrate embodiment because of the sensory representations bound into many of them, but they also demonstrate transbodiment because conceptual combination can produce representations such as *virus* that surpass the senses. Besides concepts captured in human languages by words, there are nonlinguistic concepts functioning in many other animals with complex brains.

It would be pointless to look for a strict definition of concepts, but a three-analysis is easy to produce, summarized in Table 4.1. First, exemplars of concepts range from sensory ones like *red* to attributes of objects like *box* to relations

TABLE 4.1

Three-Analysis of *Concept*, According to the Semantic Pointer Theory

Exemplars	Dog, car, song, happy, atom, virus, god
Typical features	Exemplars, typical features, explanations, embodiment, transbodiment
Explanations	Explains: thought, language
	Explained by: neural mechanisms—semantic pointers

among objects like *parent*. Second, the typical but not universal features of concepts include having corresponding words and being learned from experience or conceptual combination. Third, concepts explain important mental functions like categorization and sentence generation, and these operations of concepts are best explained by viewing them as semantic pointers. The semantic pointer theory of concepts has no problem applying *concept* to itself, which would be difficult for empiricist theories that cannot say how *concept* can be derived from the senses.

The behaviorist B. F. Skinner argued that discussion of mental representations like concepts is pointless, because their only function is to describe relations between behaviors and environments, so it is better just to talk about those relations. But concepts have many important purposes including learning, categorization, problem solving, explanation, and language. The justification of the hypothesis that minds employ concepts is by inference to the best explanation: concepts help to provide better explanations of many psychological phenomena than alternative views. Advances in theoretical neuroscience now permit the explanations furnished by concepts to be based on neural mechanisms involving semantic pointers as well as psychological mechanisms.

The importance of concepts will be reinforced in the rest of this book, because they help to explain how people use rules, analogies, metaphors, and meaningful language. Concepts also contribute to the understanding of consciousness, creativity, and the self. Concepts help to determine what unconscious aspects of neural processing break through into consciousness. Creativity often results from putting concepts together in ways that are new, valuable, and surprising. Important functions of the self result from the application of personality concepts such as *extraverted*.

Mind–Society explores the social importance of concepts and conceptual change in topics that include personal relationships (chapter 4), prejudice (chapter 5), politics (chapter 6), religion (chapter 8), medicine (chapter 10), and education (chapter 12). *Natural Philosophy* (chapter 3) shows that the neural understanding of concepts and beliefs provides a unified explanation of three kinds of knowledge: declarative knowledge that something is the case, procedural knowledge how to do things, and perceptual knowledge of what is sensed.

NOTES

To find your approximate vocabulary size to guess roughly at how many concepts you have, go to http://testyourvocab.com.

On behaviorism, see Skinner 1976. For the skeptical idea that no unified theory of concepts is possible, see Machery 2009.

Surveys of the psychological evidence for different theories of concepts include Murphy 2002; Smith and Medin 1981; and Rips, Smith and Medin 2012. For diverse views of concepts, see Margolis and Laurence 1999, 2015. In philosophy, there is much confused debate about the nature of nonconceptual content. But content should not be taken as equivalent to meaning, which is a process (like running) rather than a thing; see chapter 10. Moreover, "conceptual" should not be used as contrast to "perceptual," because many concepts such as *squirrel* are perceptually embodied.

On concepts based on typical features rather than definitions, see Putnam 1975, Minsky Minsky 1975, Rosch and Mervis 1975, and Wittgenstein 1968. Medin 1989 emphasizes the role of explanation in concepts, which is sometimes called the "theory theory" or "knowledge view." This primarily concerns how concepts serve to provide explanations, but explanations of what makes something fall under a concept are also important, as people tend to think that concepts have an underlying essence: Prentice and Miller 2007. Scientific explanations invoke evidence-based mechanisms rather than mysterious essences.

On concepts as perceptually grounded and embodied, see Barsalou 1999, 2008, 2016. Barsalou contrasts modal approaches to representing knowledge that retain sensorimotor information with amodal approaches that transform and abandon that information. Images are conscious modal representations, but there are also unconscious ones.

For the semantic pointer view of concepts as neural processes, see especially Blouw, Solodkin, Thagard, and Eliasmith 2016, as well as Eliasmith 2013 and Thagard 2012c. Other neural network accounts of concepts include Rogers and McClelland 2004. Schröder and Thagard 2013 explain conceptual priming in terms of semantic pointers. Quiroga 2012 discusses concept cells such as the Jennifer Anniston neuron.

Explanatory identities are analyzed by Thagard 2014b.

Fodor's claim that all concepts are innate is in Fodor 1975 and subsequent works. Carey 2009 discusses core concepts that are candidates for innateness. Frank, Vul, and Johnson 2009 describe infants' preference for faces. Stiles 2008 provides a biological perspective, arguing that development depends equally on processes that decode genetic information and on environment change as the product of development. See also Mandler 2012. Klein 1998 discusses expert decision making using schemas, as do Nokes, Schunn, and Chi 2010.

On computational and neural mechanisms for conceptual combination, see Thagard 1988 and Thagard and Stewart 2011. On emergent properties in conceptual combination, see Kunda, Claire, and Miller 1990.

For more on conceptual change, see, for example, Carey 2009, Nersessian 2008, and Thagard 1992, 2012d, 2014b. Replacement of whole systems of concepts goes hand in hand with revisions of systems of beliefs by coherence processes that operate by parallel constraint satisfaction, described in Thagard 2000 and Thagard and Findlay 2011.

As an approach to conceptual analysis, three-analysis is superior to the traditional philosophical attempt at definition because the latter (a) always fails because of counterexamples or circularity, (b) often leads to dogmatism in the form of insistence that concepts like *good* and *knowledge* need to be taken as primitive, and (c) can lead to excessive metaphysics such as Plato's heavenly forms or David Lewis's possible worlds. Philosophical methods are scrutinized in *Natural Philosophy*.

PROJECT

Develop a semantic pointer simulation of conceptual combination leading to storage and ongoing use of newly generated concepts, including emergent properties. Determine whether nonhuman animals are capable of conceptual combination. Do a dynamic three-analysis of the concept of *concept*, showing how it changes from the traditional definitional view to the semantic pointer theory.

5

Rules

WHY RULES MATTER TO MIND AND SOCIETY

The American General Douglas MacArthur said that rules are mostly made to be broken and too often are for the lazy to hide behind. Contrary to MacArthur, rules are not just for the lazy. Simple entities like rocks and clouds do not need to have rules and other representations, because they do little. Similarly, primitive biological organisms such as bacteria and plants perform such simple actions that they also do not need representations. For a flower to turn toward the sun, it only needs mechanisms for detecting light and shifting its orientation toward it, without any internal way of representing light and the act of movement. In contrast, animals can perform more complicated actions in the world based on assessments of their situations. Sensations, images, and concepts are very useful in representing the world and guiding actions in it, but animals including humans also need more dynamic representations called rules.

When most people hear the word "rule," they think of the simple social rules they began to learn as children. Don't chew with your mouth open. If you can't say something nice, then don't say anything at all. Wash your hands after going to the toilet. If you don't clean your room, then you can't go to the movie. In cognitive science, however, the term "rule" is used to apply to a much wider set of representations. Rules can be about physical objects: *If water drops in temperature below 0°C, then it freezes.* There are also rules about biological objects: *If something is a tiger, then it has stripes.* Social rules can concern not only normative actions such as not chewing with your mouth open but also descriptions of what is common in the social world, such as the stereotype that Canadians are polite. Rules are not sentences but rather mental representations, which is why I indicate them by italics rather than quotes. The goal of this chapter is to show how mental rules can be understood as neural processes.

Rules are mental representations with an *if–then* structure. Some of the previously mentioned rules already have an *if–then* structure, and others can easily be translated. For example, the Canadian stereotype becomes: *If a person is Canadian, then he or she is polite.* From the cognitive perspective, rules are not just sentences, but they are processes in the mind that can describe the world. From the neural perspective, rules are processes in the brain built out of semantic pointers, patterns of firing that explain thinking as the result of binding of multimodal representations. It is important not to think of rules as just structures sitting around doing nothing but rather as playing active roles in mental and neural mechanisms. Rules enable people to conduct more complicated kinds of behavior than what they could do by simply working with sensations, images, and concepts, let alone by simply responding to their environments.

As the Canadian stereotype and other social rules illustrate, rules are important both for the operations of individual minds and for explaining how people interact with each other. If you learn that someone is Canadian rather than Elbonian (from the mythical country of Dilbert cartoons), you may be more inclined to be polite to them. This chapter describes ways in which rules are important for explaining thinking in individuals, ranging from problem solving to language use. *Mind–Society* considers many domains in which rules are crucial for understanding social behavior, including economic decisions, political actions, and religious rituals. *Natural Philosophy* shows the importance of rules for understanding know-how, causality, and morality. To understand how people think with rules, we need first to specify their psychological operations, and, second, to identify the neural mechanisms that underlie the psychology.

MENTAL MECHANISMS FOR RULES

The psychological importance of rules was appreciated in the early days of cognitive science in the 1950s. A major part of Noam Chomsky's critique of behaviorism was the argument that explaining language use requires much more mental apparatus than the simple behavioral patterns that B. F. Skinner advocated. Chomsky hypothesized that people have an internalized grammar consisting of rules that enable them to generate and comprehend an enormous variety of sentences, including ones that have been never been uttered before. Probably no one has ever said before that Australian waffles smell like asparagus cocktails, but you can understand it nevertheless.

Problem Solving

The first computational theories of problem solving, developed by Alan Newell and Herbert Simon, took rules as their basic form of representation. Newell and Simon claimed that problem solutions result from people's ability to chain together numerous rules, all of which have an *if–then* structure. For example, consider the rules that you use to buy a book, perhaps ones like the following. If you want to get a book, then you can buy it. If you want to buy a book, then you can order it online. If you want to order a book online, then you can go to the Amazon web page and search for it. If you want to make an order on Amazon, then you use a credit card. If you want to use your credit card, then you need to find your credit card number and type it in. Chaining these rules together in a series of *if–then* reasoning steps will enable you to buy the book. Of course, there are other series of rules that might obtain the same result. For example, you could use rules to figure out how to get the book from a library or how to steal it from pirate sources online.

Rules as mental representations are also sometimes known as productions, production rules, or condition–action rules, where the condition is the *if* part and the action is the *then* part. The basic mechanism for using rules is to match the condition against a representation of the current situation and then execute the action, expanding the current situation. For example, the rule to brush your teeth after meals translates into *If you just ate a meal, then brush your teeth*. Matching the condition that you ate a meal executes the action of brushing your teeth. In complex problem solving, however, we need to do more than just match one condition and execute the action, because we may need to select and chain together a whole series of rules, as in my example of buying a book. A series of matchings and executions leads to a sequence of actions that accomplishes the goal: find the website, use your credit card, and get the book. A problem solution is often an emergent result of the interaction of many rules, no one of which is sufficient to accomplish the goals of the problem.

Since the 1980s, the most prominent account of rule-based thinking has been John Anderson's ACT theory, where ACT stands for "adaptive control of thought." Anderson expanded Newell and Simon's account of representation to include concept-like nodes whose activation helps to explain how memory can affect which rules are matched. The relationship between concepts and rules is complicated. At first glance, it seems that rules are made out of concepts, because you need words and their associated concepts to express the conditions and actions in rules. For example, the rule *If something is a giraffe, then it has a long neck* seems to depend on the concepts *giraffe, neck, long,* and *having*. On the other hand, chapter 4 shows how concepts can play roles in inference and problem solving that depend on having associated rules that express their typical features. So the concept *giraffe* includes the rule that giraffes have long necks. This puzzle about concepts being part of rules and rules being part of concepts can be resolved by seeing how both operate through neural mechanisms, as described later in this chapter.

Nonverbal Rules

A major limitation of psychological theories of rule-based problem solving is that they rely on verbal representations in the conditions and actions of rules. Cognitive architectures such as ACT-R (which stands for "adaptive control of thought—rational") can accept perceptual inputs, but they translate them into verbal representations rather retaining their sensory character. But animals besides humans are also capable of sequential problem solving, even though they lack syntactically complex language. Rats, for example, can learn behaviors such as avoiding foods they have only tried once, applying the rule *If you eat a new food and you get sick, then avoid it.*

In the absence of verbal representations, the representations of the conditions and actions of rules are better expressed as sensory and imagistic structures. For example, a possibly innate rule for a mouse could be expressed as *If smell-of-cat, then run-away.* Here *smell-of-cat* is an olfactory representation, and *run-away* is a motor representation. These nonverbal representations can be understood as patterns of neural firing as described in chapter 2 and displayed using the notation introduced in chapter 3 to indicate semantic pointers: <smell-of-cat> → <run-away>. With conditions and actions represented by semantic pointers, multimodal rules can incorporate sensory, motor, and emotional information. As with images and concepts, rules on this interpretation are capable of modal retention, preserving some of the character of sensory and motor inputs.

Even for humans, such rules are important, for example, when you infer that someone is friendly by means of the visual and emotional rule: <*smiles*> → <*friendly*>. People's many habits can be expressed as verbal rules, but they usually have motor and sensory components that are better captured by multimodal expressions such as <*shower*> → <*apply-soap*>. Here <*apply-soap*> is not just words, but a composite that is motor, visual, tactile, and olfactory.

No one disagrees that human and animal minds have sensations, but arguments for images, concepts, and rules are more complicated. Just as a theory of mind needs images and concepts to explain the varieties of thinking described in chapters 3 and 4, psychology needs to expand mental processing to include rules. The justification is that otherwise we cannot explain various aspects of human behavior such as language, problem solving, and habits.

Many important observations can be explained by the supposition that people have rules in their minds and procedures that work with rules such as the following.

Physical: *If an object is unsupported, then it falls.*
Biological: *If an animal goes without food for weeks, then it dies.*
Technological: *If you want to write a computer program, use a high-level pro-gramming language like Python.*
Psychological: *If you get a cut, then you feel pain.*
Social: *If you insult people, then they get angry at you.*
Language: *If you want to make a word plural in English, then add* s.
Legal: *If people are insane, then they are not responsible for their actions.*
Medical: *If people have an infection, then they get a fever.*

All of these rules require concepts that can rely on visual, kinesthetic, and other sensory representations, not just words. The rules are not universal gener-alizations, for they can have exceptions, such as hibernating bears that can go without food.

Rules are excellent for encoding procedural knowledge about how to do things (knowledge how) as well as declarative knowledge about the world (knowledge that). Human activities usually require both kinds of knowledge. For example, brushing your teeth uses declarative knowledge that toothbrushes are instru-ments used to clean teeth and also procedural knowledge how to move a brush in your mouth.

Systems of rules that include nonverbal representations can provide mental models like the imagistic ones described in chapter 3. You can capture your under-standing of how bicycles work with simple verbal rules like:

If the pedal moves, then the crank turns.
If the crank turns, then the chain moves.
If the chain moves, then the back wheel turns.
If the back wheel turns, then the bicycle goes forward.

But a richer understanding comes from having visual and possibly kinesthetic representations of concepts like *pedal, moves, crank,* and *turns.* People who have watched bikes work can use these images to produce dynamic nonverbal rules that have the general form: <*image1*> → <*image2*> is the nonverbal version of "if-then," perhaps based on the sensory–motor understanding of causality described in chapter 3. Mental modeling of a bicycle can then amount to running a movie in your head rather than a series of verbal inferences.

Logic

Verbal inferences can also be carried out by rules. Putting rules to work usually requires matching the condition and executing the action, a kind of forward inference corresponding to the logical rule modus ponens, which has the general form *If P then Q, and P, therefore Q.* But forward inference can be much more complicated than modus ponens when there are competing rules that can yield different conclusions, such as both:

> *If people have an infection, then they get a fever.*
> *If people have an infection and they take aspirin, then they don't get a fever.*

Deciding which of these rules to apply in a current situation depends on numerous factors such as how well each rule fits the current situation and how well it has performed in the past. For example, if you see a bird that is black, white, and upright, then it is better to apply the rule *If something is a bird and it is a penguin, then it does not fly* than the more general rule that birds fly.

In addition to forward inference, rules can also contribute to reverse inference that works backwards from a result to figure out how to produce it. Rules can be run backwards to generate explanations, a procedure that psychologists sometimes call "attribution" and philosophers call "abduction." For example, a physician might infer that a patient with a fever has an infection because the infection would explain the fever. This kind of inference is obviously risky, because alternative hypotheses and additional evidence should also be taken into account. Before a physician concludes that a patient has an infection, there needs to be an inference to the best explanation with the form: Given all the symptoms and all the hypotheses generated from all the relevant rules, the best explanation of the patient's symptoms is an infection. Abductive inference can operate with nonverbal rules such as <*pushed*> → <*fall*>, which can enable you to imagine that a falling person was pushed using visual and motor representations rather than words.

The meaning of rules as mental representations is different from the interpretation of *if–then* in formal logic, which construes it as a function of the truth values of the *if* part and *then* part. *If P, then Q* is taken to be false when P is true and Q is false, and otherwise true. This analysis has the peculiar result that *If P, then* Q comes out true whenever P is false or Q is true. For example, consider in following: *If Justin Bieber is Prime Minister of Canada, then marmalade is sour* and *If Justin Bieber is not Prime Minister of Canada, then marmalade is sweet*. On the usual interpretation of *if–then* in formal logic, both of these odd statements come out true.

In contrast, ordinary understandings of *if–then* usually assume some causal or semantic connection between the *if* part and the *then* part. The two sentences about Justin Bieber are anomalous because there is no apparent connection between him and marmalade. Chapter 3 mentions that the typical features of causality include manipulative ability: A causes B when controlling A changes B. The truth-functional semantics for *if–then* completely loses the natural psychological assumption of a causal connection between the parts.

Logicians have tried to deal with these semantic anomalies by introducing modal notions such as necessity and possible worlds. They supplement the truth-functional *if–then* by specifying that P strictly implies Q when Q is true in all possible worlds in which P is true. Unfortunately, this move into *possible worlds* semantics takes logic even farther into the realm of psychological implausibility and metaphysical extravagance. There are elegant formal treatments of possible worlds but no sensible interpretation of what they are and how they are related to each other and the real world in which we live.

The reason that formal logic painted itself into this semantic corner is the pursuit of the syntactic dream, the assumption that inference is primarily a matter of logical form so that meaning and pragmatics are subsidiary. The semantic pointer interpretation of rules smoothly integrates logical syntax with semantics and pragmatics.

Memory

Memory is another mental mechanism important for thinking with rules. How many rules do people have in their minds? Chapter 4 estimated that people have at least 10,000 concepts, each of which is associated with multiple rules. For example, the concept *cat* is associated with numerous rules such as that cats are mammals, have four legs, and eat birds. Most rules are dormant in memory most of the time, so how do they become available for matching? If you have not thought about aardvarks for years, then the rule that aardvarks have scaly skin may not be immediately accessible for inferential use. Spreading activation among concepts explains how rules can become available for the matching operation: Thinking of dogs may make you think of cats, which makes available rules about cats.

Causality

Explanation and problem solving require causal rules to figure out why things happen and what will happen in the future, but what is causality? Chapter 2 described the origins of understanding of causality in sensory–motor–sensory patterns, which allows infants and animals to have a rudimentary appreciation of cause and effect. But understanding of causality becomes much more sophisticated with experience and education. No simple definition of causality is obtainable, but the three-analysis of *cause* shown in Table 5.1 illustrates a sophisticated understanding of causality. People who think a lot about causal relations in the world can go beyond simple examples and sensory–motor patterns to appreciate the importance of regular rules, manipulations that intervene in the world, statistical relationships, and networks of multiple interacting causes.

NEURAL MECHANISMS FOR RULES

To describe how rules might work in the brain, we need to go beyond verbal descriptions that have been used in psychological theories. To approximate the neural nature of rules, think of them as having the structure: *If representation1, then representation2.* Representations can not only include words, as in *If something is a dog, then it is furry,* but also the whole diversity of sensory representations described in chapter 3, ranging from vision to pain. These representations could also include emotions such as anger and happiness. What unifies all of these from a brain perspective is that they all are patterns of firing in neural groups.

TABLE 5.1

Three-Analysis of *Cause*

Exemplars	*Pushes, pulls, motions, collisions, actions, diseases*
Typical features	Temporally ordered events, with causes before effects
	Sensory–motor–sensory patterns
	Regularities expressed by rules
	Manipulations and interventions
	Statistical dependencies, with causes increasing the probabilities of effects
	Causal networks of influence
Explanations	Explains: why events happen, why interventions work
	Explained by: underlying mechanisms

In the structure *If representation1, then representation2,* the representations are neural patterns, but what is the *if–then* relation? Naturally, this has to be a pattern also, but what kind of pattern is it? Chapter 2 shows how semantic pointers can manage relations as well as properties. Properties such as *red* and *furry* are simple features of a single object, whereas relations concern multiple objects, as in "The dog chased the cat," which expresses the relation of chasing between a dog and a cat. Properties can be represented in the brain by simple patterns, but ascribing a property to an object to form a belief requires binding the property to the object. With relations, the binding is more complicated because relations always involve multiple roles. In the relation of chasing, the roles include the chaser and the chased. To keep these roles distinct, there need to be bindings of *dog* to *chaser* and *cat* to *chased*, to provide contrast to the representation that the cat chased the dog.

We can understand the *if–then* relation in the same way, as a pattern of firing that binds the condition (*if* part), which is itself a neural pattern, to the action (*then* part). Keeping the condition and action separate is crucial because *If P, then Q* is different from *If Q, then P*; dogs are mammals, but not all mammals are dogs. The neural pattern that produces the rule *Dogs are mammals* comes about by recursive binding:

$$bind\,[(bind\; if-then\,relation)\,(bind\,dog\,condition)\,(bind\,mammal\,action)].$$

Figure 5.1 shows this structure as a semantic pointer of the sort described in chapter 2.

The simplest rules connect only two representations, but people are capable of incorporating more patterns into rules with multiple conditions and multiple

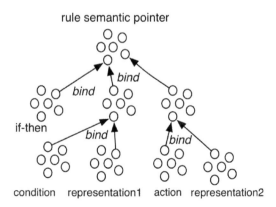

FIGURE 5.1 Neural representation of a rule *if representation1 then representation2* as a semantic pointer that binds two or more representations, each of which is a semantic pointer. Binding of *if–then* to *relation* is omitted.

actions, as in *If something is a dog that is foaming at the mouth, then it is rabid and you should run away*. All that is required for a neural process to produce these more complicated rules are more bindings. Figure 5.1 shows rules where the *if–then* relation, the condition, and action are explicitly represented by different patterns in neural groups, but the Semantic Pointer Architecture also accommodates rules that are compiled into processes capable of more direct operation without explicit *if–then* inference.

Figure 5.1 should help to clarify the relations between rules and concepts. Unless they are images, *representation1* and *representation2* are concepts, which are themselves patterns of neural firing—semantic pointers. Chapter 4 described how the bindings that go into these semantic pointers operate on (a) representations of sensory and motor experiences—the exemplars; (b) representations of typical features, usually other concepts; and (c) representations of rules used in explanations. So, concepts are partly made out of rules just as rules are partly made out of concepts. This is not circular, because, at bottom, both rules and concepts, understood as semantic pointers, are made out of neural processes.

Figure 5.1 shows how the semantic pointer interpretation of rules not only handles their syntactic complexity but also points toward integrations with semantic and pragmatic aspects. The representations that go into the rule get their meaning from relations to sensory experience and with other representations. The *if–then* relation is usually causal, so it inherits meaning from the sensory–motor–sensory schema that underlies causality. Pragmatic aspects of rules include context, which is managed by having the condition of the rule match the current situation, and purpose, which is managed by the contribution of goals to rule-based inference and the incorporation of emotions discussed in chapter 7. Hence the semantic pointer construal of rules avoids the syntax-first approach that has bedeviled logic and linguistics, as discussed in chapter 10.

The basic psychological process for working with rules is to match the condition and then execute the action. Matching a condition to a stimulus such as a sensory combination of shape and color can operate with the same mechanism that chapter 3 described for matching concepts: reactivating the original pattern of firing. Once the condition is thereby matched and there is not a rule with a better match, the rule can be applied by executing the action. For example, a mouse might have a multimodal rule to run away from cats: <*cat*> → <*run away*>. Applying this rule requires reactivating the mouse's sensory patterns of the smell and look of cats and then executing the motor action to run away. Hence even something as simple as the nonverbal rule of a mouse to run away if a cat is present can involve the representation of multiple modalities, including emotions such as fear.

Making the case that rules are neural processes requires three steps, two of which have been taken. First, I sketched how to encode rules with their *if–then* structure as neural processes. The conditions and actions are as easily encoded as images and concepts were in chapters 3 and 4. Producing the whole *if–then* structure requires the ability of semantic pointers to bind representations of conditions, and actions into combined neural patterns. Second, I sketched how the matching and firing operations of rules can be performed by neural trans- formations, using the matching and instantiation operations already applied for images and concepts. Third, it remains to be shown that this neural under- standing of rules is powerful enough to explain psychological phenomena that motivated rules in the first place. Let us examine how the semantic pointer interpretation of rules applies to innateness, learning, problem solving, and language.

USES OF RULES

The explanatory identity that rules are neural processes, specifically semantic pointers of the kind illustrated in Figure 5.1, needs to be evaluated with respect to how well it explains available evidence. The two key claims are (a) that rules are an important kind of mental representation in humans and (b) that rules can be identified as semantic pointers. Both claims can be justified by showing how construing rules as neural processes provides superior mechanisms for explaining psychological facts.

Innateness

The semantic pointer interpretation of rules shown in Figure 5.1 assumed that there is a neural pattern for the overall *if–then* relation, but what is its origin? Because rules are such a general component of animal thought, it is plausible that the general *if–then* relation is innate, but particular rules may be either innate or learned. A rule is innate if it has become part of human genetics as a result of evo- lution by natural selection. For a rule to be innate, it does not have to be active at birth, because there may be a developmental period before the rule can be put into use. For example, children have an innate capacity to develop the ability to walk, but walking usually does not appear until toward the end of a child's first year. The standards for judging that a rule might be innate will be the same standards ap- plied to the question of the innateness of concepts, including cultural universality, dedicated brain areas, animal precursors, adaptive contribution, and absence of alternative explanations.

In assessing the innateness of rules, it is important to distinguish between rule-based inference and simple reflexes. If you are hit on the knee, your lower leg will swing out, but that does not mean you have a rule that says *If your knee is tapped, then swing your leg*. Swinging your leg out is just a simple physical response to the stimulus of tapping the knee. Similarly, people do not need to learn a rule *If something is coming toward your head, then duck*, because that also may be a simple physical response. So what are the best candidates for rules that might be innate?

Since the 1950s, language is been a showpiece for postulating innate rules, because of the influence of Noam Chomsky. In all cultures, children learn to speak and understand the local language within a period of a few years. Chomsky argued that this capability is best explained not by general learning mechanisms but by a genetically inherited capacity to learn specific types of grammar. Children can learn any of the thousands of human languages because all languages have a common, universal grammar acquired genetically. For example, all human languages have ways of structuring sentences into subjects, verbs, and objects, even though they do this in different ways. So perhaps children have an innate, unconscious rule to guide them in learning a local language, with a structure something like *If you are trying to learn a language, then detect its structure for subject, verb, and object*.

The rules of particular languages such as English and Chinese are not innate but must be learned through exposure to the language as spoken by parents and other people. But it may be that rules of universal grammar are built into the human brain and enable people to slot their current language into a more general framework. Unfortunately, Chomsky's research program was not successful at specifying the rules of universal grammar, and current theories claim that syntax requires only a minimal set of basic operations. For example, Merge combines two syntactic objects into a new syntactic object, analogously to the bind operation in the Semantic Pointer Architecture.

Another plausible domain in which innate rules may operate is number. All human languages have number systems, even though some are no more complicated than *one, two, many*. But chimpanzees have a rudimentary number sense, enabling them to distinguished numbers of things at least up to five or six, and young children also can make such discriminations. Other domains that might be candidates for innate rules include ones with core concepts such as *object* and *face* mentioned in chapter 4. For example, infants' ability to recognize faces at birth suggests that they might have a nonverbal rule about faces having eyes.

Assuming that there are some innate rules, the key question is how they could be genetically encoded in brains. The answer is a more complicated version of the innateness of concepts described in chapter 4. First, there needs to be an innate representation of the complex relation *if–then*. This requires a group of neurons with synaptic connections capable of generating a pattern of firing that can produce the bindings of conditions and actions shown in Figure 5.1.

Second, there needs to be a genetically encoded version of the condition and the action, so that the organism does not have to learn that the *if–then* relation applies to sets of examples furnished by the senses. The conditions and actions in an innate rule need to be innate concepts. For example, given the quickness with which infants notice and react to faces, even within an hour after birth, there may be an innate rule of the form *If you see a smiling face, then smile*. For this rule to be innate, there needs to be innate concepts *face* and *smile*, as well as an innate motor pattern for smiling. The concept of *smiling face*, as well as the action of smiling, are plausibly encoded by semantic pointers that bind together other patterns of firing in multiple modalities. Hence, Eliasmith's Semantic Pointer Architecture can explain the possibility of innate rules, although it makes no claims about how prevalent they are.

Is knowledge about causality innate or learned? Chapter 3 described how infants already exhibit some expectations about causal interactions, so it may be that they were born with a rule schema like *If sensory-state and motor-action, then different-sensory-state*. This general rule could enable easy learning of more specific rules such as *If blanket-still and move-arm, then blanket-move*. Here the sensory states and motor actions are nonverbal representations. Eventually, a person can learn much more sophisticated ideas about causality not dependent on motor manipulation, for example, ideas about probability mentioned in Table 5.1.

Learning

Even if a few special concepts and rules are innately part of the genetic equipment of all human beings, most of our representations are learned from sensory experience and interactions with other people. Hence, we need to figure out the neural mechanisms by which rules are learned. In language, for example, people learn how different languages deal with future and past tenses. In English, the typical rule for turning a verb into a past tense is to add "ed," as in "I walked to the river." In contrast, Chinese signals past tenses with adverbs like the equivalent of "yesterday," rather than by modifying the verb. English speakers also need to be able to recognize exceptions to the add "ed" rules, as in the sentence "I went to the river" instead of "I goed to the river." Physical rules (e.g., *If you drop an object, then it will fall*) and social rules (e.g., *If you insult people, then they will be angry at you*) also need to be learned from experience.

The key question then is how neurally encoded rules can be learned from experience. At the mental level, a rule has the structure *If conditions, then actions*, but at the neural level a rule needs to be interpreted as a pattern of firing built out of patterns for the *if–then* relation, the conditions, and the actions. There are various learning mechanisms that can be used to build up such patterns.

The simplest way of learning rules is by association of representations for conditions and actions through Hebbian learning. Suppose a child is becoming acquainted with an unfamiliar animal such as a weasel, which puts the child in a position to learn numerous rules such as *Weasels have fur, Weasels have teeth*, and *Weasels are vicious*. If the child sees several vicious weasels, then the neurons that collectively encode the concept *weasel* will be active at the same time as the neurons that collectively encode the concept *vicious*. Synaptic connections between the neurons in each of these possibly overlapping groups will be strengthened through the simultaneous activation of the respective neurons, in accord with the Hebbian principle that whatever fires together wires together. Then, the condition concept *weasel* can become associated with the action concept *vicious* by virtue of strengthened associations between the neurons encoding them. In this way, Hebbian learning can accomplish generalization of rules from experience. Making the Hebbian result more explicit requires binding the condition and action into the overall *if–then* structure. Chapter 7 discusses emotional learning by rule generalization, with such results as *If you eat chocolate, then you feel happy*. Such rules can be learned by reinforcement learning that associates particular behaviors with pleasure or pain.

Other kinds of rule learning are more complicated and require different kinds of binding, when rules are learned from other rules. In current psychological theories of rule-based problem solving, the primary mechanism for learning rules consists of combining rules by stringing them together. For example, suppose you have the rules *If you want to buy something, then go on the Internet* and *If you go on the Internet to buy something, then go to the Amazon website*. These rules can be strung together into a more efficient rule *If you want to buy something, then go to the Amazon website*. More generally, this learning involves taking two rules of the form *If condition1, then action1* and *If action1, then action2* and combining them into a super rule of the form *If condition1, then action2*.

Creation of new rules by stringing old rules together requires a complex transformation using unbinding and binding. First, the brain needs to unbind the condition from the first rule and unbind the action from the second rule and then rebind them into another *if–then* structure connecting the first condition and the second action. This transformation does not involve Hebbian learning but can be much faster when carried out by processes of binding and rebinding. As in Hebbian learning, combination results in new neural connections.

Like concepts and images, therefore, rules can be learned in two fundamentally different ways—by generalization from experience and by combination of other representations. Both concepts and rules can not only be learned by perceptual associations, but they can also be produced by bindings of existing representations in conceptual combination and rule combination. Learning does not have to be just the slow, incremental process that occurs with Hebbian and reinforcement learning, but it can also involve the larger leaps from generating new concepts and rules by combination.

Problem Solving

Rules are often useful for solving problems. Sometimes a single rule can solve a problem for you, for example, when you get rid of a headache by applying the rule *If you have a headache, then take an aspirin*. More complicated problems require chains of rules with multiple steps, as in the sequence *If your clothes are dirty, then wash them* and *If your clothes are washed, then dry them in a dryer*. Rule-based problem solving can operate in three different ways: proceeding from the current situation toward a goal, working backward from a goal to current resources, or working bidirectionally by starting at the beginning and also working backward, aiming to meet in the middle. Respectively, these three ways of solving problems are called forward chaining, backward chaining, and bidirectional search.

John Anderson, the main developer of the ACT theory of rule-based problem solving, has increasingly been tying it to neural processes by identifying brain areas that are plausibly involved in the key processes of applying rules. For example, he conjectures that the central process of selecting and matching rules is carried out by the basal ganglia, an area of the brain with connections to many others. Moreover, Anderson and his colleagues have been collaborating with researchers on neural network models of the sort developed by Randall O'Reilly. The resulting hybrid models provide interesting ideas about how rule-based problem solving can operate in the brain, but I think a deeper account can be developed using the Semantic Pointer Architecture.

The key question is whether semantic pointers can be used in sequential problem solving. Terry Stewart and Chris Eliasmith have used the Semantic Pointer Architecture to simulate solution of the Tower of Hanoi problem, in which a solution results from moving disks on and off of pegs. One big advantage of using semantic pointers is that the representation of the pegs and the disks need not be restricted to verbal symbols. Peoples' representations of pegs and disks can easily be visual (i.e., what they look like) and kinesthetic (i.e., what it feels like to move them). This greater representational power allows for rules in which the conditions and actions correspond to the full sensory capacity of the human brain. Similarly, the rule *If you have a headache, then take an aspirin* does not need to be understood as merely verbal. Your representation of a headache can include the sensory aspect of having a pain, and your representation of an aspirin can be of a visual and tactile entity that is small, round, white, and easy to pick up.

Despite this increased representational diversity, the usual problem-solving process of a rule-based system can still be carried out in a series of steps by matching the conditions of the rules and executing their actions. The simulations of solving the Tower of Hanoi by the Semantic Pointer Architecture provide a good fit to human performance. Hence, the theory of the brain involving binding and semantic pointers is capable of explaining inferential problem solving using rules. There is much work to be done, however, to show how rules based on semantic pointers can also be used in backward chaining and bidirectional search.

Rules can also contribute to the solution of explanation problems, thanks to the availability of causal rules with the structure *If cause, then effect*. For example, an unfortunate person's lung cancer can be explained by running backward the rule *If smoker, then gets-lung-cancer*. This rule is far from universal, but it summarizes a well-established causal connection. When the person is already known to be a smoker, then the inference is just that the particular lung cancer was the result of the smoking. However, when the relevance of the cause is unknown in a particular case, the rule can be used to generate an abductive inference: Maybe the person is a smoker, because that would explain lung cancer.

Such rule-based attempts to generate causal explanations can lead via conceptual combination to theoretical concepts like *virus* and *quark*. When there are no available rules that describe relations between observable factors, people can consider rules that introduce nonobservable ones. For example, thunder can be explained by hypothesizing the existence of thunder gods or, more recently, by the existence of electrical discharges in the form of lightning. Evaluation of which of these competing hypotheses fits best with the evidence requires parallel constraint satisfaction by semantic pointer competition.

For both explanation and planning, rules help people to imagine ways in which the world can change and be changed. Imagination produces mental simulations in which rules are run sequentially to make inferences about what can happen under different circumstances. These simulations can be nonverbal as well as verbal, for example, when crows and chimpanzees use twigs as tools to retrieve food, requiring a sequence of rules such as <*twig*> → <*retrieve-food*>. Simulations with multimodal rules are also important in a mode of empathy described in chapter 7.

Rules are not the only way to solve problems. Some problems can be solved simply by manipulating images as in chapter 3, by applying concepts as in chapter 4, and by using analogies as in chapter 6. In all of these kinds of problem solving, sensory and motor images can make valuable contributions in addition to verbal representations.

Memory

Memory for rules is an important part of problem solving. People may have tens of thousands of rules, but they will not be able to use a potentially useful rule if it never gets retrieved from memory. Long ago, I learned rules about how to make a white sauce from flour and butter, but I cannot remember them now because I have not used this kind of cooking technique for decades. Solving a problem on the fly can require quickly retrieving the relevant rule or rules and being able to put them into play. One possibility is that rules enter contention for application to current situations by spreading activation among the concepts that are used in their conditions and actions. For example, think of a headache should bring into working memory useful rules for dealing with the problem, perhaps not just by taking an aspirin but potentially by getting a head massage. Hence, the problem description about a headache should generate associations of relevant rules for getting rid of headaches.

Language

There are numerous ways in which rules are useful for explaining aspects of language such as pronunciation, spelling, grammar, and communication. The rules for pronunciation are naturally understood using auditory representations rather than verbal ones. In English, there is an approximate rule that says that the letter "c" is pronounced like a "k" if it is followed by the vowels "a," "u," or "o" (as in "cat"), but like the letter "s" if it is followed by the vowels "i" or "e" (as in "city"). Such rules can be written in words, but they can be understood at least as well in terms of the sounds that go with the pronunciation of "k" and "s." Spelling rules can usefully use spatial representations, as in the mnemonic "i" before "e" except after "c." This translates into the rules *If you are spelling words with* i *and* e *together, then the order is* i *and then* e and *If you are spelling words with* i *and* e *together following* c, *then the order is* e *and then* i. The relations of *after* and *order* are spatial relations best mapped onto a visual image.

Similarly, rules of grammar apply not merely to abstract verbal representations but also to structures that need to consider spatial and temporal order, as in the structure of a sentence that has a subject, then a verb, and then an object. Language also operates with social rules, such as *If you are speaking to someone important, then do not use profanity.* Linguistic rules expressed in sounds and spatiotemporal location benefit from the enhanced representational power of semantic pointers over words. Hence, any theory of language that employs rules can benefit from the Semantic Pointer Architecture.

How Rules Change

Like concepts, rules can change by generation, alteration, and replacement. Generation methods include not only the ones already discussed—generalization from examples and rule combination—but also less common ones. Sometimes, generalization does not require many examples because background knowledge justifies a quick inference. For example, testing an element for combustibility does not require many samples because there is little variability in how a particular element combines with oxygen. This kind of quick generalization from small samples is more like quick memory storage than like the gradual synaptic changes required for Hebbian and reinforcement learning. Similarly, abductive inference can lead to relatively fast formation of rules whose explanatory contributions are immediately evident. For example, Darwin formed the rule *If natural selection, then evolution* because of its explanatory power by a process of abductive generalization rather than generalization from examples.

Rules can be altered in many ways, for example, by specialization of a rule that turns out to be too general. You may have started out with the rule that birds fly but had to specialize it into *If something is a bird and it is not a penguin or ostrich, then it flies.* A particular rule may turn out to be so defective that it simply has to be abandoned, such as the nineteenth-century prejudice that women cannot handle university education. Sometimes whole systems of rules are replaced by other systems, as has occurred in political revolutions where the rules describe government procedures, and in scientific revolutions where the rules are theories and methods.

SUMMARY AND DISCUSSION

Rules are mental representations of the form *If condition, then action*, where matching the condition leads to execution of the action. Chaining rules together makes possible solution of complex problems, such as figuring out how to get from one city to another. Mental rules of this sort are also important for explaining people's ability to generate and comprehend language. Semantic pointers provide a valuable supplement to conventional theories of rules in two ways. First, they show how rules as mental representations can also be neural representations, through encoding and binding of *if–then*, the condition, and the action, all as patterns of firing. Second, semantic pointers show how conditions and actions can go beyond verbal information to incorporate all the kinds of sensory information described in chapter 3. For example, the useful rule *If you have to urinate, then find a toilet* is more than verbal, because having to urinate is an internal sensation, toilets are identified by their visual and tactile features, and finding is often a kinesthetic representation involving moving through space. Hence, a rule composed of semantic pointers is a more plausible representation: *<need-urinate>* → *<find-toilet>*.

In the 1980s, some enthusiasts for neural network models saw explanations based on neural connections as an alternative to symbolic, rule-based explanations. However, from the perspective of the Semantic Pointer Architecture, there is no incompatibility. Neural network theories benefit from appreciating that human brains really do work with rules, and the task then is to figure out how patterns of firing in neural groups can behave like rules. Rule theories also benefit from appreciating that the representations that go into the conditions and actions of rules are frequently multimodal, requiring the full sensory power of semantic pointers. This power shows how rules can be embodied when the conditions and actions are representations that are wholly or partly based on sensory and motor experiences. But rules can also be transbodied when they are formed from representations that transcend the senses as in the hypotheses that quarks are subatomic particles and that justice is fairness.

Another element neglected in standard theories of rule-based problem solving is the importance of emotion. Chapter 7 describes emotions as semantic pointers that bind physiological perception and cognitive appraisal. In a particular problem-solving situation, some goals are more important and pressing than others, and the difference is captured by emotional associations. Having to go to the bathroom a bit may make you emotionally uncomfortable, but a severe need to urinate can induce panic and fear of embarrassment, focusing attention on solving this particular problem. The effect of emotion on attention also influences consciousness, according to the theory proposed in chapter 8.

Later chapters in this book report additional applications of rule-based reasoning to action in chapter 9, to language in chapter 10, and to creativity in chapter 11, particularly in connection with the discovery of new methods. *Mind–Society* discusses many domains in which brain-based mental rules are important, for example, when people behave in accord with social norms.

NOTES

Major sources for rule-based theories include Newell and Simon 1972; Newell 1990; Rosenbloom, Laird, and Newell 1993; Anderson 1983, 1993, 2007. Applications of rules to numerous domains are discussed in Holland, Holyoak, Nisbett, and Thagard 1986. Spreading activation of concepts as a mechanism for retrieving rules from memory is modeled by the PI (which stands for "processes of induction") system of Thagard 1988.

In philosophy, *if–then* structures are termed *conditionals*, consisting of an antecedent and a consequent. On the use of rules and logical reasoning in the Semantic Pointer Architecture, see Eliasmith 2013.

To play the Tower of Hanoi, go to https://www.mathsisfun.com/games/towerofhanoi.html.

The role of rules in language is emphasized by Chomsky 1980 and Pinker 1991, 1999. Neural network alternatives are defended by McClelland and Patterson 2002 and Smolensky and Legendre 2006.

On the number sense, see Dehaene 2011. *Natural Philosophy* (chapter 10) discusses mathematics.

A model of abduction in neural networks is presented by Thagard and Litt 2008, reprinted in Thagard 2012d. If there are competing explanatory hypotheses, the best can be selected by using parallel constraint satisfaction to infer the best explanation: Thagard 1992, 2000.

It is currently popular to model causal reasoning by Bayesian networks, but these are psychologically limited: Jones and Love 2011, Thagard 2004. Bayesianism is like behaviorism, radical embodiment, and evolutionary psychology in blocking inquiry concerning specific neural and mental mechanisms responsible for important phenomena; see *Natural Philosophy* (chapter 3).

Model rule-based problem solving in the Semantic Pointer Architecture including bidirectional search and rule combination. Expand the architecture to include rule learning by combination and abductive generalization.

6

Analogies

Albert Einstein wrote to his son that life is like riding a bicycle—to keep your balance, you must keep moving. This analogy between living and riding provides advice about how to deal with daily difficulties. Many problems can be solved using rules, concepts, and images, but these kinds of mental representations do not provide a full account of human thought. People's experiences often go beyond what regularities they have learned in the past. Especially when we are engaged in novel and creative activities, we usually lack sets of rules, concepts, or images that we can put readily to work. Then we need to employ another kind of mental representation: analogies. The boxer Mike Tyson drew a different analogy about life's difficulties when he said that everyone has a plan until they get punched in the face.

Analogy is a kind of thinking that uses a previous case to deal with problems in a new situation. Suppose that you are going on your second date, traveling to a foreign country for the second time, or doing your income tax after a year's relief. Your experience the first time is rarely adequate for forming rules about what to expect, but your previous experience can be valuable for dealing with problems that you are likely to encounter the next time. You can deal with the new situation by adapting what worked in a previous case and by avoiding what did not work before.

Analogies can valuably contribute to decision making. Imagine you need to buy a new car but do not want to bother researching all the available brands with their strengths and weaknesses. A time-saving solution is simply to buy the same kind of car you bought previously, with your last car serving as an analog for the new problem of buying the next one. Obviously, decision making by analogy can be harmful if the situation has changed so that your previous assessment is no longer valid. Another way in which analogy can contribute to decision making is through the use of role models. You can take the behavior of another person as a model for what you should do, considering your situation as analogous to what he or she previously faced. Asking yourself what would Jesus do or, what would Gandhi do, enables you to solve a moral problem by analogy. Biblical parables are moral analogies, telling people to act, for instance, like the good Samaritan.

Teachers often use analogies to help their students understand complex new ideas, for example, by comparing the structure of atoms to the solar system. If students know that the planets rotate around the sun, then they can achieve a rudimentary understanding of invisible atoms by being told that electrons rotate around the nucleus of an atom, in much the same way that planets rotate around the sun. Generations of biology students have been told that viruses, hormones, neurotransmitters, and drugs affect cells by binding to receptor molecules on the cells much as a key enters a lock. Philosophers explain how thoughts are coherent to their students using a variety of analogs such as spider webs and crossword puzzles. Road maps are visual representations that are only analogous to actual road systems, not exact depictions. Chapter 2 uses a variety of analogies such as cooking to foster understanding of semantic pointers.

People often use analogies in attempts to persuade others, taking into account previous successes and failures. For example, when the United States invaded Iraq in 2003, supporters of the invasion invoked an analogy to Nazi Germany and Hitler to support it, but critics warned that it would become another Vietnam. Analogies can also be used largely for entertainment purposes, for example, in parodies (like *The Onion* newspaper) and jokes, as in this comparison: Men are like wine – some turn to vinegar, but the best improve with age.

Analogies can also be helpful in learning how to solve professional problems. Many business school students are trained by the case method, learning about successful companies such as Federal Express that suggest solutions to future problems. Lawyers are trained to use analogies in the form of legal precedents, enabling them to deal with new cases by analogy to old ones. The clinical training of medical professionals provides them not only with rules for how to recognize and treat diseases but also a stock of cases that can be suggestive for future patients with novel conditions that do not fall under any of the standard medical rules.

Analogy is not just a mundane activity, but it is also a contributor to many of the greatest mental leaps that humans have accomplished across different fields. Some of the most important scientific theories of all time, including Darwin's theory of evolution by natural selection and Einstein's theory of special relativity, were based on analogical thinking. Mathematicians often use analogy to develop whole new areas by analogy to previously explored ones, for example, when Galois developed group theory by generalizing symmetries in physical objects. Analogies also contribute to explanations in social sciences, for example, when economists sought to understand the economic crisis of 2008 by comparison with the great crash of 1929.

Analogies have also contributed to social innovations, for example, when new educational and health systems are developed by adapting previously successful ones. When Canada instituted its universal healthcare system in 1984, it did so by adapting what were considered to be the successful features of the British National Health Service, while trying to avoid recognized limitations. Using analogies is no guarantee of creativity and success, because the new situation may be so totally different from previous experience that any analogy with past experience will be misleading.

Analogical thinking has also made great contributions to the humanities. Many novels such as Tolstoy's *War and Peace* were partially based on analogies to the authors' own lives. Musical composers have used analogy to develop new works by adapting previously available melodies, for example, in Bach's *Goldberg Variations*. Painters have used analogy in developing creative new works that adapt previous images and methods, as in the inspiration that Picasso got from African art.

Analogy thus makes substantial contributions to human thinking, despite its limitation in basing a current solution on a single previous case. We need to understand the mental and neural mechanisms that produce both creative analogies and destructive ones.

MENTAL MECHANISMS FOR ANALOGY

Understanding analogy as a mental process can begin by contrasting analogies with perceptions, images, concepts, and rules. Analogies are always comparisons between two situations: a *source* analog resulting from previous experience and a *target* analog, which is the new situation or problem for which the source is supposed to be useful. For Picasso, the target was new paintings, and the source was African sculptures. Analogies require representations of two different situations, each of which can have considerable internal structure. For example, people who say that their job makes them feel like a ticking time bomb believe that the emotional stresses of the job make them ready to explode. The information about the source and the target analogs may well be encoded by sensations, images, concepts, and rules, but the use of the source to generate inferences about the target employs processes not found in those other kinds of mental representation. Analogies are like images in that they stand for particular situations, unlike concepts and rules, which express generalities.

Analogical thinking requires a combination of four main psychological processes: obtaining, mapping, adapting, and learning. The first process is obtaining a source analog that can suggest a solution for the target. In teaching uses of analogy, the source is simply given by the teacher, for example, when students are told that they can understand the target analog of the atom by comparison with the source analog of the solar system. However, when a problem solver is working alone, the source analog may be obtained by remembering it, if the person can retrieve a previous case that is relevant for dealing with the new situation.

Sometimes, however, a suggestive source analog comes along by serendipity. For example, Darwin got the idea of natural selection through a fortunate reading of the ideas of the economist Malthus about how a discrepancy between rapid reproduction rates and limited food availability could generate a struggle for existence. Occasionally, a problem solver will purposefully generate a source analog to help with a difficult problem, as Francis Crick and James Watson did when they built wooden models for their guesses about the structure of DNA. Hence, there are at least four ways you can obtain a source analog to put to work: by being given it by someone else, by remembering it, by stumbling across it, and by intentionally generating it.

Once a potentially useful source analog becomes available, you need to determine its relevance to the target problem through a psychological process called mapping. The source does not have to be a perfect match for the target, but it must be capable of filling in what needs to be learned about the target. For example, suppose someone makes a joke that coffee shops are spreading through a city faster than head lice through a kindergarten class. To get the joke, you have to recognize the mapping between coffee shops and lice. The mapping does not have to be complete or perfect, so long as it is sufficient to accomplish the purpose of the analogy.

When the basic mapping between the source analog and the target analog is understood, then the source can be adapted to apply to the target. The process of adapting needs to transform the target using what is known about the source. In the head lice joke, the purpose is to transfer the negative emotion of disgust from the lice source to the coffee shop target. Emotional transfer is also important in empathy, discussed in chapter 7, and in many political arguments, for example, when the American invasion of Iraq was criticized for being likely to be as disastrous as the previous war in Vietnam. But most analogies transfer cognitive representations leading to the solution of a problem, not just emotional attitudes. For example, Darwin transferred concepts about population growth from Malthus's human case to the general world of plants and animals.

Once a target problem has been solved thanks to a relevant source, you can move on to the final stage of analogical thinking—learning from the successful analogy. Chapter 5 talks about learning rules from multiple examples, but sometimes it is possible to generate a rule from just two examples when a source and target have been connected to generate a problem solution. For example, you may be able to extract generalizations from your first and second visit to a foreign country. Even if a fully general rule cannot be generated, abstraction of the source and the target can produce a schema, which is a conceptual pattern that captures what is most crucially relevant to the source and target.

How does the mind manage to carry out such complicated processes as retrieving a source from memory, mapping the source to a target, adapting the source to provide the appropriate kinds of information about the target, and learning by generalizing the source and target into a schema? In the 1990s, Keith Holyoak and I built on earlier work by analogy theorists to develop the theory that all of the stages of analogy employ the same three fundamental constraints: structure, meaning, and purpose. We called this the "multiconstraint" theory of analogy.

Structure is the relational arrangement of an analog, for example, the difference between coffee shops spreading through a city and the city spreading through coffee shops. In verbal analogies, structure is carried syntactically by grammatical structure, but in perceptual analogies structure is carried by spatial and temporal arrangement in images. Meaning concerns the similarities between the different elements of the source and target analog with respect to verbal or sensory features. According to the meaning constraint, mapping and other processes involving source and target analogs are partly based on similarities with respect to verbal or sensory encoding. For verbal analogies, this constraint looks for words that are synonyms or are more loosely connected. For perceptual analogies, this constraint looks for items that look, sound, taste, smell, or feel alike. Finally, purpose is the pragmatic constraint that the operation of analogies is always shaped by the goals that the analogy is supposed to accomplish, which might be explanation, problem solving, decision making, persuasion, or entertainment. Structure, meaning, and purpose correspond respectively to syntax, semantics, and pragmatics, which previous chapters claimed to be integrated by semantic pointers. What would a neural theory of analogy look like?

NEURAL MECHANISMS FOR ANALOGY

A new understanding of analogy based on semantic pointers should have several ingredients. First, it expands how analogies are represented, allowing inclusion of a full range of sensations and images, plus emotions. Second, it suggests new procedures for mapping between source and target analogs based on the constraints of structure, meaning, and purpose. Third, the semantic pointer approach should propose new ways of thinking of retrieval and the other processes in analogical thinking, including adaptation, transfer, and learning.

Representation

Analogy is usually discussed as a matter of words. Many analogies are indeed verbal, but others operate in different modalities such as pictures. The classic analogy between the atom and the solar system can be expressed in words as shown in Table 6.1. But it is just as natural to use diagrams to show the comparison as operating between visual structures, as in Figure 6.1. Whenever I describe this analogy to other people, I find myself waving my arm to illustrate how the planets going around the sun corresponds to the electrons going around the nucleus of the atom. The analogy is not only visual but also dynamic, requiring kinesthetic representations to show the planets and electrons in motion. Another kinesthetic aspect of the analogy is the comparison of the forces that hold the planet to the sun and the electron to the nucleus: force is often explained to beginners as a push or a pull, which are muscle movements. Motor analogies also operate in sports instructions, when a coach teaches by displaying a motion such as a tennis serve and telling a player to do it the same way.

Both verbal and visual analogs can be captured by semantic pointers of the sort shown in Figure 6.2. This figure is highly simplified, as it does not show the bindings

TABLE 6.1

Verbal Representation of Analogy between the Solar System and the Atom

Solar system (source)	Atom (target)
Sun	Nucleus
Planet	Electron
Revolves around (planet, sun)	Revolves around (electron, nucleus)
Gravitational force between (planet, sun)	Electrical force between (nucleus, electron)
Cause (force, revolves)	Cause (force, revolves)

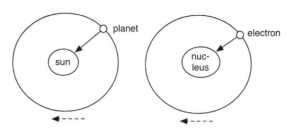

FIGURE 6.1 Visual representation of the analogy between the solar system and the atom. Dotted arrows indicate motion and solid arrows indicate the forces of attraction.

needed to mark the different relational roles of *cause, force,* and *revolves.* Moreover, the arrows from *planet* and *sun* indicate more complicated bindings than can easily be shown in a diagram, forming the semantic pointers that bind (a) *force, planet,* and *sun* and (b) *revolves, planet,* and *sun.* The significance of Figure 6.2 is that a complex semantic pointer for the solar system can result from verbal, visual, kinesthetic, or combined multimodal representations of the contributing concepts. The capability of semantic pointers for modal retention maintains in compressed form some of the characteristics of these different kinds of representations.

There are also auditory analogies that require nonverbal representations. John Lennon wrote the Beatles song "Because" as an adaptation of Beethoven's "Moonlight Sonata," after asking Yoko Ono to play it backwards. Composers often borrow aspects of the music of others, for example, when Dvořák incorporated

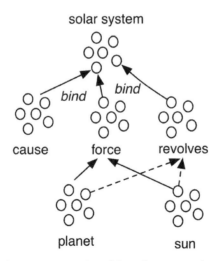

FIGURE 6.2 Semantic pointer representation of the solar system, simplified as indicated in the text. In the bottom row, the solid and dotted lines indicate two different bindings, one for *force* and the other for *revolves.*

folk melodies and when rap musicians sample parts of popular songs. In all these cases, one piece of music serves as a source analog for the target of producing a new piece of music. Modern dance is a form of art that is simultaneously musical, visual, and kinesthetic. Martha Graham developed one of her choreographies by analogy to a painting by Kandinsky. Cooking can involve analogies of taste and smell, when one imagines a new recipe by taking an old recipe and substituting different ingredients that will taste at least as good as the original recipe. Analogies based on hearing, taste, and smell all require the nonverbal images that chapter 3 explained as semantic pointers.

There are many kinds of emotional analogies. Some serve to generate emotions from verbal or visual descriptions, for example, in the saying that academics would rather use each other's toothbrushes than each other's terminology. This comparison generates pleasurable surprise, as well as some disgust. In other emotional analogies, emotions are explained in terms of verbal or visual descriptions and in the vast amount of poetry and music that explores the nature of love, as in Shakespeare:

> Love is a smoke made with the fume of sighs,
> Being purged, a fire sparkling in lovers' eyes,
> Being vexed, a sea nourished with lovers' tears.
> What is it else? A madness most discreet,
> A choking gall and a preserving sweet.

Accordingly, a full account of analogy needs to deal with emotions as well as images, not just words. Chapters 2 and 3 show how semantic pointers have full representational generality, in that a pattern of neural firing produced by binding can capture sensory as well as verbal information. Chapter 7 presents a semantic pointer theory of emotions, which shows that emotional analogies can be represented as well. *Natural Philosophy* (chapter 6) describes the ethical importance of empathy, a kind of emotional analogy. Analogy can be a comparison not just between two verbal descriptions of the source and target but also between two multimodal representations based on semantic pointers.

Mapping

Semantic pointers do not merely improve representation of analogies but also suggest new ways of accomplishing the key operations of mapping, retrieval, and adaptation. Current computational models of analogy are heavily driven by syntactic structure, although the multiconstraint theory that Keith Holyoak and

I developed allows some role for meaning and purpose also. Encoding analogs as neural processes based on semantic pointers allows mapping to be simultaneously a matter of syntax, semantics, and pragmatics. Contrary to our ACME (analogical constraint mapping engine) model of analogical mapping and other prominent models such as the structure mapping engine, analogy need not operate in a syntax-first fashion.

Semantic pointers incorporate syntax as the result of bindings sensitive to the structure of relations, and these bindings also maintain semantic information such as the sensory origins of the representations. So if *sun* is the neural representation based on visual images of a yellow sphere, and *earth* is based on a blue sea and brown land, then the relation of the Earth going around the sun incorporates those two kinds of visual representations plus a visual/kinesthetic representation of going around.

One of the advantages of incorporating semantics directly into analogical mapping should be a dramatic reduction in the search space for determining which aspects of the source compare with which aspects of the target. If the process of analogical mapping narrows its comparisons by considering meaning as well as syntactic structure, it should be able to get much more directly to a reasonable guess of what compares to what. Pragmatics can be useful in the same way, directing the brain to seek out comparisons that satisfy the purpose of the analogy such as problem solving, persuasion, and amusement.

Using neural representations rather than merely verbal ones should enable thinkers to be both more efficient and productive. Syntactic matches tend to be all or none, but patterns of neural firing are much more fluid and should be able to generate the kind of flexible slippage that Douglas Hofstadter has highlighted for creativity. The atom is only partially similar to the solar system, and more advanced students have to learn about ways in which electrons differ from planets. Neural networks that use semantic pointers to encode analogies lend themselves to approximate matching and therefore to creative flexibility. Although neural processes operate in parallel, analogical mapping should not proceed all at once but sometimes incrementally. In the atom example, you might first figure out that *planet* maps to *electron* but only subsequently realize that *gravitational force* maps to *electrical force*.

Obtaining

Similar flexibility should assist in the retrieval of analogs from memory. Some artificial intelligent systems for case-based reasoning try to perform retrieval efficiently by heavily indexing the cases with respect to their purpose. For example, if one has the problem of trying to figure out how to repair a television, a system may efficiently pull out a previous repair relevant to the current one from a database of cases indexed by the malfunction to be fixed. However, psychological experiments show that people rely less on pragmatic constraints than on more superficial semantic elements that sometimes are not good at pulling out from memory the most relevant kind of analog. Retrieval of analogs from memory should operate using the same neural mechanism of pattern completion already discussed for images, concepts, and rules.

Obtaining a source analog by serendipity or by having it given to you does not require as complicated a neural process as retrieving it from memory. But there still is a need to explain how a student recognizes an analog's relevance to the target problem. For example, a student needs to grasp that the solar system is useful for understanding atoms, which can be accomplished by doing a partial mapping as previously described. Constructing a useful source analog, as Crick and Watson did for DNA and Maxwell did for electromagnetism, is a much more complex process, requiring all the mechanisms for building new images, concepts, and rules described in previous chapters.

Adapting

The remaining question is how semantic pointers can contribute to adaptation and transfer. Once you have obtained a source analog and mapped it to a target, then the source can be adapted to produce a solution to the target through analogical inference. For example, if you want to know why the electron goes around the proton and if you know that the orbits of planets around the sun are the result of the force of gravity, then one might naturally infer abductively that there is an analogous force that keeps electrons going around protons. The result is explanatory transfer from the solar source analog to the atom target analog. This inference requires a process of unbinding and binding: taking apart the semantic pointer for gravitational force between sun and planet, doing the mappings of sun to nucleus and planet to electron, and then binding the newly generated concept of electromagnetic force to the mapped concepts of nucleus and electron.

Through such developments, the cognitive investigation of analogy can resist the syntactic dream that has tended to restrict the consideration of structure to linguistic expressions. Structure pervades sensory experiences such as vision, hearing, and touch as much as it does language. In neural mechanisms, structure is entwined with meaning, by virtue of the way that semantic pointers combine structural relations with binding of sensory and motor representations. Purpose is also incorporated through the representation of goals and the emotional connections described in chapter 7. Hence analogy provides another illustration of how the Semantic Pointer Architecture serves to integrate syntax, semantics, and pragmatics.

USES OF ANALOGIES

Innateness

The value of the Semantic Pointer Architecture account of analogy depends on how well it increases understanding of fundamental aspects of thinking, including innateness, learning, problem solving, memory, and language. Previous chapters considered innate concepts, rules, and images, but I am not aware of any evidence that there are source analogs that everybody is born with, enabling them to solve complex problems without any required learning. Carl Jung claimed that there are universal archetypes, which are events such as birth, figures such as the hero, and motifs such as the creation that are part of the collective unconscious and shape people's thinking. Such archetypes are more complicated than concepts and might be thought of as potential source analogs for understanding people's experiences. These archetypes, however, are more likely to have been learned through people's cultural experience than to have become established genetically by evolution. Analogy thus seems irrelevant to the question of innateness.

Learning

On the other hand, analogy is important for understanding two kinds of learning. The first kind is when an analogical inference adapts some piece of information about the source to generate a new conclusion about the target, for example, that there is a force making the electron go around the nucleus. The conclusion can not only be in the form a new piece of verbal information, but it can also be represented perceptually, such as a guess at what a new cooking recipe is likely to taste like. For example, when considering a recipe for a curry with lentils and rhubarb, I may infer that the result will be analogous to other curries that I have cooked but with a twist added by the unusual rhubarb ingredient.

The second kind of analogical learning generalizes from a source and target to produce an abstract schema that captures what is important to both of them. For example, someone might produce a schema for a system of attracting and revolving that generalizes from the solar and atom analogs. This schema might have other uses, for example, describing how fans cluster around movie stars. It is a question for future research how semantic pointers that represent a source and a target can be generalized into something more abstract.

Problem Solving

For problem solving, the biggest advantage of semantic pointers over previous theories of analogy is the move beyond verbal analogies to include all forms of perception and emotion. Thanks to multimodal representations, a semantic pointer approach can consider mapping and retrieval for a much wider range of analogies than previously considered, covering hearing, taste, and emotion, as well as vision. Mapping of a source to a target can be facilitated by the smooth integration of structure, meaning, and purpose. Whether a source analog is obtained by teaching, retrieval, serendipity, or construction, a mapping that is both multimodal and multiconstraint can efficiently put the elements of the analogs in correspondence to suggest useful inferences about the target problem. Justification of the claim that human analogical problem solving employs neural representations like semantic pointers requires more computer modeling than has so far been done. It especially needs to be shown that neural transformations can generate in all sensory modalities the appropriate inferences and abstracted schemas.

Memory

Analogy is important for understanding memory because it requires retrieval not only of individual perceptions, images, concepts, or rules but also of whole situations that require many representations. When I travel on a subway, I am inevitably reminded of the time when my pocket was picked in the Paris Metro. This retrieval is not of isolated concepts but of the whole package of information about me traveling in 2004 with my sons and a lot of luggage and suddenly noticing that my wallet was gone. This episode forms a package that gets retrieved largely as a whole. Hence, understanding memory requires appreciating not just particular facts but how more complicated representations of whole relational act episodes can be recovered. Understanding analogical retrieval is therefore an important part of understanding memory in general.

We have already seen a number of ways in which the semantic pointer representation of analogs is useful for understanding retrieval. Not only do semantic pointers capture the appropriate structural information, they also bring with them the relevant similarities carried by the words or sensory representations that describe the relations. So the development of a semantic pointer theory of analog retrieval should be a contribution to the theory of memory in general, covering large episodes and not just particular events.

Language

If language were mostly syntax, then analogy would not be very important. But language is also wrapped up with meaning and purpose—semantics and pragmatics. The most obvious use of analogy in language is in figures of speech. Some similes and metaphors are superficial comparisons, for example, saying that love is like a rose or that your job is a jail. But interesting similes and metaphors have rich underlying analogical structure, a whole system of matching relations, that are put into correspondence to each other by the comparison. Consider for example Shakespeare's metaphor:

> All the world's a stage,
> And all the men and women merely players;
> They have their exits and their entrances,
> And one man in his time plays many parts.

Shakespeare spells out the parts as the seven ages of a man, from puling infant to decrepit oldster. This metaphor is based on a systematic analogy between plays with numerous characters and lives multiple phases.

Traditional approaches to metaphor treated it as a defective way of not saying what is literally true. But George Lakoff and others have argued that metaphor is not merely a literary flourish but rather a fundamental way of adding meaning to utterances. Chapter 10 says much more about the contribution of metaphor to linguistic meaning, but here I emphasize the underlying analogical structure of rich metaphors. Shakespeare's stage metaphor requires the analogical mapping shown in Table 6.2. The approach to language called cognitive linguistics treats metaphorical uses of concepts as central to language, even to syntax, as chapter 10 discusses. Another literary application of analogy is allegory, which uses a systematic comparison to accomplish a practical goal such as moral illumination. For

TABLE 6.2

| Analogy between Theatre and Life | |
Theater (source)	Life (target)
Stage	World
Player	Person
Parts	Stages of life
Perform (player, parts)	Go-through (person, stages)

example, George Orwell's *Animal Farm* brilliantly depicts the failures of Stalin's Soviet Union by mapping it to a barnyard.

How Analogies Change

Changes in the behaviors of individuals and groups result from changes in the mental representations of the individuals and their prevalence in the groups. As with the previous kinds of representation discussed—images, concepts, and rules—changes in analogy operate in three ways: formation, alteration, and replacement. The formation of a new analogy can dramatically affect how people think, for example, when Darwin realized that nature can perform a kind of selection analogous to what breeders do. Formation is explained by the mechanisms for obtaining and adapting source analogs already discussed. Adapting does not have to be a one-shot process because further intellectual developments can make an analogy much deeper and more effective. Darwin's analogy was much improved when his vague ideas about how organisms inherit traits from their parents were supplanted by the theory of genetic inheritance developed decades later. Alteration of an analogy requires adding information to the source analog in a way that encourages additional or different mappings to the target.

The most radical change in analogies occurs when a new source analog replaces an old one that dominated thinking. For example, a person in psychotherapy may manage to shift from the self-images of a deer caught in the headlights or a ticking time bomb to the more positive metaphors of a car under repair or a phoenix rising from the ashes. Groups of individuals may change dramatically when different analogies become commonly used by the individuals in them. For example, American military efforts in the Middle East look desperate when they are compared to the Vietnam debacle but heroic when they are compared to the efforts to stop Hitler in World War II. These therapeutic and historical changes in analogies are highly emotional, producing shifts between positive and negative reactions to situations. Because semantic pointers readily accommodate emotions, they are well placed to explain the operations of these passionate analogies.

SUMMARY AND DISCUSSION

Analogies contribute to many kinds of human thinking, including problem solving, decision making, explanation, persuasion, and entertainment. An

analogy is a systematic comparison between a source analog and a target analog, where information about the source is used to generate inferences about
the target. The major stages of analogical thinking are obtaining source analog
by memory retrieval or other means, mapping the source to the target, adapting
the source to inform the target, and learning by generalizing source and target
into a schema.

Most theories of analogy have used verbal representations, but a much broader
appreciation of analogical thinking can be gained with semantic pointers. Analogies
often use words, but they can also operate with visual, auditory, and other sensory
modalities, all of which can contribute to all stages of analogy. Emotion can also
be an important component of analogical thinking, for example, in empathy and
humor. The theory of emotions as semantic pointers in chapter 7 completes the
account of how analogies can be multimodal as the result of neural processes.

The semantic pointer theory enhances understanding of analogy in several
ways. First, it explains how neurons can represent complex relations, including the
relations among relations required for analogies. Second, it avoids the syntax-first
bias by showing how to integrate meaning (semantics) and purpose (pragmatics)
with syntactic structure. Third, it handles multimodal analogies because of representation of sensory, motor, and emotional information.

Analogies from the semantic pointer perspective support both embodiment and
transbodiment. Analogies are embodied when they incorporate sensory–motor
and emotional representations. But embodiment is less relevant when analogies
use abstract concepts distant from bodily operations, as in the unfair analogical
insult that philosophy is to science as ornithology is to birds. Analogies contribute
valuably to transbodiment when they help to generate theoretical concepts such as
natural selection and *light wave* that far surpass sense experience.

The paradox of analogical thinking is that sometimes its use is astonishingly
creative and productive, but at other times it can be misleading destructive or
drudgingly conservative. Two of the most successful technology companies were
built on productive analogies. Google's search algorithm was inspired by academic
citation practices: Just as academics appraise published papers by how often they
are cited by other papers, Google rates Web pages by how often they are linked
to by other pages. Many of the best ideas in Apple's first graphical interface for
Macintosh computers were adapted from ideas invented but not developed by
Xerox, which preferred to stick with its established copier business. Productive
analogies have emergent properties, generating unexpected solutions that could
not be gained by aggregating existing ideas. Once Steve Jobs began thinking of a
computer screen as a desktop rather than as a command line, Apple could begin

to develop drawing programs and word processing that deals with a whole page at once.

On the other hand, generals typically prepare for the last war, rather than developing strategies more suitable for new kinds of conflict. Analogizing to familiar cases can similarly be a conservative force in industry, medicine, and academia, making analogical thinking destructive rather than productive. In online discussions, a sure sign of intellectual degeneration is when one side starts to accuse the others of being like Nazis. Analogies always need to be assessed for their productivity or destructiveness. Intellectual and practical progress can result from analogical change that replaces outmoded analogies (a car is a horseless carriage) with exciting ones (a car is a computer on wheels).

The same disparity can be found in all other kinds of representation, including images, concepts, rules, and emotions, which often contribute to mental goals but can also get in their way. The history of science is full of concepts that seemed promising but have needed to be abandoned, such as *ether, phlogiston, vital force,* and *psychoanalysis.* Some emotions are productive when they encourage goal-accomplishing actions, but others are destructive when they lead to paralysis or bad results.

Philosophers tend to think of analogy as a form of argument, but analogies on their own provide little evidence for their conclusions. The main use of analogies should be to suggest and support conclusions, not to stand alone. Here is some advice for using analogies. First, do not use them in isolation, but rather integrate analogical considerations with other forms of reasoning such as inference to the best explanation. Second, consider multiple analogies, comparing the current situation to many previous cases, some of which may reveal problems with a single analogy. Third, make sure there is a coherent mapping between the source problem you have chosen and the target problem, not a selective mapping that picks aspects of the source to distort how the target is viewed. Fourth, avoid emotional distortions of analogies of the sort discussed in chapter 7 in connection with motivated inference and fear-driven inference.

While appreciating the contributions that analogies make to human thinking, it is important not to exaggerate their centrality. Douglas Hofstadter and Emmanuel Sander consider analogy to be the "fuel and fire of thinking" and claim that analogy is the "core of cognition." They set up a false dichotomy about whether analogy or categorization is the core of cognition, claiming that all categorization involves analogical comparison so that analogy is fundamental. But the discussion of concepts in chapter 4 shows that analogy is not the same as categorization, a much simpler kind of inference in which an object is classified by applying a concept. It is a mistake to try to reduce all of cognition to just one elementary sort of procedure when the multifarious mind is capable of operating with perceptions, images, concepts, rules, analogies, and emotions. What these forms of mental representation have in common is an underlying set of neural mechanisms using patterns of neural firing, binding, and transformations.

Putting analogies into the cognitive mix helps explain human thinking, but the story is still far from complete. Chapter 7 adds emotions and shows how they contribute to important kinds of analogical inference such as empathy. Chapter 10 describes further the analogical contribution of metaphor to language, and chapter 11 expands on the common but nonexclusive contribution of analogy to creativity. *Mind–Society* and *Natural Philosophy* display the importance of analogy for domains as diverse as politics, history, law, and philosophy.

NOTES

On the Einstein quote about life, see https://quoteinvestigator.com/2015/06/28/bicycle/.

General works on analogy include Gentner, Holyoak, and Kokinov 2001; Holyoak 2012; Holyoak and Thagard 1995.

For many examples of creative analogies, see chapter 11, as well as Hofstadter and Sander 2013, Jiang and Thagard 2014, and Thagard 2012d, 2014a. *Mind–Society* (chapter 13) discusses the role of analogies in engineering design.

On metaphor, see Lakoff and Johnson 1980 and references in chapter 10.

Bartha 2010 discusses philosophical uses of analogy. Thagard 2014d and *Natural Philosophy* (chapter 1) critique the use of analogical thought experiments in philosophy.

Thagard and Shelley 2001 (reprinted in Thagard, 2006) discuss emotional analogies. Shelley 2003 analyzes the use of multiple analogies. The psychodynamic concept of transference concerns emotional analogies, for example, when a patient transfers feelings from a parent to a therapist.

For the structure mapping engine, see Gentner 1983; Falkenhainer, Forbus, and Gentner 1989; and Forbus, Ferguson, Lovett, and Gentner, 2017.

Rasmussen and Eliasmith 2014 present a neural network model of solving Raven's matrices, a kind of analogical problem solving.

Models of visual analogy include Croft and Thagard 2002; McGreggor, Kunda, and Goel 2014; and Lovett, Tomai, Forbus, and Usher 2009.

On case-based reasoning in artificial intelligence systems, see Kolodner 1993. The major use of analogy in artificial intelligence today is recommender systems that advise people of things similar to what they already like.

Eliasmith and Thagard 2001 describe a convolution-based integration of structure and meaning in analogical mapping. For mapping using neural synchrony, see Hummel and Holyoak 1997, 2003. On neural correlates of creative analogy, see Green et al. 2012, Green 2016.

Thagard 2011 explains allegory as emotional analogy.

PROJECT

Construct Semantic Pointer Architecture models of analogical mapping, retrieval, transfer, and learning. Show that neural transformations can generate the appropriate inferences and abstracted schemas in all sensory modalities.

7

Emotions

Ralph Waldo Emerson said that nothing great was ever achieved without enthusiasm. If he was right, then thinking requires more than the kinds of mental representation so far discussed. Great thinking, from science to politics to art, also needs to include emotions such as enthusiasm, excitement, hope, impatience, and fear of boredom.

Traditionally, emotions are viewed as impediments to greatness, as detrimental to rationality. In the early days of cognitive science, the focus on representation and computation led to neglect of emotions, under the assumption that they are peripheral to the most important kinds of thinking. More recently, however, there has been a growing appreciation among psychologists, neuroscientists, and philosophers that emotion is a central part of human thinking. Evidence has accumulated that emotions are pivotal for core cognitive functions such as decision making, problem solving, creativity, and language. The usual division of the brain into newer, high-level cognitive areas and ancient emotional limbic ones is seriously defective. Most cognition is infused with emotion at the same time that emotion, at least in humans, has a substantial cognitive component. Hence, neglecting emotions in the investigation of mind would be as serious as neglecting images, concepts, rules, or analogies.

The importance of emotions is even clearer in society. People not only interact verbally with sentences and visually with gestures, but they also interact emotionally. Emotional communication is crucial for social relationships, ranging from romantic involvements to mass activities such as religious rituals, sporting events, political rallies, and riots. Broad social phenomena like economic crashes, political ideologies, and religious movements are all intensely emotional.

This chapter first explains emotions as mental processes involving a combination of cognitive, physiological, and social aspects. Then, it shows how viewing emotions as semantic pointers synthesizes previous theories of emotions that turn out to be compatible rather than competing. The neural theory that emotions are semantic pointers unifies a wide range of phenomena about emotions and sets the stage for elucidating their social significance.

PSYCHOLOGICAL THEORIES OF EMOTION

Suppose you are crossing the street when a large truck turns the corner and you are barely able to jump out of the way. This experience naturally generates many emotions: initially fear that you might be killed by the truck, then relief that you survived, then anger that the driver was so careless, and perhaps finally happiness that you managed to get through the day without being squashed like a cockroach. What are these emotions of fear, relief, anger, and happiness?

Historically, there have been three major theories about the nature of emotions. The oldest is the theory of cognitive appraisal, which says that emotions are judgments that evaluate your current situation with respect to your goals. This theory goes back to the ancient Greek Stoics and is still maintained by philosophers such as Martha Nussbaum and psychologists such as Klaus Scherer. On this view, your fear results from an evaluation that the truck seriously threatens your fundamental goals of being healthy and alive. Your happiness results from the appraisal that escaping the truck supports these goals. Your anger comes from the evaluation that the truck driver was responsible for threatening your goals.

An alternative theory of emotions, proposed by William James more than a century ago, says that emotions are physiological perceptions tracking changes in bodily states. When the truck nearly runs you over, your body undergoes major changes such as increases in heart and breathing rate, sweating, elevation of the stress hormone cortisone, and possibly digestive changes too embarrassing to mention. The common-sense view is that first you have an emotion and then you have bodily changes, but the physiological perception account says that this is backwards: You have the emotions because you have the physiological changes. This theory is today advocated by neuroscientists such as Antonio Damasio and philosophers such as Jesse Prinz.

A third approach to emotions emphasizes their social dimensions, the ways in which our expectations about behavior are shaped by our cultural environments. How we react to situations such as nearly being run over by a truck may be influenced by our social expectations, for example, the belief that drivers ought to operate their vehicles carefully. Then, anger would be socially sanctioned in a way that might not occur given other beliefs, for example, that everything that happens does so because of God's will or physical determinism. The view that emotions are primarily social constructions derived from our cultural experiences has been advocated by philosophers such as Rom Harré and sociologists such as Émile Durkheim.

The cognitive, physiological, and social accounts are not competing theories because they each point to a different dimension of emotions that needs to be encompassed within a unified theory. Compare perception, which sometimes has been interpreted as a bottom–up process of transforming sensory stimuli into perceptual experience and at other times interpreted as a top–down process where expectations lead to acceptance of hypotheses about what is being perceived. As chapter 3 indicated, the current consensus is that perception is both bottom–up and top–down, requiring an interaction of sensory and interpretive processes. This integrated interaction is quickly and naturally performed by the brain by virtue of its capacity for parallel processing. Similarly, emotion can be understood as an integrative process of combining physiological perceptions with cognitive appraisals and social interpretations. This integration is performed by neural mechanisms using semantic pointers, patterns of firing that bind representations of both physiology and appraisal.

Emotion is obviously too complicated to succumb to a definition, but a three-analysis is useful to integrate the many facets built into the semantic pointer theory. Table 7.1 shows that there are standard examples of emotions and a wide range of typical features across physiology, cognition, social relations, neural patterns, and conscious experiences. Emotions already make major contributions to explaining people experiences and behaviors, including self-reports. But cognitive science is still at the early stages of identifying all the multilevel mechanisms that produce emotions.

Moods, such as feeling generally good or bad for hours, differ from emotions in several ways. Moods last longer, usually do not have specific causes, and are more general experiences not associated with a specific situation that they are about. In contrast, emotions such as happiness are usually prompted by an occurrence or memory that they represent and may last only a few seconds.

A theory of emotions has to satisfy demanding requirements. First, it should apply to the relatively simple emotions that occur in all humans and many animals,

TABLE 7.1

Three-Analysis of *Emotion*

Exemplars	Happiness, sadness, fear, anger, disgust, surprise, shame, embarrassment, pride
Typical features	Physiological changes, cognitive appraisals, social influences including linguistic ones in humans, neural patterns in multiple brain areas, enjoyable or painful experiences
Explanations	Explains: experiences, behaviors, reports
	Explained by: molecular, neural, psychological, and social mechanisms

such as happiness, sadness, fear, anger, and surprise. Second, it should apply to the full range of social emotions in humans that require an understanding of interpersonal relations, such as shame, guilt, pride, embarrassment, gratitude, and resentment, all the way up to nested emotions such as fear of humiliation and desire for love.

Third, a theory of emotions should be able to explain how emotions interact with other forms of mental representation, from sensations to analogies. Emotions naturally attach to concepts and beliefs, generating values and attitudes. For example, valuing democracy requires a positive emotional reaction to it, and having the attitude that racism is horrible requires a strong negative emotion. Perceptions can generate emotions, for example, when the sight and sound of a truck bearing down on you generates fear. Similarly, images retrieved or constructed from memory may carry the same emotional character, for example, when you later remember the truck that almost ran you over or construct the even more horrific image that it actually hit you.

Concepts usually carry with them emotional values, for example, the positive emotions that most people attach to the concept of food and the negative emotions that most people attach to the concept of vomit. Emotional values can also be attached to more abstract concepts like justice and loyalty. A powerful kind of emotional change occurs when social goals produce shifts in the emotional values attached to concepts, for example, when *queer* shifted from being derogatory for homosexuals to being a sign of pride. Rules are also often emotional in ways that were neglected in chapter 5, for example, when rules about how to behave carry with them the threat of fear from a previous failure that produced anxiety or embarrassment. Rules can also have positive emotional associations, as in the democratic principle that governments should be elected.

Chapter 6 described how emotions can be generated by analogies, for example, in persuasion and jokes. Analogies often use cases that have already been emotionally interpreted, for example, when you base a decision on a previously successful case that generated happiness or on a previous failed case that generated disappointment. The empathic use of analogies to understand the feelings of other people is usually targeted at getting a grasp of their emotions. Empathy is emotional imagery sometimes carried out by analogy, but there is also a more direct, automatic mode of empathy resulting from perceptual processes, for example, when you flinch when seeing a football player get tackled. A third mode of empathy results from unconsciously simulating someone's mental state using multimodal rules.

Fourth, a theory of emotion needs to explain why various emotions feel differently. Fifth, a comprehensive theory of emotions should indicate the strong link between emotions and actions and explain why different emotions lead to different kinds of behavior. For example, the natural reaction to fear is running away, whereas anger may prompt an attack.

NEURAL MECHANISMS FOR EMOTIONS
Emotions in the Brain

Providing a neural account of emotions would be much easier if there were a one-to-one relationship between particular emotions and particular parts of the brain. It might have turned out, for example, that fear is firing of neurons in the amygdala and that happiness is firing of neurons in the nucleus accumbens. It has long been known that amygdala activity is associated with fear and that the nucleus accumbens is associated with pleasure. However, decades of brain imaging using functional magnetic resonance imaging has made it clear that every emotion is associated with multiple brain areas, and every emotion-related brain area is associated with multiple emotions. As with other mental operations, the correspondence of function with brain areas is many-to-many rather than one-to-one.

Luiz Pessoa has amassed evidence that challenges common views of the relation between cognition and emotion. He rejects the belief that cognition and emotion are separate processes occurring in different parts of the brain. The amygdala has long been known to be important for emotions such as fear, but it has connections with dozens of brain areas including ones often thought of as cognitive in the prefrontal cortex. Emotion influences perception as a result of projections from the amygdala to visual cortex. Emotion can also influence perception because of other regions involved in the assessment of value such as the orbitofrontal cortex.

Like other cognitive processes, perception operates with limited capacity, and motivation serves to increase the salience of some elements, which makes it more likely that they will win the competition over other representations. Chapter 3 mentioned wishful seeing, in which people perceive their environments in ways that conform to their desires. Hence, it would be a mistake to think of the brain as having strictly separate cognition areas and emotion areas.

Brain imaging alone does not even begin to suggest an adequate theory of emotion. Instead, we can develop a theory of emotions as patterns of neural firing derived from bindings that integrate mental representations such as concepts and images with a combination of cognitive appraisals, physiological perceptions, and social interpretations conveyed by language. Once these mechanisms are specified, it becomes possible to see how emotions play important roles in problem-solving, learning, language, and social interactions.

Emotions as Semantic Pointers

Explaining emotions within Eliasmith's Semantic Pointer Architecture requires demonstrating how they result from the familiar neural mechanisms: representation by patterns of neural firing, binding, transformation, and competition. Figure 7.1 shows how to construe an emotion as a semantic pointer resulting from binding several kinds of representation. The circles indicate large neural groups, and the arrows represent transformations of neural activity in those populations through interactions with other groups that perform binding.

Unlike moods, which can be diffuse and not tied to any identifiable representation, emotions are attached to specific cognitive representations of a situation using images, concepts, and rules. What connects these representational patterns of firing with emotions?

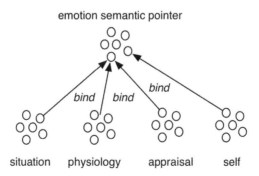

FIGURE 7.1 A semantic pointer for an emotion binds the representations of a situation, physiological reaction, cognitive appraisal, and self.

Representations of situations using images and concepts need to be bound with neural representations of physiological states. States of the body are encoded by neural groups found in parts of the brain such as the insula and the amygdala, both of which receive signals from various body parts. But having these signals and the patterns of firing that result from them is not sufficient for emotions, because the physiological states need to be tied to the representations that indicate what the emotion is about. Fear of a dangerous truck connects the visual or verbal representation of the truck and the bodily reaction to it. The pattern of firing of the neural population that represents the truck needs to be bound with the pattern of firing that sums up the bodily changes that are taking place in heart rate, breathing, and so on.

Physiology alone is not enough to distinguish among different emotions—the bodily changes that take place with different emotions such as fear and anger are not sharply different. Further refinement of emotions requires a process of cognitive appraisal that evaluates the relevance of a situation to a person's goals. For example, anger is differentiated from fear not by any specific physiological signature but by an appraisal that identifies some person or thing as responsible for a threat to goals and therefore deserving of anger. Appraisal is even more clearly important for complex social emotions such as shame, guilt, and pride, where there needs to be an evaluation of the situation with respect to people's social connections and goals. Basic binding of representations of situations, physiology, and appraisal is enough to explain simple emotions such as happiness and sadness, but complex emotions such as pride and gloating require incorporation of the self and its social relations.

In sum, the semantic pointer theory of emotions consists of the following hypotheses.

1. Emotions are semantic pointers, which are patterns of firing in spiking neurons that integrate information of different sorts by neural bindings.
2. The information bound into semantic pointers for emotions includes external stimuli, physiological changes, stored concepts, and linguistic knowledge.
3. Emotional reactions occur when stimuli generate semantic pointers that combine physiological perception, cognitive appraisal, and social context.
4. Emotions become conscious when semantic pointers cross a threshold by outcompeting other semantic pointers.

Chapter 8 explains consciousness as resulting from semantic pointer mechanisms.

Self and Language

Complex emotions can occur in humans thanks to our capacities for self-representation and language. The standard way for testing whether an animal has a sense of self is to put a mark on it and see whether the animal recognizes itself in the mirror as being marked. Humans can so recognize themselves by two years of age, but so far only members of a few other species have passed the mirror test: chimpanzees, bonobos, orangutans, gorillas, dolphins, killer whales, elephants, pigs, and magpies. In humans, and a few other species of animals, emotions involve an additional kind of binding to a representation of oneself. For a rat, there is fear associated with a stimulus, but for a human there is fear that belongs to the self.

Language is not essential to emotions, which also occur in nonhumans, but linguistic representations can enhance differentiation of emotions by facilitating appraisal. Cognitive appraisal theories of emotion often seem to require too much cognitive work. If a truck is bearing down on you, your emotional reaction of fear should not depend on a complex calculation of the relevance of the truck to all of your goals, ranging from survival and health to interpersonal relationships. A big part of the psychological advantage of emotions is that they contribute to fast reactions to events that need to be dealt with in real time. Physiological changes are rapid and are one of the ways in which fast responses can be produced. But there is another way in which cognitive appraisal can be fast and frugal rather than slow and deliberate.

Fast appraisal results from how our verbal mental representations come prepackaged with emotional association thanks to our linguistic experiences. As the discussion of values and attitudes described, many of our concepts are associated with emotional reactions. For example, if you hear about a truck that caught on fire, some of your appraisal can be shaped by your previous associations of the concepts *truck* and *fire*. Knowing from your previous personal and linguistic experience that fire is dangerous, part of your semantics of fire is therefore an association with fear. Figure 7.2 expands on Figure 7.1 to show more of the bindings of the representations relevant to emotion: sensory information, physiological changes, appraisal with respect to goals, and value-carrying semantic information connected with the linguistic concepts involved in the representation of the situation. For example, even children who have never seen a house on fire are likely to have picked up from other speakers that fire is emotionally negative.

Hence, the semantic pointer theory of emotions incorporates social information in two ways: via linguistic encodings and via cognitive appraisal with respect to goals that can include social motivations such as belonging to groups and being respected by others. Because the formation of emotional semantic pointers includes

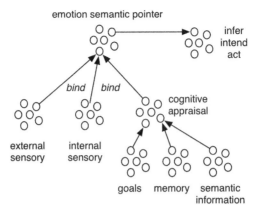

FIGURE 7.2 Expanded semantic pointer for emotion, with external sensory representations for the situation, internal sensory representations for physiology, and an expanded depiction of cognitive appraisal. The self is omitted, but a connection with action is shown.

bindings of encodings of physiological states, semantic pointers smoothly integrate all three dimensions of emotion—physiology, appraisal, and social—that often have been treated as competing theories. Emotions such as feeling happy, sad, angry, and afraid are emergent results of the interactions of neural groups capturing all these dimensions.

The semantic pointer theory of emotions makes it easy to understand the neural basis for values, attitudes, and desires that result from recursive bindings. Because emotions are semantic pointers, they can be bound with other representations (images, concepts, beliefs, rules) to produce new semantic pointers with the general structure: bind (representation emotion). For example, my desire to finish a draft of the book by Christmas results from (a) the binding of the concept *finish* with *book, Christmas,* and *future* and (b) the binding of *physiology* with *appraisal* to produce a positive emotion akin to happiness. Desire is not an attitude that an abstract person has toward an abstract proposition but rather a brain state corresponding to the following binding:

bind (object-of-desire wanting)

Here, *object-of-desire* indicates the neural representation of an object such as a piece of cake or of a more complicated state of affairs corresponding to a sentence like "I eat the cake." According to Kent Berridge, wanting is a pattern of firing in brain areas such as the ventral pallidum and nucleus accumbens that is physiologically different from liking.

Empathy

Empathy is the ability to share and understand the emotions of others. It is important for personal relationships and politics (*Mind–Society*) and for ethics and literature (*Natural Philosophy*). If I have been hospitalized because of a car accident, you can try to grasp my emotional state by remembering similar experiences you have had of accidents or hospitalization. This effort requires a combination of three mental processes that together enable you to put yourself in my shoes: analogy, emotion, and imagery. Empathy is a kind of analogy because you need to understand my situation as analogous to your own experiences, which provide a source for appreciating me, the target of explanation. This understanding is not a matter of abstract causal explanation, however, because the empathizer aims to have feelings similar to the target. Hence, empathy requires the generation of mental images, for example, when you imagine what it might be like to have been in my car accident. These images are emotional, for example, when you imagine how I might be sad and afraid as the result of the accident. Empathy is analogical emotional imagery.

Chapter 3 explains perceptual images as retrieval and transformation of semantic pointers, and the same operations apply to emotional images. After you experience an emotion as a binding of a situation, physiological state, and cognitive appraisal, you can store this experience in memory as neural connections. When you hear of a similar event, you can retrieve the memory and re-experience the emotion by reactivating approximately the pattern of neural firing you had before, producing an emotional image.

Emotional images are subject to the same kinds of transformations as perceptual ones: intensification, focusing, combination, juxtaposition, and decomposition. You may infer that my situation is even worse than what you have experienced and intensify your imagined emotion accordingly. Depending on how I describe my situation, you may focus on a particular aspect of it, such as distressing pain. Creative empathy may require combination of emotions resulting from juxtaposition of situations, for example, if your past experience includes a car accident and a hospitalization at separate times. Then, you can juxtapose the two events and mentally combine the emotions that resulted to better imagine my experience. Finally, you may need to decompose the emotional experience to separate some irrelevant aspect such as a religious dimension that you had but I did not.

Like all analogical mapping, empathy requires a process of unbinding and rebinding when you take an experience of your own and transfer it to another person whose experiences have been similar. This process requires that your emotional experience includes a representation of your self, bound in with the external, internal, and appraisal representations shown in Figure 7.1. To empathize with me, you modify your retrieved emotional image by replacing the binding with your self by the binding with your representation of me. Putting yourself in somebody else's shoes is then a matter of emotional imagery and analogical transformation by substitution of bindings. Empathy is not just the simple aggregate of the firing of neurons that perform representation, binding, and mapping but rather an emergent result of interactions of diverse neural groups. Thus, semantic pointer accounts of imagery, analogy, and emotion combine to produce a general theory of empathy.

This theory applies not only to the relatively slow, conscious, and deliberate kind of empathy that takes place when you actively try to understand me but also to the fast, unconscious, automatic empathy that can result more directly from perception and mirror neurons. If I actually see you hit by a car and writhing in pain, then without elaborate analogical mapping I may have neurons in my brain firing for pain, emotion, and body movements that are roughly the same as the ones that would fire if I were the one hit by a car. The result is still analogical emotional imagery using semantic pointers, but the processes are less subject to complicated transformations like juxtaposition of situations and combination of emotions.

A third mode of empathy consists of figuring out what others are feeling by using your nonverbal unconscious rules to simulate them. This process is more dynamic than simply recognizing their situations by neural mirroring or analogical inference because you can use a chain of embodied rules to make inferences about their ongoing experiences. For example, if you have the embodied multimodal rules <rejected> → <withdraw> and <withdraw> → <relief>, then you can unconsciously chain them together to feel something like rejection, withdrawal, and relief yourself, analogous to what the other person may be experiencing. This process is the embodied simulation mode of empathy.

The analogy, mirroring, and simulation modes of empathy can be complementary: A good friend or skilled psychotherapist can use all of them to develop a rich understanding of another person. You can feel someone else's pain by reasoning about it analogically, perceiving it via mirror neurons, or by using your unconscious embodied rules to simulate it. These deliberate, automatic, and dynamic modes of empathy can all help you to understand other people by putting yourself in their shoes, in ways illuminated by viewing emotions as semantic pointers. Modal retention of the sensory aspects of pain and emotions enable people to be empathic, not just verbally but with feelings that approximate those of others.

In sum, emotions are semantic pointers, a special kind of pattern of neural firing that results from binding representations of sensory, verbal, internal bodily, and evaluative information. But, as with semantic pointers in general, what matters is not just how they get put together but also what they can be used to do. When the whole package of information gets bound into a pointer, it constitutes an emotion that can be used for many purposes, including inference, action, and explanation.

Chapter 8 addresses the crucial question of how emotions and other mental states can become conscious. Attention is a mechanism by which the brain's resources are focused on what is important to the organism. Assessing importance would be an enormous cognitive task if it required a lot of inference, but emotions do a quick and often effective assessment of importance by combining information about the situation, changes in physiological states, goals, and linguistic usage. Emotions help to guide attention by increasing firing rates in neural populations for some semantic pointers, thereby enabling them to outcompete other representations less important to the goals of the organism. For example, if you have an emotional attachment to dogs, you will be more likely to pay attention to pictures and stories about them. This emotional effect on attention boosts some semantic pointers toward consciousness, as described in chapter 8.

Not only do emotions help to focus on what is important to think about, they also provide strong guidance about what to do. Positive emotions such as happiness and pride lead to actions that approach something desired, whereas negative emotions such as fear, anger, and sadness tell us about situations to avoid. Chapter 9 provides more details about how emotions can lead to action.

USES OF EMOTIONS

As with other kinds of mental representation, a neural theory of emotions should help to make sense of important psychological phenomena concerning innateness, learning, memory, language, problem solving, and decision making. Each of these can be illuminated by considering emotions as semantic pointers.

Innateness

Are emotions innate or learned? Putting the question in this way is crude, because some aspects of emotions may be innate while others are learned from cultural experience, so it is better to apply the criteria for innateness sketched in chapter 2. First, are emotions culturally universal? Among the thousands of cultures investigated by anthropologists, none have been identified as having people who lack emotions. Paul Ekman claims that there are at least six culturally universal emotions: happiness, sadness, fear, anger, surprise, and disgust. He showed pictures of facial expressions to people in New Guinea who had limited exposure to Western culture but who had no difficulty identifying the six emotions. However, other cross-cultural research has challenged the claim that facial expressions of emotion are culturally universal.

Even if there are basic emotions across cultures, there is much cultural variation in how emotions are expressed behaviorally and linguistically. In some cultures such as Japan, public physical display of emotions is discouraged, and languages vary greatly in the varieties of words that they use to describe emotions. For example, Russian makes discriminations about different kinds of sadness not found in English. Moreover, the mere fact that all cultures use emotions does not conclusively imply that emotions are universal, because there are learned cultural practices such as dancing and sports that turn up in all cultures. Hence, we need to consider additional criteria for whether emotions are innate.

My second criterion for innateness is whether there are specific brain areas dedicated to supporting a behavior. This criterion does not require that there be one specific brain area for emotion, and indeed emotions are clearly distributed across many different brain areas, including the amygdala, the striatum, the insula, and various parts of the prefrontal cortex, especially ventromedial and orbitofrontal. Nor does this criterion require that there be specific brain areas for particular emotions, for example, fear in the amygdala. I already stressed that the relation between psychological functions and brain areas is many-to-many, not one-to-one. Nevertheless, some evidence that emotions are innate derives from seeing that the brain areas that support emotions are found universally in all humans. In the absence of biological calamity, everyone is born with an amygdala, striatum, and the other brain areas mentioned. There therefore appears to be a biological basis for the cultural universality of emotions, in a way that there is not for the cultural universality of sports and dancing.

The third criterion for innateness is whether there are precursors in animals from whom humans evolved. Neural precursors are indeed easy to find for brain structures such as the amygdala, which is even found in fish, and for fear circuitry, which is common to all mammals. Behavioral precursors are also easy to find for joy, anger, and other simple emotions. More complex emotions however, such as shame, pride, embarrassment, and gratitude, are not to be expected in other animals with more limited cognitive resources.

My fourth criterion for judging a behavior to be innate is whether it was adaptive during the evolutionary period when that species developed. This criterion is often hard to apply because of lack of knowledge of evolutionary history. Modern humans seem to have evolved around 100,000 years ago, and we have no detailed information about the environments in which they evolved that could tell us the extent to which emotions were adapted. Nevertheless, it is easy to see how, in humans and in other animals, simple emotions such as happiness and fear could contribute to basic biological goals of survival and reproduction by encouraging mating, social cooperation, and the avoidance of predators. It seems plausible therefore that emotions may well have been and continue to be adaptive, despite the inferential and behavioral mistakes that they sometimes provoke.

Finally, the fifth criterion for innateness is the absence of other factors, innate or learned, of which the behavior in question might simply be a side effect. The culturally universal practice of sports, for example, is plausibly a cultural side effect of the biological human need for exercise. However, I have not seen any plausible hypotheses about how emotions might result as biological or cultural side effects.

Overall, even though there are no conclusive arguments to show that emotions are innate, the evidence points to an innate component to emotion with respect to simple, nonsocial emotions. However, this component is compatible with a large component of cultural learning that allows for considerable variation in behavior and language in different groups of people. We saw the same pattern for concepts and rules, some of which are plausibly built into the human brain by evolution, but with enormous room for cultural accumulation and variation.

The semantic pointer theory of emotions can explain both innate and learned aspects of emotions in ways analogous to the similar explanations for concepts and rules. Semantic pointers can be innate when there are genes that organize neurons and the synaptic connections between them to generate patterns of firing that bind diverse representations contributing to action. Most semantic pointers however are learned by mechanisms such as Hebbian adjustment of synaptic connections that result in representations and bindings congruent with experience and goals.

Learning

Emotions are relevant to learning in various ways. First, there is the question of how emotional responses are learned, going beyond the biologically innate aspects of emotion. Second, there is the question of how emotions contribute to learning in general, showing that learning is not a narrow cognitive process but can be influenced by emotions.

It is evident from cross-cultural studies that many aspects of emotion are learned rather than biologically innate. Although some facial expressions such as smiles and frowns may be part of universal biological expressions of emotion, there are other emotional gestures that vary from culture to culture. Most Europeans express agreement by nodding their heads up and down, but Bulgarians express agreement by shaking their heads side to side. Americans insult people and display anger by raising their middle finger, whereas Italians raise their fists while grasping their biceps. Linguistic variation is even greater, as languages range widely in their expressive capacity for describing different emotions. In English, there are hundreds of different words for emotions, but other languages have fewer. Some languages have words for emotions not found in English, such as the German "schadenfreude" (glee at the misfortune of others) and the Danish "hygge" (comfortable coziness). Clearly, therefore, there is a large learned component to emotion based on people's cultural experiences.

Individually, people engage in evaluative learning to figure out what makes them happy and sad. I know, for example, that bananas usually bring me pleasure, whereas liver makes me retch. Evaluative learning can be viewed as a special kind of rule learning of the form *If you do X, then you feel Y*, where Y is an emotional reaction. Evaluative rule learning can operate both with simple emotions such as happiness and disgust and with complex social emotions such as guilt and pride, when they become associated with particular behaviors such as slacking off or working hard. The mechanisms of rule learning described in chapter 5, ranging from basic Hebbian learning to rule combination, could also be responsible for evaluative learning where the action (the *then* part) of the rule is an emotion expressed as a semantic pointer.

Going in the other direction, emotions can contribute to learning because of the roles they play in attention and motivation. There is an unlimited number of concepts and rules that people might learn, but people need to acquire representations that will be useful to their biological and cultural goals. Emotions provide the focus of attention, leading people to concentrate on things that really matter to them. Even science, which is sometimes viewed as a cognitive enterprise that is supposed to be dispassionate, requires emotions such as enthusiasm and excitement to motivate scientists to work hard and keep focused. At the molecular level, pleasurable experience and learning both involve mechanisms using the neurotransmitter dopamine. Other neurotransmitters (e.g., serotonin, norepinephrine) and hormones (e.g., cortisol, oxytocin) also influence emotional states. *Mind–Society* (chapter 10) discusses molecular mechanisms for medical depression, along with mental, neural, and social mechanisms that interact to cause sadness.

Memory

Memory interacts with emotions in at least two ways. First, emotions are an important part of what is remembered. When it has been years since I saw a particular movie or read a particular book, often all I can remember about the book or movie is whether I liked it or not. Memory of a situation leads to recall of emotions such as happiness, excitement, annoyance, or boredom associated with the experience. These emotions can influence future decisions, such as whether to read another book by the same author or see another movie by the same director. An account of memory needs to include not just recall of images, concepts, rules, and analogies but also of the emotions that are associated with them. Activating a cognitive representation naturally activates the associated emotion because of the nature of the bindings that go into semantic pointers. Revival of mental representations bound into semantic pointers will also reactivate some of the physiological states and cognitive appraisals that go into associated emotions. Usually, therefore, memories of events are also memories of emotions.

But memory can also be an effect of emotions, not just a cause. Psychologists have studied the phenomenon of mood-congruent memory: If you are in a particular emotional state, then you are more likely to remember situations associated with that same emotional state. For example, if you are feeling happy, you are more likely to remember other happy situations then if you were depressed. This kind of memory can prolong depression, when feeling sad makes you primarily remember sad experiences, which then make you even more depressed. The effect of emotions and moods on memory is natural from the perspective of the semantic pointer theory of emotions. A firing pattern that results from binding a representation of a situation with the physiological states and cognitive appraisals associated with it will naturally lead to reactivation of similar firing patterns. Hence, the semantic pointer theory of emotions can explain the operation of mood-congruent memory.

Language

There are contributions of language to emotions and of emotions to language. Language influences emotions by virtue of the influence of semantic information on cognitive appraisal displayed in Figure 7.2. Animals that lack language can derive their emotions from binding of nonverbal representations with physiological perceptions and appraisals performed without the benefit of linguistic inferences or associations. But for humans, more complex and differentiated emotional states can arise as a result of the ability of language to make fine distinctions.

For example, the difference between shame and guilt depends on the contrast between violating social expectations and contravening some more abstract moral code. In addition to *schadenfreude* mentioned earlier, German has emotion words for concepts not verbalized in English: *weltschmerz* is depression about the state of the world; *kummerspeck* is excess weight gained from emotional overeating; and *torschlusspanik* is fear that time is running out as one gets older.

Emotion also has a powerful influence on language. What you say and how you say it depends heavily on the effect of your current emotional state on the motivation for linguistic communication and the execution of it. If you are angry at people rather than happy with them, then what you say and how you say it will be dramatically affected, for example, the use of profanity rather than polite language. One explanation of why people often use metaphorical expressions is that they are more emotionally engaging than their literal counterparts, as shown by greater activation of the amygdala. The ubiquity of emotion in language is illustrated by the increasingly popular technique of sentiment analysis applied to social media such as Twitter, using tools such as SentiWordNet, which indicates the emotional positive and negative associations of thousands of words.

Problem Solving

The influence of emotions on problem solving is not always advantageous, because strong emotions such as anxiety, depression, or mania can interfere with the accomplishment of people's goals. Such emotions can make it difficult to focus on the task at hand, distracting from the concepts, images, rules, and analogies that might be most relevant to generating a problem solution.

But emotions also have valuable roles to play in effective problem solving because of their contributions to motivation, attention, and evaluation. As we saw earlier, emotions attached to specific goals provide priorities that ensure that you are accomplishing what matters most to you. Without emotion, human problem solving would be aimless, because you need positive emotions such as happiness to steer you in some directions and negative emotions such as fear to avoid danger. Problem solving by other computational systems such as robots employs nonemotional mechanisms for motivation, attention, and evaluation.

In addition to providing motivation, emotions serve to focus attention on the most relevant path to a problem solution, helping you to put your cognitive resources to work at points more likely to be useful. At any time, there are unlimited deductive inferences that are logically valid but utterly pointless to make, for example the inference from P to P & P and P & P & P and so on to eternity. Making these inferences would rapidly exhaust the memory of any animal or machine.

Inductive inference also needs to be constrained by the needs of the thinker. The evaluation and attention functions of emotion provide crucial ways in which inferences can be focused on what actually matters to the organism. Good inference is not just a matter of syntax and semantics but also requires pragmatic concerns about making inferences that are worth the mind's time and effort.

Despite the importance of emotions for good cognition, the influence of emotion on cognition is not entirely beneficial. Emotions can distort our inferences when there are things that we strongly want or things that we strongly fear. Motivated inference occurs when people reach conclusions based more on harmony with their goals rather than with available evidence. Using emotions to shape inferences is legitimate in decision making but not in determining what is true or false. People are entitled to their own opinions but not to their own facts. If you decide that you should spend all your money on lottery tickets because it makes you excited to think that you are going to win the lottery, then you are succumbing to motivated inference that flies in the face of the evidence that the probability of your winning the lottery is very small. People are prone to motivated inference in all the domains that are important to them, including finances, careers, relationships, health, and religion. For example, budding entrepreneurs are often excessively confident that their new ventures will take off, even though most new companies fail. Somebody coined the term "hopium" to describe the addictive effects of emotion-driven overconfidence.

Semantic pointers help to explain why people are so prone to motivated inference and associated errors, including wishful thinking, positive illusions, optimism bias, and self-deception. Emotions influence all mental representations because of bindings of images, concepts, and rules with emotions, including physiological states and cognitive appraisals with respect to goals. Hence, everything in the mind potentially has an emotional component that encourages goal relevance. Such highlighting is important for problem solving to ensure that mental resources serve goals but can have the unfortunate effect of distorting inferences about what is true rather than desired.

Another way in which emotions can interfere with good thinking is fear-driven inference, the opposite of motivated inference. Whereas motivated inference biases you to believe what you want to believe, fear-driven inference goes in the other direction, leading you to believe something that makes you unhappy. Like motivated inference, fear-driven inference operates in all domains where people have strong emotional concerns, including finances, careers, relationships, and health. For example, some people panic when it looks like there is going to be a setback in the stock market, because they cannot stop thinking that there is going to be a crash, which they obviously do not want to occur. In relationships,

some people become unduly suspicious about the fidelity of their partners, even
though it makes them unhappy to think that their partners might be unfaithful.
The psychological mechanism of fear-driven inference is that the emotional salience of negative events leads a person to think that they are much more likely
than they actually are. The neural mechanism of fear-driven inference is competition among semantic pointers. Intense fear and anxiety pump activation
to semantic pointers bound to them, so that inferences supporting negative
thoughts are prone to be made in the absence of strong evidence. *Mind–Society*
shows how motivated and fear-driven inference play important roles in diverse
social phenomena, including economic cycles, political ideologies, and religious
observances.

Decision Making

Emotions are enormously important for deciding what to do. Inference about
what to believe can be based on coherence with evidence, but inference about what
to do unavoidably requires assessing the relevance of actions to different goals.
Suppose you are trying to decide whether to buy cheap sunglasses from a drug-
store or expensive ones from an optical store. Both sunglasses would offer some
protection from the sun, but you have to decide whether the increased cost of the
expensive sunglasses is justified by their superior appearance and durability. How
you balance these competing goals will depend on your emotional attitudes toward spending money versus looking good and impressing your friends. Contrary
to the assumptions of economists, these goals, attitudes, and beliefs cannot easily
be reduced to the mathematical utilities and probabilities needed for so-called rational choice, because people rarely have enough information about the present
and future to specify these quantities.

The traditional view that emotions just get in the way of making decisions was
challenged effectively by Antonio Damasio, who gave neurological reasons why
emotions should be viewed as integral to good decisions, not contrary to them.
Emotions serve as inputs to decision making because they provide an assessment
of the relative value of different goals, for example, how much you care about
the cost or appearance of sunglasses. In semantic pointer terminology, each of
your goals has a binding with emotions that in turn bind both to physiology and
appraisal. Emotions are also outputs from decision making when goal-based assessment of actions results in them becoming bound with emotions that govern
what will actually be done. If you end up wanting the expensive sunglasses because of your emotionally important goals, then you have a positive emotion attached to the action of owning those sunglasses. The multimodal (verbal, visual,

kinesthetic) representation of buying becomes bound to a combination of physiological state (gut feeling) and cognitive appraisal (relevance of goals, semantic
associations). Damasio uses the term "somatic marker" for the physiological representations that contribute to emotions, but semantic pointers are richer than
somatic markers because they can also include binding of information about appraisal and the self.

Many practical problems require decisions between alternative actions. On the
assumptions of most economists, decision making is and ought to be based on
maximizing expected utility, calculated by combining estimates of probabilities
and quantifiable utilities. Experiments from behavioral economics suggest that
this account of economic decision making is not psychologically accurate. For example, merely framing a decision in terms of losses rather than gains can dramatically shift people's choices.

An alternative account of decision making views people as making their decisions based on the emotional coherence of actions and decisions. The theory of
emotional coherence can be summarized in three principles:

1. Representations have positive or negative emotional values.
2. Representations can have positive or negative emotional connections to
   other representations.
3. The emotional value of a representation is determined by the values and
   acceptability of all the representations to which it is connected.

Decision making then is adjusting actions and goals in relation to each other, in
an emotional version of the process of parallel constraint satisfaction described in
chapter 2. Actions and goals can be represented by semantic pointers, and choices
among competing actions result from semantic pointer competition.

The produced decision is a kind of emotional gestalt—a whole impression of
what is the best action to perform, analogous to the perceptual gestalts discussed
in chapter 3. This gestalt is the emergent result of the interplay of many goals and
actions carried out by the interactions of various neural groups with millions of
neurons. A chosen action ends up bound to a positive emotion, unless it has significant downside that results in binding to a mixture of emotions. If you are having
trouble with an important decision, you are probably experiencing emotional gestalt shifts, which are transitions between different states that are each emotionally coherent with some of your goals.

Consider the following application of emotional coherence. Many students
face the decision of what to do after graduation, which is difficult because it
involves conflicting goals. Choosing to get a job would contribute to practical

goals such as having money and placating parents. But taking a year off to travel would satisfy other goals such as having fun, relaxation, and self-understanding. A third alternative might be going to graduate school in a program that contributes to long-term goals of getting a better job as well as short-term goals such as learning interesting material. Some students find themselves flipping between one inclination and another because of slight changes in experiences. For example, an interesting class session might incline a student toward the emotional gestalt of pursuing graduate school, but encounters with annoying university bureaucracy can tip the student in the other direction. Emotional coherence shifts the decision based on the way in which current experiences make different kinds of goals more or less salient.

Decision making by emotional coherence fits well with semantic pointers. Every node in a network of emotional coherence, including positive goals such as having fun and negative ones such as being poor, can be understood as a semantic pointer that binds a combination of verbal or imagistic representation, physiological perception, and cognitive appraisal. The support and conflict links between nodes in a coherence network can be captured in a more realistic neural network implementation by large numbers of excitatory inhibitory links between the neurons in one semantic pointer and the neurons in another pointer. Parallel constraint satisfaction is accomplished by semantic pointer competition, for example, between getting a job and keeping on studying, even though each of these is represented by thousands or millions of neurons.

This account allows for both good and bad decisions because the appraisal component of emotions shows how they can be rational or irrational. If emotions were just physiological reactions, then they would have no connection with reasons. However, appraisals of a situation with respect to one's goals can definitely be subject to judgments of rationality. If your emotion reflects a thorough evaluation of the extent to which your situation does in fact contribute to or conflict with your goals and if those goals are themselves compatible with your needs, then the emotion can be judged to be rational. There are important cases where emotions fail these tests, for example, when a person has an unrealizable goal such as living to be 1,000 years old and false beliefs that taking dangerous drugs will increase longevity. Then, the person is irrational to be taking the drugs. In contrast, if a person has the nearly universal need to be in social relationships, and the well-founded belief that spending time with a friend or lover helps to accomplish this goal, then it is perfectly rational for the person to be happy about spending time in this way. The hazard is that motivated and fear-driven inferences sometimes encourage people to stay in dangerous relationships.

How Emotions Change

Decisions often result in emotional changes, for example, from anxiety to relief. More generally, emotions construed as semantic pointers can change in several ways. The binding of an emotional reaction to a representation results from bindings with both cognitive appraisals and physiological reactions, so changing either of these may revise the emotion. Physiological characteristics such as heart and breathing rates can be changed by interventions such as drugs (e.g., beta blockers, tranquilizers), exercise, meditation, and social interactions ranging from hugs to psychotherapy. Cognitive appraisals can be changed by adding new representations such as goals, actions, and details about the relevance of actions to goals. Such additional information can alter the results of parallel constraint satisfaction to generate a different emotional gestalt.

Emotional changes can be local, for example, going from liking the idea of going to graduate school to finding it repugnant. But changes can also involve whole systems of beliefs and attitudes, for example, when a person shifts from being emphatically left wing in politics to being aggressively conservative. Emotional changes can include major alterations in social norms, for example, away from the 1950s attitudes that smoking is fun and homosexuality is evil. Emotional shifts in emotions include mood changes, which are more diffuse and long-lasting than emotional reactions to specific events. *Mind–Society* describes how emotional depression and recovery can be explained by a combination of the cognitive–emotional mechanisms in this chapter and equally relevant social mechanisms.

SUMMARY AND DISCUSSION

No comprehensive account of human thinking can ignore emotion. Emotions are important mental representations because they serve not only to stand for things in the world but also to indicate their value. Decision, action, and many kinds of problem solving require determining how the world should be, not just how it is. Perhaps robots could do their evaluations by purely mathematical calculations like the expected utilities favored by economists. But humans and other animals evolved with emotions as part of their innate biological machinery to guide action and inference.

Semantic pointers provide a neural theory of emotions that synthesizes psychological approaches usually taken as contradictory. Emotions are patterns of neural firing that result from binding three different factors that are complementary rather than conflictive. A verbal or sensory representation of a situation can be bound both with a representation of the physiological states that the situation elicited and with a cognitive appraisal of the import of the situation. Cognitive appraisal can also incorporate social factors because of the contributions of social goals and the culturally established associations of emotional words. Thus, semantic pointers provide a unified theory of emotions that integrates physiological perception, cognitive appraisal, and social interpretation.

Semantic pointers for emotions can feed into neural mechanisms for inference, problem solving, and decision making, all of them potentially leading to action. Decisions are not mathematical calculations of expected utility but rather parallel processes that aim to satisfy conflicting emotional constraints. The result of a decision is an emotional gestalt, a whole set of coherent actions and goals that can guide actions that may be rational or irrational, depending on how the available information is used.

Irrationality arises when emotional coherence (resulting from value-driven parallel constraint satisfaction performed by semantic pointer competition) biases the brain to be unduly optimistic or unduly pessimistic. Motivated inference encourages positive illusions that things are better than they are, whereas fear-driven inference encourages negative illusions that things are worse than they are. Sour grapes and rationalization also result from emotional inferences where estimates of value (utility) and estimates of truth (probability) interact inappropriately. Specifically, the relations are:

Motivated inference: high utility→ high probability (e.g., I really want that job, so I'm sure to get it).

Fear-driven inference: high disutility → high probability (e.g., I'm terrified that my mole is cancerous, so it must be).

Sour grapes: low probability → low utility (e.g., I can't afford a BMW, but it's too unreliable anyway).

Rationalization: high probability → high utility (e.g., I have to go to Moose Jaw, so it should be a fun city).

These interactions make no logical sense but follow naturally from emotional coherence resulting from ongoing interactions of cognition and emotion in the brain.

In the semantic pointer theory, emotions are both embodied (tied to physiology) and transbodied (going beyond the senses). Embodiment comes through binding of the full range of internal sensory representations from heart rate to cortisol levels. Transbodiment comes from bindings that also incorporate complex

cognitive appraisals that include social aspects, making emotions capable of contributing to abstract attitudes such as that democracy is good and slavery is odious.
Such attitudes and other values and desires are not only connected with visceral
reactions but also go beyond them to incorporate all the nonsensory power of
some concepts and rules.

The semantic pointer theory of emotion has implications for chapters to
come. Chapter 8 describes a new theory of consciousness that naturally applies
to the many emotional aspects of conscious experience, such as feeling happy
and sad. Chapter 9 on intention and action provides a more detailed account
of how emotions motivate people to do things and why people sometimes fail
to do what they intend. Emotion also contributes to the accounts of language,
creativity, and the self in chapters 10 to 12. *Mind–Society* and *Natural Philosophy*
identify emotions as a major unifying factor in answering important questions
in social sciences, professions, and humanities. In all of these cases, emotions
are central to human thinking, not peripheral annoyances. Both the potential
rationality and potential harm of emotions contribute to social explanations
and ethical evaluations.

NOTES

The Emerson quote is from Wikiquote. Similarly, Hegel said that nothing great in
the world has been accomplished without passion.

Useful general works on emotion include Barrett, Lewis, and Havilland-Jones
2016; Davidson and Begley 2012; de Sousa 2013; and Keltner, Oatley, and Jenkins
2013. I avoid use of the psychological term "affect," which sometimes is used for the
composite of emotion, mood, and motivation and sometimes for the experience
(feeling) of emotion. What I mean by "emotion" is given by the three-analysis in
Table 7.1. On moods see https://www.psychologytoday.com/ca/blog/hot-thought/
201805/what-are-moods.

Proponents of appraisal theories of emotion include Nussbaum 2001; Oatley
1992; and Scherer, Schorr, and Johnstone 2001.

Proponents of physiological theories of emotion include James 1884, Damasio
1994, 2012; Prinz 2004; and Niedenthal, Barsalou, Ric, and Krauth-Gruber 2005.
Kreibig 2010 reviews autonomic nervous system activity in emotions. For bodily
maps of emotions, see Nummenmaa, Glerean, Han, and Hietanen 2014. The integration of appraisal and physiological aspects of emotion was proposed by Schacter
and Singer 1962, whose experiments were modeled by Wagar and Thagard 2004.
Panksepp 1998 is a pioneering work in affective neuroscience.

On social theories of emotion, see Harré 1989 and Fisher and Chon 1989. Emotions promote social interaction by synchronizing brain activity across individuals: Nummenmaa et al. 2012. Because emotions result from the interaction of molecular, neural, psychological, and social mechanisms, they exemplify multilevel emergence as explained in chapter 12. *Mind–Society* (chapter 3) describes social mechanisms for emotion transmission.

For evidence that emotions are distributed over many brain areas, see Lindquist, Wager, Kober, Bliss-Moreau, and Barrett 2012 and Pessoa 2013. Also consult neurosynth.org. Emotional imagery engages brain areas including the nucleus accumbens, amygdala, and medial prefrontal cortex: Costa, Lang, Sabatinelli, Versace, and Bradley, 2010. Distributed neural signatures for identifying emotions can be produced by a combination of brain imaging and machine learning: Kassam, Markey, Cherkassky, Loewenstein, and Just, 2013.

The semantic pointer theory of emotions is defended in Thagard and Schröder 2014 and Kajić, Schröder, Stewart, and Thagard forthcoming. This theory builds on earlier neural theories including Thagard and Aubie 2008. The semantic pointer theory of emotions is broadly compatible with the "psychological construction" approach of Barrett 2012, 2017, but is far more specific about the neural mechanisms that generate emotions through a combination of physiological perception and cognitive interpretation.

For evidence that emotions attach generally to concepts, see Fazio 2001 and work on sentiment analysis: see the Wikipedia article "Sentiment Analysis" and http://sentiwordnet.isti.cnr.it. Spering, Wagener, and Funke 2005 discuss the role of emotions in problem solving.

Emotions also attach to representations of objects: Lebrecht, Bar, Barrett, and Tarr 2012. Sadness impairs color perception: Thorstenson, Pazda, and Elliot 2015.

On self-recognition in mirrors, see: Broom, Sena, and Moynihan 2009; Prior, Schwarz, and Güntürkün 2008. Gieling, Mijdam, van der Staay, and Nordquist 2014 challenge pigs' use of mirrors. Macaque monkeys have been trained to respond to mirrors, but it is not clear whether this constitutes self-recognition: http://www.nature.com/news/monkeys-seem-to-recognize-their-reflections-1.16692.

Berridge, Robinson, and Aldridge 2009 discuss the neural differences between wanting and liking.

On empathy, see Bernhardt and Singer 2012, Decety 2014, Thagard 2010, and *Mind–Society*. On mirror neurons, see Iacoboni 2008 and Hickock 2014. *Natural Philosophy* (chapter 6) discusses the relevance of empathy to ethics.

Discussions of the importance of emotions for decision making include Damasio 1994; Thagard 2006; and Lerner, Li, Valdesolo, and Kassam 2015.

On questions about emotions, culture, language, and emotions, see Ekman 2003, 2016, Lomas 2016, Smith 2015, and Wierzbicka 1999. Ekman's claims about the cultural universality of facial expressions of emotion are challenged by Jack, Oliver, Yu, Caldara, and Schyns 2012 and by Gendron, Roberson, van der Vyver, and Barrett 2014. For an online review, see http://www.wwu.edu/culture/altarriba2.htm. Niedenthal and Brauer 2012 discuss the social functions of emotions.

On the emotional appeal of metaphorical expressions, see Citron and Goldberg 2014.

On motivated inference, see Kunda 1990, 1999 and Hughes and Zaki 2015. On fear-driven inference, see Thagard and Nussbaum 2014. Simon, Stenstrom, and Read 2015 provide experimental evidence for emotional coherence.

For more on emotional coherence construed as parallel constraint satisfaction, see Thagard 2000, 2006. For experimental critiques of rational choice theory, see Kahneman and Tversky 2000; Litt, Eliasmith, and Thagard 2008. *Mind–Society* provides examples of irrationality in politics and economics.

PROJECT

Connect semantic pointer models of emotion more directly to models of action and consciousness. Simulate emotional imagery, decision making and indecisiveness. Model deliberate, automatic, and dynamic empathy as analogical emotional imagery. Figure out how molecular mechanisms (e.g., serotonin) interact with cognitive appraisal and physiological perception.

8

Consciousness

Stuart Sutherland wrote in 1989: "Consciousness is a fascinating but elusive phenomenon; it is impossible to specify what it is, what it does, or why it evolved. Nothing worth reading has been written on it." Thinkers such as William James and Sigmund Freud made some interesting remarks on consciousness, but in 1989 there were no good theories, in psychology or philosophy or neuroscience, that could tell us much about it. I propose to fill this lamentable gap with the theory that consciousness results from competition among semantic pointers.

Some important features of mind and society require an account of consciousness. All the kinds of mental representations so far discussed have conscious components, especially perceptions, images, and emotions. Perceptions such as colors, shape, sounds, and pains are experienced, not just had. When perceptions are turned into images, they recreate conscious experiences, for example when I remember the wretched cauliflower I had for dinner yesterday and imagine how it could have been cooked much more satisfactorily. Chapter 7 discussed the physiological and cognitive aspects of emotions such as happiness, fear, and anger, but emotion without consciousness is like summer without sunshine. There may well be unconscious emotions, but far more important are the conscious experiences that usually go along with them.

Consciousness is also often associated with concepts, rules, and analogies. At any given moment, most of our concepts are unconscious, but we sometimes become aware that we are thinking about cauliflower, giraffes, or sex. Similarly, rules can be used without awareness, but there are times when you become aware of a particular rule, for example when you realize that you are violating the traffic rule about driving above the speed limit. Analogies are usually conscious: even though you might not be aware that you are thinking analogically, you are at least aware of the source and target analogs. For example, if you are metaphorically analogizing that your life is a train wreck, then you may be aware of aspects of your life and aspects of train wrecks, both visual and emotional. Hence consciousness is important for understanding all forms of mental representation.

Consciousness is also vital for understanding how societies work, because people influence each other's consciousness in ways that lead to changes in social behaviors. Conscious experiences can spread among groups of people, for example when the enthusiasm or anxiety of one person is communicated to others. Emotional communication that propagates similar conscious experiences among members of a group is important for understanding social phenomena ranging from stock market panics to religious fervor. Consciousness is also crucial for the interpersonal process of empathy discussed in chapter 7. The goal of empathic understanding is not just an intellectual explanation of what someone is feeling but actually to feel something like what the other person is experiencing. So empathy is inherently conscious as well as social.

Another important social phenomenon that often benefits from consciousness is teaching. If you are a skilled musician, athlete, or artist, you may not need much conscious experience to execute your own accomplishments. But becoming consciously aware of what you do can help you to teach others how to do it. Although imitation is found in chimpanzees and other nonhuman animals, intentional instruction is confined to our species, with possible rare exceptions such as meerkats teaching their offspring what to eat. Because of the importance of emotional communication, empathy, and teaching in the development of human societies, a theory of consciousness is desperately needed for explanations in social science, the professions, and the humanities.

PSYCHOLOGICAL THEORIES OF CONSCIOUSNESS

Can anyone talk about consciousness without a definition of it? According to the discussion of concepts in chapter 4, the demand for a definition of consciousness is futile. But a three-analysis of the concept of consciousness using exemplars, typical features, and explanations is easy to do, as sketched in Table 8.1. I have already mentioned important standard examples of consciousness that are familiar from

TABLE 8.1

Three-Analysis of *Consciousness*

Exemplars	External perceptions such as colors; internal perceptions such as pain; emotions, thoughts, self-awareness
Typical features	Experience, awareness, attention, shifts, starts and stops, unity
Explanations	Explains: behaviors, reports, experiences
	Explained by: neural mechanisms including semantic pointer competition

experience with colors, sounds, pains, emotions, and so on. These can serve as the exemplars of consciousness that need to be explained by a theory of consciousness.

The typical features of consciousness include feeling, awareness, and attention. Perceptions, images, and emotions are all experiences that we feel, not just have. Sometimes in addition to experiencing feelings, you are also aware that you are having them, and sometimes you are also aware of yourself having these experiences. Feeling, awareness, and self-awareness are increasingly complex features of consciousness that need to be explained by a comprehensive theory. Conscious experience also involves shifts in attention, because at one moment you can be conscious of one thing in your environment, such as this text, but then suddenly start thinking instead about something else such as a song you recently heard at a concert. Given the current state of understanding of consciousness, it would be folly to try to provide a set of necessary and sufficient conditions for consciousness in terms of feeling, awareness, and attention, but we can usefully note that these are typical features of consciousness.

Finally, a three-analysis of the concept of consciousness indicates how it figures in explanations. People invoke consciousness to explain many aspects of human behavior, for example the difference between conscious actions and involuntary ones. Consciousness is also important for explaining the difference between being asleep and awake, focused and distracted, and even dead and alive. People behave differently when they are consciously aware of what they are doing, as recognized in everyday life and the law. These everyday explanations would be more solid if they were based on a good theory of the mechanisms of consciousness, which I will provide using semantic pointers. This theory can explain feeling, awareness, and attention, the typical features of consciousness, as they occur in exemplars from imagery to empathy.

There are, however, prominent alternatives to neural explanations of consciousness. The commonsense view of consciousness is dualism, which says that a person combines two fundamentally different things, a body and a non-material mind—a soul. Dualism is increasingly rare among psychologists, neuroscientists, and even philosophers, but it is by far the most popular view of mind worldwide. Of the 7.5 billion people in the world, around 6 billion are adherents of religions that believe in an afterlife. Christians, Muslims, Hindus, Buddhists, and members of many other religions believe that you do not die when your body dies but can survive after death because your soul goes on. If survival after death actually happens, then consciousness has to be something nonphysical rather than the result of brain mechanisms. A nonmaterial soul is beyond the reach of scientific explanation, so cognitive science would simply have to give up on explaining consciousness.

The neural mechanism approach to consciousness is materialist but not in the everyday sense of being excessively concerned with money. Rather, materialism is a philosophical view that nothing exists except for the kinds of things studied by science, namely matter and energy, which are convertible into each other. Materialism is monistic, claiming that there is only one kind of thing that exists, in contrast to the dualist view that matter and mind are two fundamentally different things. Another monistic view is idealism, not in the everyday sense of being concerned only with lofty values. Idealism in philosophy is the view that ideas and consciousness are all that exists. From this perspective, mind is fundamental, and matter is only a manifestation of it. Idealism puts consciousness at the center of the universe.

Another view of consciousness is panpsychism, which says that everything in the universe has at least a bit of consciousness to it. Whereas neural mechanism accounts claim that consciousness is a special kind of brain process, panpsychism says that consciousness can be a property of anything, not just animals but also plants, rocks, and maybe even atoms. The main support for panpsychism comes from the argument that consciousness is so mysterious that we could not understand where it comes from unless everything in the universe has a little bit of it that could eventually add up to the full-blown consciousness found in humans. This argument fails if mechanisms can be identified that show how consciousness emerges from the interactions of neurons.

At another extreme, some scientists and philosophers have been skeptical about the whole idea of consciousness. From the 1920s to the 1960s, the dominant view in psychology was behaviorism, which claimed that a scientific approach to the mind should avoid talking about theoretical abstractions such as consciousness and concern itself with merely identifying patterns of observable behavior. This restriction is based on a faulty view of science. Sciences such as physics, chemistry, and biology legitimately theorize about nonobservable entities such as atoms, chemical bonds, and genes because doing so provides well-justified explanations of observations. Similarly, psychology can go beyond behaviorism and take consciousness seriously by trying to explain it, not just explain it away.

One way of providing a psychological explanation of consciousness is to see it as resulting from purely computational processes in which algorithms are applied to representations. This was the predominant form of psychological explanation from the 1960s until the rise of neural network models in the 1980s. The computational approach differs from the neural approach in that it allows for the possibility of consciousness in computers that have sufficiently complex algorithms. But robots have yet to achieve consciousness, and it is not at all clear from a purely computational perspective what it would take for them to get there.

What are the grounds for concluding that an entity is conscious? You know that you are conscious because you are aware of experiences such as pain, happiness, and hearing music. But how can you conclude that other people are conscious, let alone that consciousness extends to other mammals, birds, reptiles, fish, or robots? There are several kinds of behavioral evidence that make it reasonable to assume that other people are conscious.

First, there are verbal reports, when people describe their own experiences and feelings as conscious. Second, there are behaviors that you know from your own experience are closely connected with consciousness, such as smiling when you are happy or grimacing when you are in pain. From your own happy smiling and painful grimacing, you have the rules that happiness causes smiling and pain causes grimacing. When you see other people smiling or grimacing, it is easy to explain these behaviors by supposing that they have the same conscious states as you. This inference is not mere analogy but rather an inference to the best explanation that builds on both the analogies between you and other people and on the systematic causal explanations that you can give of the behavior of others. The best explanation of the behaviors of other people, including their bodily movements and verbal reports, is that they are conscious just like you.

Extending this inference to nonhuman animals is tricky, because they are not able to provide verbal reports. But when a chimpanzee bares its teeth, or when a rat frantically tries to escape a trap, we observe behaviors that can be plausibly explained by supposing that the chimp or the rat has feelings that are like the anger or fear familiar in human beings. In addition to facial expressions and approach-avoidance behaviors, there is other evidence that suggests similarities in consciousness between humans and other animals. For example, injured fish have diminished ability to accomplish tasks such as learning to run mazes but regain some capacity when they are given painkillers.

The inference to the best explanation that attributes consciousness to other people and at least some animals is supported by increased understanding of the neural causes of experiences. We saw in the last chapter that the neural circuitry for basic emotions like happiness and fear is similar across mammals, which supports the view that similarities in behavior result from similarities in experiences. The inference that nonhuman animals are conscious is supported both by how this explains their behavior but also by how the presence of consciousness is explained by neural mechanisms that are found in all animals, not just humans.

What about robots? Despite impressive advances such as Google's driverless cars, which drive on their own around California, there are still no robots capable of sufficiently complex behaviors to license inferences that they are conscious. We should put aside the question of whether robots can be conscious until they begin to show the kinds of behaviors that lead us to attribute consciousness to humans and other animals.

Any acceptable theory of consciousness must explain important phenomena observed in humans. First, there is qualitative experience, the different feelings that come along with perception, emotion, and cognition in general. Second, consciousness begins and ends, most frequently with people's going to sleep and waking up, but also as the result of other causes such as anesthetics and blows to the head. Third, there are shifts in experiences, where people go from experiencing one aspect of consciousness to another aspect. When I taught, I prohibited the use of laptops by students, because I know that if they are paying attention to the websites on their laptops, they rarely shift their attention to my lecturing.

Fourth, even if nonhuman animals are also conscious, consciousness may differ across species. Chapter 7 on emotions described differences between the simple emotions such as happiness, sadness, and fear that all mammals are capable of and the complex social emotions such as shame that require a sense of self and its place in society. A theory of consciousness should deal with feeling, awareness, and self-awareness that may vary across species. Fifth, a remarkable aspect of consciousness in humans is that there is a kind of unity to it. We usually do not perceive life as a disjointed mixture of disconnected sensations and emotions but rather as unified into particular combined experiences such as feeling happy that the coffee smells good. On the other hand, consciousness can sometimes become disjointed as a result of hallucinations brought on by hunger or drugs.

Suppose that theoretical neuroscience can describe brain mechanisms for all of these phenomena. This description would provide solid evidence that consciousness is a brain process so that there is no need for dualism, idealism, or panpsychism. Moreover, the behaviorist worry about consciousness being unobservable and therefore unscientific would be removed, because consciousness would be as theoretically legitimate as gravity. Let us now see how far semantic pointers can go in providing plausible explanations of features of consciousness.

NEURAL MECHANISMS FOR CONSCIOUSNESS
Hypotheses

The semantic pointer competition theory of consciousness consists of the following hypotheses:

> H1. Consciousness is a brain process resulting from neural mechanisms.

> H2. The crucial mechanisms for consciousness are: representation by patterns of firing in neural groups, binding of these representations into semantic pointers, and competition among semantic pointers.

> H3. Qualitative experiences result from the competition won by semantic pointers that unpack into neural representations of sensory, motor, emotional, and verbal activity.

The restriction of consciousness to brains in H1 is merely a recognition that all the entities so far known to be conscious have brains. Hypothesis H2 breaks down into three claims about neural representation, semantic pointers, and competition, all of which were presented in chapter 2. Neural groups represent the world because neurons that interact with the world and each other become tuned to regularities in the environment. A semantic pointer is a special kind of neural representation—a pattern of firing in a group of neurons—that is capable of operating both as a symbol and as a compressed version of sensory and motor representations. For example, people's neural concept of chocolate unpacks (decompresses) into sensory representations of sweetness, texture, and so on, while allowing the semantic pointer to figure in inferences such as that you should not eat too much chocolate because it is a kind of candy. Semantic pointers are formed by binding together simpler representations, where binding is a neural process that compresses information into a more compact form suitable for manipulation.

According to H2, the third mechanism of consciousness is competition among semantic pointers. Semantic pointers do not by themselves explain consciousness, because there are countless neural representations being formed all the time, most of which do not enter consciousness. For example, context enables you to interpret the sentence "The pen is in the bank" as meaning that a writing device is in a financial institution rather than that a pig enclosure is by a river. Doing this requires the construction of various complex representations, only some of which become conscious. Attention is a psychological process that selects a small subset of candidate representations as worthy to enter consciousness. I propose that the specific kind of representations engaged in the competition for attention are semantic pointers.

As a first approximation, consider the struggle for attention in Figure 8.1, which shows an extreme case of someone who is both texting and thinking about work while driving. Much evidence shows that driving while texting or talking on the phone is dangerous, because drivers fail to pay attention to what is happening on the road. Unlike the similar Figure 4.2, which shows competition among concepts to categorize sensory input, the competition in Figure 8.1 is for attention. The human mind is limited in its capacity to attend to more than a few items at once, so driving can easily lose out if texting or working becomes more salient. A more detailed version of Figure 8.1 would show texting, working, and driving as a host of perceptions, images, and concepts captured by semantic pointers.

Semantic pointers can compete with each other even when they are being represented by the same neurons, as was shown in Figure 2.6. A group of neurons forms a distributed representation of a concept; that is, each concept is ideally some pattern of activity across all these neurons. So those same neurons can represent multiple semantic pointers via a pattern of activity that amalgamates the two patterns of activity for the two concepts. In order to have them compete, we add recurrent connections among the neurons.

Hypothesis H3 proposes that qualitative experiences—all the sensations, feelings, and thoughts that people are aware of—result from competition among semantic pointers, as described in chapter 2. Whether semantic pointer competition or some other theory of consciousness is most plausible needs to be decided on the basis of which theory provides the best explanation of the full range of known

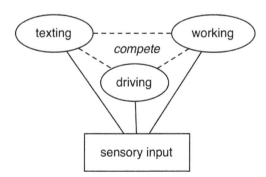

FIGURE 8.1 Competition for attention among texting, working, and driving. Solid lines indicate excitatory connections among neural groups, and dotted lines indicate inhibitory connections.

facts about consciousness. The classes of facts to be explained include the qualitative experiences mentioned in H3, onset and cessation, shifts of attention, different kinds of consciousness, and unity in diversity.

Many cognitive scientists have noticed the importance of attention for consciousness and suggested that competition among representations is the key to
attention. But competition and attention alone cannot explain why different representations lead to different experiences, which requires the theory of representation provided by semantic pointers.

Qualitative Experience

The biggest challenge for theories of consciousness is to explain the occurrence of
subjective, qualitative experiences such as the pain of a headache, the taste of a
beer, and the joy of a victory. I propose that these are neural processes that result
from the formation and competition of semantic pointers.

A theory of conscious experience must answer two basic questions: (a) Why are
there different experiences such as pains, tastes, sounds, and emotions? (b) Why
do these experiences feel like anything at all? The first of these is answerable
because of the different neural representations that get bound into a semantic
pointer, as described in chapter 3. Consider pain, which typically results from stimulation of sensory neurons (nociceptors) that respond to crushing, tearing, heat,
cold, or chemical irritation. In humans, the conscious experience of pain usually
arises from such stimulation plus bindings in the brain that integrate the nocicep-
tive signals with locations, emotions, and self-conceptions, producing in humans
complex semantic pointers like "I have an annoying pain in my toe."

Other perceptual experiences such as taste, touch, sound, hearing, smell, kinesthesia, balance, temperature, time, and bladder fullness result from different
patterns of neural firing generated from diverse receptors that produce signals
combined into different semantic pointers. Perceptual experiences do not always
result directly from perceptions, because the brain can store neural patterns and
reactivate them in memory, imagination, and dreaming.

Chapter 2 described how semantic pointers are capable of modal retention,
retaining in partial, compressed form the information resulting from the particular sensory or motor modality that produced them. In contrast, verbal symbols such as "cat" discard modal information, whereas the semantic pointer for
the concept *cat* can retain some of the visual, tactile, and auditory characteristics
that went into its formation. These characteristics contribute to the diverse conscious experience of cats. Competition among semantic pointers is different from

competition among mental representations in other explanations of attention, because semantic pointers perform modal retention.

As chapter 7 argues, emotions such as happiness, sadness, fear, and anger result in part from sensory inputs, especially ones for internal bodily states but also from appraisals of the implications of the current state of an organism for its goals such as surviving and reproducing. Semantic pointers bind together neural representations of a situation, physiological changes, and cognitive appraisals to produce a combined representation. Different combinations produce different qualitative experiences because of the different neural firings that contribute to the resulting semantic pointer.

Situations can be represented purely perceptually, or by verbal sentences, which can be neurally constructed by the same kinds of binding operations that produce semantic pointers. Semantic pointers explain why we can talk about our consciousness experiences, because semantic pointers can function as symbols that can be bound into verbal reports such as "My toe hurts" or "I see a blue sky." In nonhuman animals, however, semantic pointers can have symbolic functions in inference without being encoded verbally. Specific conscious qualities result from specific patterns of neural firing and binding, making it easy to differentiate among the many different kinds of conscious experience.

Incorporating the self into representations of pain and emotions requires further binding discussed later in relation to kinds of consciousness. The question of what it is like to be conscious is too obscure to pursue, but differences in neural representations easily handle the more particular question of why there are differences in what it is like to be in pain, in love, and in the desert.

Binding of different kinds of inputs into semantic pointers explains the differences among various sensations and feelings, but why do these experiences feel like anything at all? The best available explanation is that qualitative experience is an emergent property of the three mechanisms that operate in organisms capable of neural representation, binding, and semantic pointer competition. We have already seen that there is nothing mysterious about emergent properties, which belong to wholes, do not belong to any of their parts, are not aggregates of properties of the parts, and result from the interactions of the parts. Such emergence is common in complex systems, and chapters 3 to 7 describe its occurrence in perception, imagery, concepts, rules, and emotions. Representation, binding, and competition are each emergent results of the interactions of many neurons, not the aggregate of bits of representation, binding, or competition that are properties of individual neurons.

Then consciousness is an emergent outcome of the interaction of three mechanisms with emergent properties. No wonder it has been so difficult for people to accept that consciousness is a biological process, since emergence is not easy for people to understand, and emergence from emergence is even more challenging.

There are several available explanations of why consciousness has evolved. It may be an adaptation that increases the ability of organisms to survive and reproduce (like emotions), a byproduct or side effect of other processes that are adaptive (like mathematical ability), a chance result (like diseases caused by mutations), or a cultural artifact (like rock music). Given the apparent commonality of consciousness in humans and other animals, the chance and cultural explanations are implausible, but current evidence is not sufficient to decide between the adaptation and byproduct explanations. It is possible that consciousness makes attention, learning, and action more effective, but it also possible that consciousness resulted as a side effect from sufficiently complex processes of neural representation, binding, and semantic pointer competition.

The side-effect and adaptation explanations might turn out to be complementary. Perhaps consciousness originally was only an accidental emergent result of neural activity in simple organisms such as fish and mice but then turned out to be useful for the survival and reproduction of the highly social animal, *Homo sapiens*.

Onset and Cessation of Consciousness

There are more straightforward facts than qualitative experience that must be explained by any plausible theory of consciousness. Humans and other animals experience the cessation and onset of consciousness every day when they go to sleep and wake up. Stopping of consciousness can also result from unusual occurrences such as anesthetics, concussions, strokes, seizures, and death.

Most kinds of consciousness reduction involve increases in neural inhibition, decreases in neural excitation, or both, interfering with processes of representing, binding, and competition that all depend on a balance among excitation and inhibition. In sleep, the accumulation of the neurotransmitter adenosine (which can be blocked by caffeine) acts as a direct negative-feedback inhibitor of neural firing. Anesthetics work by enhancing inhibitory transmission and/or blocking excitatory conduction. Concussions cause several kinds of metabolic disturbances including lactate buildup that hinders neurons. Death brings total elimination of neural firing and hence the end of consciousness, and less severe events such as strokes and heart attacks can also dramatically reduce excitation. In sum, decreases in excitation and/or increases in inhibition produce disruptions in representation, binding, and competition that remove consciousness in sleep, anesthesia, injury, disease, and death.

It is easy to see how the mechanisms of semantic pointer competition can explain loss of consciousness from increases in neural inhibition and decreases in excitation. If neural firing decreases, there will be less formation of representations and less binding of representations into semantic pointers. Moreover, in the semantic pointer competition, there will be fewer semantic pointers that achieve a minimal threshold required for conscious experience. Once loss of consciousness occurs because of sleep, anesthetics, or concussion, a drop in sensory input further decreases neural activity required for the formation, binding, and competition of representations. Dreaming revises consciousness by replacing sensory inputs by internally generated neural activity arising from memory.

Seizures and epilepsy are more complicated in that they seem to involve hyperactivity of neurons rather than inhibition. How can an excess of excitation disrupt representation, binding, and competition to an extent that eliminates consciousness? One possibility is that, when uncontrolled excitation floods a neural network, it saturates the network of competing semantic pointers so that none are able to exceed a threshold that corresponds to entry into consciousness. The operation of a threshold explains why neural firing, binding, and competition among semantic pointers can all operate in unconscious processes.

Shifts in Consciousness

As people go through their days, their consciousness naturally moves among many different kinds of experiences, for example when a doorbell rings to shift attention away from working. Semantic pointer competition inherits from other competition theories of attention the natural ability to explain these shifts. At one moment, some representations are winning the battle for the limited resources of consciousness, but incursion of new stimuli such as the doorbell has two effects. First, new semantic pointers are formed, binding the stimuli together and connecting them with other representations such as the verbal representation that a parcel is being delivered and the emotion of excitement. Second, if the resulting semantic pointers develop more powerful patterns of firing than those already dominating consciousness, then the new semantic pointers will suppress and replace the old ones, unless there is sufficient mental capacity that the new and old can coexist.

How such competition works is most clear in simple neural networks that associate one artificial neuron with one representation. If a neuron for doorbell receives activation from input neurons and thereby inhibits a neuron for coffee, then attention shifts from coffee to doorbell. The situation is more complicated in biologically realistic networks where doorbell and coffee are each represented by

patterns of firing in large numbers of neurons with many excitatory and inhibitory connections. Nevertheless, computer simulations show that neural networks
with semantic pointers can accomplish the more complicated activation and sup-
pression needed to produce competition between representations.

Moreover, the competing semantic pointers have the huge advantage over local
representations that they incorporate sensory, motor, emotional, and verbal information by virtue of their compression and decompression functions. Simple
models of competition cannot explain why attentional shifts bring different kinds
of experience because they lack the connections to sensory and motor processes
that are bound into and unpacked from semantic pointers.

Competition among semantic pointers is useful for explaining important psychological phenomena such as binocular rivalry and inattentional blindness.
Binocular rivalry occurs when different visual images are presented to each eye
and the brain fails to integrate them, so that the brain switches between the interpretations suggested by each eye as the result of competition between incompatible construals. Inattentional blindness occurs when people fail to notice obvious
events. I conjecture that such failures result from the ignored events being out-
competed by other representations encoded as semantic pointers.

Kinds of Consciousness

The semantic pointer approach can accommodate the view that there are various
kinds of consciousness associated with organisms of different levels of neural
complexity. Different kinds of consciousness all require neural representation and
semantic pointer competition but differ with respect to the extent of binding.

First, consider fish, the simplest organism for which behavioral evidence currently suggests the attribution of consciousness. It is plausible that fish feel pain
because their anatomy includes detectors for tissue damage whose stimulation
is transmitted to the trigeminal nerve and alters behavior such as avoiding novel
objects. Such alteration of behavior can be eliminated by a dose of morphine that
affects the fish's opioid system. It therefore seems that the attention of fish is affected by pain, just like the attention of humans, suggesting that for fish pain is a
conscious experience.

Semantic pointer competition can explain these results by supposing that the
fish have a representation of pain that competes with their representations of
novel objects such as a tower. Fish do not have a lot of neurons to work with,
roughly a million, so they are unable to produce complicated bindings and incapable of holding many representations in consciousness. Nevertheless, the pain
caused by a noxious substance such as vinegar is enough to distract them, even

though their semantic pointers may be built out of no more complex representations than *pain* or *tower*.

Mammals have a lot more neurons, approximately 50 million in a rat and hundreds of millions in a cat, enabling them to produce much more complex semantic pointers. A rat may be able to bind together complexes of sensory representations for smell, taste, and pain, enabling it to perform one-trial learning as occurs in taste aversion resulting from nausea. Mammals show many of the same pain behaviors as humans, such as eye closing, aggression, and writhing.

Finally, *self*-consciousness requires millions or billions of neurons to enable representations of self. Chapter 7 lists the few species so far shown experimentally to recognize themselves in mirrors. These organisms have enough neurons and neural processing to produce bindings that include the self. For example, the semantic pointer representing that you have an unpleasant pain in your toe can require binding together representations of pain, toe, unpleasantness, and yourself. Unpleasantness is an emotion that binds physiological information with cognitive appraisals, and the representation of yourself binds representations of your body, your memories, self-concepts, and current experiences. Semantic pointer competition can easily explain how consciousness operates at different levels of complexity corresponding to different capacities for producing semantic pointers by binding. With around 86 billion neurons, people can be self-conscious about complex situations that generate social emotions such as pride and embarrassment.

Unity and Disunity of Consciousness

Philosophers have tried to explain the unity of consciousness, for example when drinking a cup of coffee produces an integrated experience of taste, smell, touch, and vision. I maintain that unity results from mechanisms of binding and competition, whose infrequent failure can then explain the occasional disunity or disjointedness of consciousness. There are mental disorders that disrupt the unity of consciousness, such as schizophrenia (where experience is sometimes fragmented) and hemispatial neglect (where people fail to be aware of items on one side). Even in everyday life, consciousness can be fragmented when one is attending to multiple stimuli, so a theory of consciousness needs to be able to explain disunity as well as unity.

Unity of consciousness results from the binding of representations into semantic pointers. Consciousness overcomes confusion of unconnected experiences because neural mechanisms bind separate perceptual representations into ones that combine different modalities. For example, representation of a cup of coffee can consist of a pattern of firing in a neural group that draws on patterns of firing for coffee's color, taste, smell, and feel and also for the weight of the cup, the pleasure associated with drinking the coffee, and even the representation of the self as the owner of all these experiences. See chapter 12 for more on self-representation.

Although a high degree of unity is a common property of consciousness, semantic pointers can also explain why consciousness is sometimes fragmented. Binding usually produces multiple semantic pointers that compete for consciousness, but that process need not result in exactly one winner. Semantic pointer competition, like some lotteries, can have multiple winners, with several unified representations entering consciousness. For example, you can be conscious of your cup of coffee, your computer screen, and radio music all playing at once. Competition is not a winner-take-all process but rather one that allows for a small number of semantic pointers to outcompete other representations to surpass a threshold.

Hence consciousness is sometimes disorganized even in normal brains and can become even more so when brain functioning is disrupted by drugs or disease. For example, drugs like LSD (which disrupts serotonin) and diseases like schizophrenia (with excessive dopamine activity) interfere with normal binding and competition operations and hence produce abnormally disorganized conscious experiences.

It remains an open question why human consciousness is limited to a relatively small number of representations. The small capacity of consciousness may be an adaptive feature that encourages effective action, but it may also be an unfortunate bug arising as a side effect of insufficient numbers of neurons to produce large numbers of simultaneously active semantic pointers. In computer simulations, the mechanisms of neural representation, binding into semantic pointers, and semantic pointer competition all require large numbers of neurons—tens or hundreds of thousands. Forming more complex semantic pointers by recursive binding and allowing more of them to enter consciousness would require more neurons in the convergence zones where competition occurs.

Why has the brain not evolved to produce richer kinds of representations, for example relations among more than just three or four objects, and to allow more representations to be active in consciousness? The answer probably involves several factors, such as limitations on metabolism resulting from the energy needed to run many neurons, limitations on head size resulting from the challenges of childbirth, and lack of advantage for survival and reproduction of larger brains during the period around 100,000 years ago when modern humans evolved.

USES OF CONSCIOUSNESS

Consciousness challenges cognitive science as a major phenomenon to be explained. Identifying its neural mechanisms shows how to connect it with other important issues concerning innateness, learning, and change.

Innateness

Assuming against the behaviorists that consciousness exists, we can ask whether it is innate or learned. Consider again the criteria for innateness used in previous chapters: cultural universality, specific brain areas, animal precursors, adaptiveness during the evolutionary period, and absence of alternative explanations based on learning and culture.

No studies directly address the question of whether consciousness occurs in all human cultures, but there is an indirect argument based on emotion. As chapter 7 described, there is considerable debate about whether specific emotions are culturally universal, but no one challenges the view that emotions of some sort are part of every human culture. Because emotions are usually conscious, conscious experience is culturally universal. Different languages vary in the richness of their vocabulary for describing states of consciousness, but no one has identified a culture where people are incapable of describing their mental experiences. Hence cultural universality does seem to support the innateness of consciousness.

One contrary view was proposed by Julian Jaynes in a popular book from the 1970s. He claimed that high-level consciousness (awareness of awareness) was a cultural development that only occurred when the Ancient Greeks became sufficiently literate that they could attribute their experiences to their own minds rather than to messages from the gods. However, Jayne's hypothesis has little direct evidence for it, and it runs contrary to the commonness of emotion and sensation words in nonliterate societies.

Innateness would be supported by the existence of specific evolved brain areas, but there is no one brain area responsible for consciousness. There do, however, seem to be various brain areas that are strongly involved in consciousness including the dorsolateral prefrontal cortex and the cingulate cortex. There is no specific organ of consciousness that was selected for in the way that the heart or the liver evolved as organs with identifiable functions.

Did consciousness provide survival value during the period when humans or other animals evolved greater thinking capacity? It is difficult to say because of lack of historical evidence and uncertainty about the functionality of consciousness. It is possible that consciousness provided greater effectiveness in problem solving and learning, and it might also have contributed to human functioning in complex social groups of 50 to 100 people.

According to the social brain hypothesis, intelligence and human brain size increased because of their social advantages. Perhaps conscious experiences such as empathy helped people to understand the emotional states of others and thereby to predict, control, and coordinate their behaviors. But it is also possible that consciousness evolved much earlier, perhaps even in fish. Pain is adaptive in fish and other animals, because of its contribution to avoiding harm. But is feeling pain more adaptive than merely having pain? Does a cognitive bottleneck that requires competition for attention based on emotional significance increase the ability of fish and other organisms to survive and reproduce? I do not know.

Applying the fourth criterion for innateness, animal precursors, is similarly uncertain. Nonhuman animals lack verbal reports, but they show other kinds of behavior that seem to indicate consciousness in humans: writhing in pain, leaping with joy, and crying with grief as has been reported in elephants. If nonhuman animals are conscious, then humans could have inherited the capacity to be conscious along with the brain structures that they share with other mammals.

Finally, the claim that consciousness is innate should be evaluated with respect to alternative hypotheses, such as cultural learning. Although culture undoubtedly affects what people are conscious of, for example images on computer screens, little learning is required for newborn babies to have emotional experiences such as pain, distress, and satisfaction. Overall, therefore, it seems reasonable to speculate that the capacity for consciousness is innate.

Learning

Learning influences consciousness by providing new sensations and images, along with new concepts to interpret them. Enhanced sensory experiences of colors, taste, and sounds make people conscious of things that they were not aware of before. Moreover, acquiring new concepts like the color *chartreuse*, the taste *hamburger*, and the sound *saxophone* results in different conscious experiences. Learning can also produce new connection strengths that will enable some concepts to outcompete other ones to become more frequently conscious. For example, parents of a new baby become much more attuned to crying than they were previously.

Going in the other direction, consciousness affects learning because you are more likely to learn things to which you are paying attention. But consciousness is not the same as attention, and we can wonder what having a sensory or emotional experience adds to learning. Michelene Chi and her colleagues found that people who attack problems by explaining out loud to themselves what they are doing gain several advantages. They learn better, make more accurate assessments of what they understand, and use analogies more effectively.

Cognitive psychologists distinguish between two kinds of mental processes: ones that are fast, automatic, and unconscious and others that are slow, deliberate, and conscious. For example, brushing your teeth is not something you usually think about much, unless you have just been to the dentist who told you how to do a better job of it. Chapter 9 uses semantic pointer competition to explain how people switch between automatic and deliberate modes, which is important for failures of intention.

How Consciousness Changes

Changes in what you are conscious of can result from all the changes in perceptions, images, concepts, rules, and analogies described in previous chapters. For example, introducing a new concept or rule provides a new candidate for inclusion among the small class of mental representations that at any one moment can break through into consciousness.

The metaphors of "breaking through into" and "entering" consciousness misleadingly suggest that consciousness is a place or space that things go into. Rather, consciousness is a complex process involving large numbers of semantic pointers that are themselves processes of neural activity. Competition is also a process in which the excitatory and inhibitory interactions of hordes of neurons result in a few semantic pointers crossing a threshold of activation because their neurons are firing frequently.

What does it mean for a semantic pointer to cross a threshold? Recall that a semantic pointer is a pattern of firing in thousands or millions of neurons that can fire at different rates. Neurons fire slowly if they do not receive many inputs from other neurons that are firing rapidly, because of strong inputs from other neurons that are stimulated by sensation, memory, or cognitive evaluations. If many of the neurons in a semantic pointer are getting strong inputs, then their rapid firing enables a semantic pointer to outcompete other semantic pointers and contribute to conscious experience.

This consciousness threshold is analogous to the boiling threshold that occurs in water and other liquids. A pot of water consists of molecules, whose thermal energy (heat) results from their motion. In cool water, there are few molecules moving rapidly, but when water reaches the boiling point threshold of 100°C, the increases in motion of molecules turn the water into a gas, which has different properties from a liquid such as that escaping pots. Similarly, the increases in firing of numerous neurons in a semantic pointer can take it across a threshold into consciousness.

Consciousness changes more locally by shifts between different representations that result from new sensory information or internal reflection. For example, you may be mostly conscious of a text you are writing when a swerving car suddenly drags your attention back to driving. The emotional gestalt shifts described in chapter 7 are good examples of consciousness change, for example when you go quickly from feeling happy to feeling sad when you get some bad news.

SUMMARY AND DISCUSSION

Consciousness is one of the most challenging problems in all of science, but substantial progress is being made in understanding how brain mechanisms generate conscious experience. Simple conscious experiences such as sensations of colors, shapes, and sounds require only neural representations as patterns of firing that result from sensory inputs and internal processing. More complicated conscious experiences, such as your awareness that you are reading this text in a chair in a room, require the amalgamation of sensations and images into more complex representations through binding into semantic pointers. Recursive binding— bindings of bindings of bindings—can produce the most complicated kinds of conscious experience of which humans are capable, taking us from feelings to awareness to self-awareness. Consciousness is limited because recursive binding and competition among the resulting semantic pointers depend on processing by many neurons.

If consciousness had unlimited capacity, then humans could be consciously aware of all neural representations currently active. But such a broad range of experiences would be confusing and would interfere with the need to focus thought sufficiently to execute actions that are needed to accomplish goals. Hence consciousness requires a third mechanism beyond representation and binding: competition among semantic pointers determines which subset of them is sufficiently important to break through to the privileged territory of conscious experience.

The three mechanisms of neural representation, binding by convolution, and semantic pointer competition combine to explain important phenomena about consciousness. These phenomena include qualitative experience, onset and cessation, shifts of attention, different kinds of consciousness, and unity in diversity. The semantic pointer theory of consciousness also sheds light on phenomena concerning innateness, learning, and mental change.

Semantic pointers are crucial for these explanations because they show how neural mechanisms can account for all the mental representations that enter awareness, including perceptions (chapter 3), thoughts (chapters 4–6), and emotions (chapters 7). Although my descriptions in this book have been qualitative and metaphorical, many technical articles show that the mechanisms for semantic pointers such as binding and competition can be described with mathematical precision and used in computer simulations that generate expected results.

Other neural theories of consciousness have been proposed. Stanislas Dehaene has presented an impressive array of evidence to support his view that consciousness is the global availability of information encoded and broadcast in a neuronal workspace. This view appears complementary with the semantic pointer competition theory, because winning a competition can automatically broadcast information across numerous brain areas. Broadcast occurs through axonal connections from the neurons in the group for the winning semantic pointer to neurons in brain hubs such as the dorsolateral prefrontal cortex. Semantic pointers go beyond Dehaene's account in two main respects: specifying neural mechanisms for encoding information in ways that result in diverse qualitative experiences and using competition to explain what information is important enough to broadcast.

The semantic pointer theory of consciousness is also much more specific than "higher order" theories that maintain that consciousness results from representations of representations. Semantic pointers explain (a) the nature of first-order representations that result from neural activity and binding, (b) how representations of representations emerge from bindings of bindings, and (c) why some higher order representations rather than others become conscious because of the process of competition.

Explanation of consciousness as a neural process resulting from identifiable mechanisms avoids the ontological extravagance of dualism and panpsychism. The hypothesis of nonmaterial souls is simply not needed to explain conscious experience. Attribution of consciousness can reasonably be restricted to entities such as humans and other animals that exhibit behaviors that indicate the operation of attention and experience. The issue of machine consciousness can be set aside until computers and robots begin to be capable of behaviors best explained by ascription of internal experience.

Like emotion, consciousness on the semantic pointer account is both embodied and transbodied. Many of people's conscious experiences result from our internal and external senses and therefore depend heavily on the kinds of bodies we have. But recursive binding can also generate semantic pointers that valuably transcend the senses, enabling people to be consciously aware of attitudes attached to abstract ideas from the Ebola virus to black holes.

A plausible neural theory of consciousness is useful for issues to come. Chapter 9 shows its relevance to intentional action and the difference between thinking fast and slow. Chapter 12 extends it to a theory of self-consciousness as part of a general account of the self. In *Mind-Society*, consciousness resulting from neural mechanisms contributes to explanation of social phenomena such as religious experience and professional issues such as leadership. The relevance of neural theories of consciousness to refuting dualism is discussed in *Natural Philosophy* (chapter 2).

NOTES

This chapter includes excerpts from Thagard and Stewart 2014 (reprinted by permission of Elsevier) which provide much more technical detail about mathematical foundations and computer simulations that support the semantic pointer theory of consciousness. That paper also systematically criticizes the view of Tononi 2012 and Koch 2012 that consciousness is information integration. See further *Natural Philosophy* (chapter 2), which also considers philosophical objections to consciousness as semantic pointer competition. Semantic pointers integrate information but also encode it in multimodal ways and support competition for attention.

The opening quote is from Sutherland 1989 (p. 90). Freud was brilliant at generating hypotheses about emotions and the unconscious but inept at testing them. His ideas about drives, infantile sexuality, repression, the significance of dreams, and the efficacy of psychoanalysis have been superseded by developments in psychology and neuroscience.

For overviews of consciousness, see Blackmore 2012 and Bayne, Cleermans, and Wilken 2009.

For arguments that only humans teach, see Csibra and Gergeley 2011. Safina 2015 provides counterexamples such as killer whales. *Mind–Society* (chapter 11) explains teaching as the result of neural and social mechanisms.

For psychological theories of consciousness see Baars 1988, 2005. Philosophical discussions include Dennett 1991, 2017, Chalmers 1996, 2010, and Prinz 2012. For arguments against dualism, see Thagard 2010 and *Natural Philosophy*.

Important works on the neuroscience of consciousness include Crick 1994, Damasio 2012, and especially Dehaene 2014. Naci, Cusack, Anello, and Owen 2014 used functional magnetic resonance imaging to determine that participants watching a movie and reporting similar conscious experiences all displayed synchronized brain activity in the same frontal and parietal regions that support executive function. Koch, Massimini, Boly, and Tononi 2016 review research on the neural correlates of consciousness. MacDonald, Naci, MacDonald, and Owen 2015 discuss anesthesia and consciousness. Feinberg and Mallatt 2016 hypothesize about the evolutionary origins of consciousness. LeDoux and Brown 2017 present a higher-order theory of emotional consciousness.

Many cognitive scientists have maintained that attention functions by means of competition among representations: Crick and Koch 2003; Desimone and Duncan 1995; Maia and Cleeremans 2005; Slagter et al. 2010; Smith and Kosslyn 2007. Kang, Petzschner, Wolpert, and Shadlen 2017 provide evidence that consciousness involves crossing thresholds.

Chi 2005 describes the difficulty students have in understanding emergence. Because consciousness is affected by social interactions as well as molecular, neural, and psychological processes, it exemplifies multilevel emergence as explained in chapter 12.

Klauer et al. 2014 provide evidence that distracted driving is dangerous.

Braithwaite 2010 argues from behavioral experiments that fish feel pain, but Rose et al. 2012 challenge the arguments.

Jaynes 1976 claims that consciousness is a cultural development. Dunbar 2009 defends the social brain hypothesis, which is challenged by DeCasien, Williams, and Higham 2017.

On self-explanations, see Chi, deLeeuw, Chiu, and LaVancher 1994.

PROJECT

Show the application of the semantic pointer competition theory of consciousness to specific psychological phenomena such as inattentional blindness and the attentional blink. Extend the computational model to explain broadcast of information across different brain areas.

9

Action and Intention

Bertrand Russell joked in 1927: "Animals studied by Americans rush about frantically, with an incredible display of hustle and pep, and at last achieve the desired result by chance. Animals observed by Germans sit still and think, and at last evolve the solution out of their inner consciousness." From the previous chapters, it might seem that cognitive science views humans and other animals on the German model, mostly occupied with what goes on in their heads and only subordinately interested in acting in the world. But people perform hundreds of actions every day, from getting out of bed in the morning to turning off their lights at night. Much of our thinking in between is devoted to figuring out what actions to perform, for example what to wear, what to eat, what to say, and where to go. A full theory of mind needs to explain the connection between thoughts and actions.

Some of our actions are directed toward basic biological goals of survival and reproduction, for example drinking water when thirsty and flirting with potential mates. But humans also take actions in pursuit of many acquired goals, such as career success and artistic creation. For behaviorists, it would be enough to merely observe behaviors and connect them to environmental reinforcement, but cognitive science seeks to explain these behaviors by understanding the mental and neural processes that produce them. We need to know how actions arise from the various mental processes so far discussed, from sensation and imagery to emotions and consciousness.

Explanation should extend to the delightful range of activities listed by Robert Heinlein:

> A human being should be able to change a diaper, plan an invasion, butcher a hog, conn a ship, design a building, write a sonnet, balance accounts, build a wall, set a bone, comfort the dying, take orders, give orders, cooperate, act alone, solve equations, analyze a new problem, pitch manure, program a computer, cook a tasty meal, fight efficiently, die gallantly. Specialization is for insects.

Unfortunately, action and motor control are often ignored as central issues in cognitive science. Much thinking and feeling is directed toward doing things in the world, and a full theory of mind needs to show intimate interrelations among cognition, emotion, and action. Mechanisms involving semantic pointers provide the crucial connections.

In everyday psychology, the understanding of action is based on familiar concepts such as belief, desire, and intention. If you want to explain why your friends went to a concert, you may mention their desires to hear the bands that are playing, their beliefs that the concert is a good place to hear those bands, and the intentions they formed to buy tickets for the concert. But these concepts of intention, belief, and desire are too superficial to provide scientific explanations of people's actions.

Neural mechanisms can do better, if they serve to connect mental representations such as concepts, rules, analogies, and emotions to actions. Crucial to the connection are intentions, which can be understood as a special kind of semantic pointer, analogous to the semantic pointers that constitute beliefs (chapter 4) and desires (chapter 7). The result is a brain-based account of action roughly consistent with the everyday belief-desire-intention account but capable of deeper and broader explanations of important phenomena such as the frequent failure of good intentions.

One of the most disputed questions in philosophy is whether people have free will. Does a neural account of the relation between thought and action eliminate the idea of will, or does it suggest new ways of understanding it? I argue that something like conscious will may contribute to human action, but will and action lack central properties historically associated with free will.

Action is not just for individuals but often involves groups of interrelated people. Group actions are important for understanding social phenomena such as boardroom decisions in economics, government policies in politics, and family dynamics in sociology. A cognitive theory of action should explain not only the behavior of individuals but also the operations of whole groups. Many actions in the professions are social, for example when a hospital board implements a new practice, a jury declares an accused criminal guilty, or a school board decides to implement a new curriculum. Humanistic endeavors can also result from group actions, for example when musicians collaborate in a band or orchestra. Hence for social as well as psychological reasons, we need a comprehensive theory of the connections between thought and action.

PSYCHOLOGICAL THEORIES OF ACTION, INTENTION, AND WILL

In Western societies, people often explain actions by character traits such as kindness or meanness. Not all cultures are so psychological in their explanations, paying more attention to social environments. For example, in east and south Asia, people are more inclined to explain actions as resulting from social situations and responsibilities, rather than from psychological conditions like personality. In that respect, Asian attitudes are more behaviorist, looking for direct connections between environments and actions, without mediation by internal psychological states. Experimental results by psychologists show that Westerners tend to overestimate the role that personality plays in affecting behavior and underestimate the role that situations play.

In psychological explanations of behavior, people often invoke intentions, and philosophers and legal theorists have also noticed their importance. Many legal systems distinguish between homicides that are intentional from ones where the killer did not actually mean to kill the victim, which can be the difference between murder and involuntary manslaughter. The assumed role of intention might be captured by rules such as: *If a person desires an outcome and believes an action will produce the outcome, then the person will form the intention to perform the action; if a person forms the intention to perform an action, then the person performs the action.* These rules provide a connection from belief and desire to action, but they have far from universal accuracy, as everyone knows who has ever formed an intention and not followed through on it.

Common examples of intention breakdown include failures such as losing weight, exercising, working harder, treating family members better, and avoiding alcohol and drugs. Psychologists call the failures intention-action gaps, while philosophers describe them as resulting from weakness of will, also known by the Greek term *akrasia*.

In psychology, the most influential approach to action has been the theory of planned behavior of Fishbein and Ajzen, who say that behaviors result from intentions arising from a combination of attitudes, subjective norms, and perceptions of control. This account relies on experimental correlations among those factors, without any account of the psychological or neural mechanisms by which beliefs and attitudes cause intentions. Researchers in artificial intelligence have built programs that simulate behavior as the result of beliefs, desires, and intentions but follow philosophers in treating these as attitudes toward linguistic propositions, with little attention to nonverbal representations for images and emotions.

In everyday psychology, people assume that they are able to accomplish what they intend to do because of their willpower. But some psychologists and neuroscientists have been skeptical of the idea of the will, arguing that the widespread assumption that free conscious will produces actions is merely an illusion based on ignorance of psychological and neural causes. Resolving this question requires an evidence-based theory of the relation of intention, action, and will.

A strong theory of intention and action should be able to answer numerous questions. What are the beliefs, desires, and intentions that contribute to action? What role does consciousness play in determining actions? Why do intentions so frequently fail to produce desired actions? Do actions result from anything like will and willpower? How can people overcome intention-action gaps by changing their way of thinking about action? Can people increase self-control and self-regulation? A neural theory of intention and action can go a long way to answering these questions.

NEURAL MECHANISMS FOR ACTION AND INTENTION

Tobias Schröder, Terry Stewart, and I have defended the following theoretical claims:

1. Intentions are semantic pointers, which are patterns of activity in groups of spiking neurons that function as compressed representations by binding together other patterns.
2. Specifically, intentions bind representations of situations, emotional evaluations of situations, the doing of actions, and sometimes the self.
3. Intentions can cause actions because of neural processes that connect semantic pointers with motor instructions.

4. Intentions can fail to cause actions because of various kinds of disruptions affecting any of
   (a) Evaluation of the situation and doing.
   (b) Binding of the evaluation, situation, and doing.
   (c) Processes that connect the intention semantic pointer with motor processes.

Semantic pointers have already been thoroughly described, but the other claims require exposition.

Figure 9.1 displays how intentions can be construed as semantic pointers, patterns of neural firing that bind representations of situations and their evaluation along with actions and the self. All of these components are semantic pointers, that is, patterns of neural firing on their own. The binding operation relies on neural pattern transitions embedded in the connection weights between the respective groups of neurons. Bindings of semantic pointers are recursive, allowing bindings of bindings of bindings as long as there are enough neurons to produce a new pattern of firing.

Representations of situations include the physical features of the current environment, processed primarily through visual areas of the brain but sometimes also by olfactory, auditory, and tactile areas. In addition to all the sensations and images described in chapter 3, situations can also be represented by verbal beliefs construed as semantic pointers as in chapter 4.

As chapter 8 describes, people constantly evaluate situations with the emotion mechanisms of the brain, and these evaluations are an important building block of intentions. Brain areas with a prominent role in processing emotional evaluation

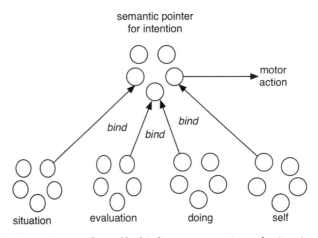

FIGURE 9.1 How intentions are formed by binding representations of a situation, evaluation, doing, and self. The sets of circles indicate neural groups. The arrows indicate flow of information performed by neural firing.

include (but are not limited to) the amygdala, insula, ventromedial prefrontal cortex, and the nucleus accumbens. The evaluations that get bound into intentions are emotions, which are themselves semantic pointers that bind appraisals and physiological perceptions.

Intentions also require representations of the intended actions, understood not as linguistic descriptions but as patterns of activation in areas of the brain involved in processing motor instructions. Neuroscientific evidence corroborates the notion of a nonverbal action vocabulary in premotor cortex, consisting of abstract representations of underlying motor programs in relation to goals.

Finally, intentions sometimes involve representations of the self, when people explicitly think of themselves as planning to do something. Intentions are about one's own actions in specific situations. Self-representations are semantic pointers that result from binding together self-related information in various modalities, from abstract verbal characterizations such as *student* to the associated emotional meanings to kinesthetic representations such as *shoveling snow*. Some of the components of self-representations are self-concepts, emotional memories, and the sensory-motor experience of agency.

Operation of intentions in the brain requires interactions among numerous areas, as shown in Figure 9.2. Relevant brain areas include sensory cortex, the thalamus, the prefrontal cortex, the basal ganglia, the amygdala, the anterior cingulate cortex, and the supplementary motor area. The connections shown are consistent with neural anatomy. The input to the system is through sensory cortex, with different patterns of firing for different stimuli. Output is from the motor area, where different patterns of neural firing represent the different actions the model can take.

Combining Figures 9.1 and 9.2, we get a model of actions as resulting from brain processes in many areas capable of forming and storing intentions as bindings of representations of situations, evaluations, doings, and sometimes the

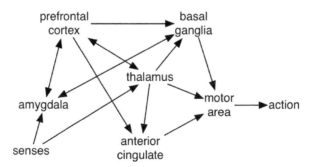

FIGURE 9.2 Model of intention with interactions of brain areas leading to action.

self. Contrary to simple explanations of action, emotions play an important role through the conduct of evaluations and the operation of the amygdala and interconnected brain areas. Actions may result from conscious processes if areas such as the dorsolateral prefrontal cortex and anterior cingulate are contributing, but consciousness is not required for action in routine behaviors such as driving a car.

Goals can be understood as semantic pointers similar to desires described in chapter 7. My goal to eat chocolate is a neural process that binds together my representation of myself, chocolate, eating, and the emotional state of wanting, which is a neural process that integrates appraisal and physiology to produce patterns of neural firing in the basal ganglia and other areas. The rules that govern action can sometimes be expressed verbally as in the statement *if I eat chocolate then I am happy*. But many actions result from rules and goals that operate without words because actions and goals can be neurally represented by multimodal semantic pointers, as in <*eat-chocolate*> → <*happy*>, supported by modal retention of sensory characteristics of chocolate and feeling happy.

What do semantic pointers add in this account of action? First, they provide a way of understanding intentions as plausible neural mechanisms, not just verbal descriptions. This understanding is sufficiently precise to generate mathematical analysis and computer simulations presented elsewhere. These simulations include an experiment where participants intentionally choose among six specific finger gestures; a situation where a person deliberately drinks alcoholic beverages; a case where a person resists temptation to smoke a cigarette; a case where intentions fail because of cognitive load; and an employment of an intention that takes an environmental cue and turns it into a course of action. The last simulation shows how neural representations can be combined, stored, and replayed.

Second, because this account of intention uses the same mechanisms invoked in all the other chapters of the book, they show how intention and action can be part of a unified neural theory of mind. Third, understanding intentions as semantic pointers displays both their embodied aspects tied to sensory-motor processes and their transbodied aspects tied to abstract representations of goals and the self.

USES OF ACTION AND INTENTION
The Causes of Action

The first question that a theory of action must answer is: How do mental states such as beliefs, desires, and intentions lead to action? A behaviorist would say that this is a dumb question, because there are no such things as mental states: actions result from the environment because of past contingencies of reinforcement. A dualist would say that beliefs, desires, and intentions provide reasons for action but do not cause actions, because the operations of a nonmaterial mind are not causal. An economist who believes that humans are always rational decision makers would say that beliefs, desires, and intentions contribute to calculations of expected utility, which people maximize in choosing actions. Neural mechanisms offer a scientific alternative to behaviorism, dualism, and rational choice.

The neural model presented in Figures 9.1 and 9.2 claims that beliefs, desires, and intentions contribute to action through their realization in semantic pointers. Senses supply information about the current situation, leading to perceptions through processing performed by brain areas such as the thalamus and visual cortex. Contrary to behaviorism, there are no simple rules relating sensory representations to actions, unlike George Foreman's "seafood diet": if I see food, I eat it. Instead, sensory representations of situations lead to action in ways that are dependent on cognitions and emotions, requiring interactions among brain areas such as the prefrontal cortex and the amygdala. The basal ganglia also play an important role in helping to evaluate situations. The results of all this processing are signals sent to motor areas that can command the muscles to carry out actions.

Making decisions requires predicting your emotional reactions to possible outcomes, for example whether you will be happy or frustrated by a job offered to you. Such forecasts require constructing an emotional image of yourself in the new situation, which requires remembering similar situations. But memory retrieval is influenced by your current emotional state, so remembering, imagery, and hence the forecasting of emotions may be biased by your current emotions. Decisions about major life changes are dependent on how bad you think things currently are and on how good you expect things to get. Both these evaluations depend on emotional judgments resulting from a neural process that combines cognitive appraisal and physiological perception to favor some actions over others.

The actual choice of what to do at a particular time is a matter of parallel constraint satisfaction with positive constraints determined by the extent to which different actions contribute to goals and negative constraints determined by the incompatibility of actions. For example, in work choice the positive constraints are the extent to which a job contributes to goals such as income and career success, and negative constraints are between alternatives such as taking a different job or retiring. When I made the major decision to retire from teaching in 2016, the positive constraints included accomplishing goals such as having more time to work on this *Treatise* and avoiding bureaucratic chores. The negative constraints included being unable at the same time to teach and to devote full attention to writing.

Hence actions are caused, but the process is extremely complicated, involving millions or billions of interacting neurons. On the cognitive side, sensory representations can be built up into more abstract beliefs, including verbal representations in humans. Nonverbal sensory representations and mental maps are all that animals need to generate their actions, but humans can operate with a combination of multisensory representations and verbal beliefs. Nonhuman animals lack language, but advanced ones such as mammals can also have multisensory representations that combine vision, smell, and touch.

Intentions, beliefs, and desires are all semantic pointers that are simultaneously cognitive and emotional, with the result that actions are caused by interactions of multiple semantic pointers across multiple brain areas. Observable actions such as walking across the room or speaking to somebody require muscle movements resulting from motor commands, but the motor commands are caused by the process shown in Figure 9.2.

Actions can also have social causes, because much of the perceptual information that contributes to human behavior involves interactions with other people, and many of the beliefs and desires that contribute to actions result from communication. Chapter 12 outlines how individual and social mechanisms interact.

Consciousness and Action

On the dualist commonsense view, consciousness is an essential contributor to action. For example, when you are making an important decision such as whether to accept a job offer, you are usually consciously aware of at least part of the process. You will most likely be thinking of some of the alternatives such as taking the job or going after another one. You may weigh the pros and cons of different actions by taking into account various goals such as salary and benefits. From the neural perspective in chapter 8, consciousness is only a small part of the process of decision making, because the semantic pointer representations of potential actions based on specific goals only become conscious when they outcompete other representations.

Many actions that we perform are the result of much less deliberative, automatic processes that do not need consciousness at all. Unless you are a beginner, you do not need consciousness to wash your hands, brush your teeth, or drive a car. These actions are the result of habits encoded in your brain by simple sensory-motor rules that do not require much cognitive and emotional processing. Because all action results from many interacting brain areas, it is more accurate to speak of automatic and deliberate *modes* of thinking, rather than of two systems or dual processes.

The modes of empathy described in chapter 7 are another example of the difference between thinking that is deliberate and conscious rather than automatic and unconscious. Which mode you are in at a particular time depends on both internal circumstances (firing patterns in groups of neurons for semantic pointers) and on external circumstances (sensory inputs from the environment including other people).

All decision making requires competition among competing actions performed by parallel constraint satisfaction, but this competition is not always sufficient for consciousness. Mundane winners of action competition such as turning left at the end of the street may not generate enough neural activity to enable the relevant semantic pointers to outcompete other semantic pointers for the limited resources of consciousness. A major contributor to such neural activity is emotion, the process of evaluating situations through a combination of cognitive appraisal and physiological perception. Ordinary unemotional decisions about how to act result from parallel constraint satisfaction but lose out in the competition for consciousness to semantic pointers more relevant to important goals such as survival and personal relationships.

Intention-Action Gaps

To explain why people so frequently fail to follow through on their intentions, we need to combine the semantic pointer account of intentional action with the semantic pointer competition theory of consciousness. Intention-action gaps (weakness of will) result from a mismatch between conscious deliberations and unconscious processes leading to action. Suppose, for example, that someone offers you a big piece of chocolate cake. On the conscious side, you may be thinking that the cake has too many calories and too much cholesterol to be compatible with your goals of looking good and being healthy. But the sight and smell of the cake activates other, more basic goals, such as eating food that is tasty because of the fat and carbohydrates. Consciously, you may think that the goals of health and attractiveness should outweigh the goals of eating fatty and sweet food, but what wins out in the neural process of constraint satisfaction does not always depend on conscious deliberation.

Identifiable circumstances distract mental processing away from the deliberate mode toward the automatic mode. Suppose you are tired, hungry, stressed, or under cognitive load with too much to think about at once. Then conscious deliberation carried out by areas such as the prefrontal cortex will not have the opportunity to vanquish more biologically basic goals such as eating sugar and fat. Intention-action gaps are simply the result of neural processes in which physically powerful goals dominate socially acquired goals that are verbally expressed.

Some philosophers have been puzzled at how weakness of will can even be possible, because it seems that a rational agent would naturally do whatever is in his or her own best interests. Rational choice theorists have the same problem: How could people fail to maximize expected utility? In contrast, psychologists recognize the frequency of intention-action gaps where people act against their overall best interests. A more realistic neural account of decision making does not assume that the psychological process is inherently conscious or optimal but rather sees conscious deliberation as vying with more automatic processes that can easily triumph under conditions such as fatigue, hunger, stress, or cognitive load. Working-memory capacity, which is crucial for conscious decisions, shrinks under conditions of stress. From this perspective, conscious deliberation is by no means the norm, just one of various processes that has to compete for scarce cognitive resources. Amazingly, people sometimes actually manage to do the right thing: to lose weight, reduce consumption of alcohol and drugs, stop gambling, avoid infidelities, and get work done rather than engage in multislacking activities such as watching TV, surfing the Web, and nibbling high-calorie food.

The semantic pointer theory of intention and action can readily explain procrastination, where people delay working on their tasks despite their deliberate commitment to get those tasks done. Procrastination is caused by the unpleasantness of the task along with inability to override the resulting negative emotion. To overcome procrastination, the initial negative emotion associated with a task needs to be replaced with more positive appraisals of the long-term consequences of tackling the task, requiring cognitive effort in the deliberate mode.

Implementation Intentions

One of the few techniques known to help people overcome intention-action gaps is employment of implementation intentions, which are rules that people form to behave in particular ways under specific circumstances. For example, if you are going to a restaurant or dinner party where you suspect that tempting cake will be served, then you can form the explicit intention to act in accord with this rule: *If someone offers cake, then say NO and look for something healthier to eat.* There is of course no guarantee that this implementation intention will actually be carried out once the cake arrives. But forming the implementation intention and rehearsing it may help you to remain in conscious mode and enable your reflectively preferred goals of health and attractiveness to overcome the automatic goals of gobbling tasty but fattening food. Having conscious implementation intentions can help people to acquire healthy habits represented in multimodal rules such as *⟨hungry⟩ → ⟨eat-carrot⟩*.

Changing Intentions

Adding implementation intentions is a simple kind of intention change, but there are additional kinds such as deleting old intentions, changing the strength of an intention, and replacing one intention by another. For example, you may intend to work hard next month, then adopt a new intention of taking a vacation. How does this work?

One major source of intention change is goal change. If you abandon your goal of having lots of money and adopt a different goal of having fun, then your intentions will quickly change to concern new actions that help to accomplish the new goals. Even if you keep your old goals, you may change your intentions when you realize that different actions are better for accomplishing the goals, so that belief revision produces new intentions. Both belief revision and goal adjustment result from parallel constraint satisfaction in which many representations interact to form a coherent system. This process is unconscious, but conscious processing can also affect behavior, for example when people reflectively decide that they need implementation intentions to overcome intention-action gaps. How do people move between conscious and unconscious processing?

Thinking Fast and Slow

Dual process "theories" of cognition are popular in cognitive and social psychology, distinguishing between two "systems" that are (1) fast, automatic, involuntary, and unconscious versus (2) slow, deliberate, controlled, and conscious. This distinction is useful for classifying mental phenomena, such as the difference between driving a car without thinking about what you are doing and driving with conscious attention. But the distinction does not constitute a theory, because it lacks the mathematical specifications found in theories in physics and the descriptions of mechanisms found in theories in biology and cognitive science. Justifying the postulation of two systems would require specifying different brain mechanisms, for which there is currently no evidence. Hence it is better just to speak of two modes of thinking, fast and slow, rather than two processes or two systems.

The Semantic Pointer Architecture can explain the differences in the operation of the fast and slow modes when it includes the theory of consciousness from chapter 8. The crucial theoretical questions are

1. What are the mechanisms that explain the fast mode?
2. What are the mechanisms that explain the slow mode?

3. What are the mechanisms that produce transitions from the fast to the slow mode?

4. What are the mechanisms that produce transitions from the slow to the fast mode?

Answering these questions provides an explanation, not just a description, of the difference between automatic and deliberate behaviors.

The first question is easy, because the fast mode is accomplished by the basic Semantic Pointer Architecture described in chapter 2, especially Figure 2.7. Action selection takes place because of interactions among brain areas that perform functions such as interpreting sensory inputs, evaluating rewards, and limited access to working memory. Thinking is fast because all of these processes are performed by billions of neurons operating in parallel, without conscious will.

What makes the slow mode different is readily explained by the mechanisms for consciousness described in chapter 8. Competition among semantic pointers carried out through inhibitory links among the neurons that compose them allows only a few of them to cross the threshold of consciousness, which results from the firing rates of the neurons in the semantic pointers. The slow mode draws much more heavily on working memory than the fast mode. Working memory contains only a small fraction of the representations stored in long-term memory, and consciousness is achieved by only some of the representations in working memory. The result is a bottleneck that dramatically slows down processing to operating with a small number of representations. Conscious awareness gives people the feeling that they are acting deliberately and voluntarily and that they are in control of their actions. The next section on the will raises the question of whether these feelings are accurate.

Transitions between fast and slow modes occurs because of the same mechanisms that produce and eliminate consciousness. If you are in a dreamless sleep, you are in neither mode, because no actions are being selected. Waking brings some amount of consciousness, although many activities such as putting on your socks can be done automatically. If you are in fast mode, and the combination of external stimuli and internal processing increases the firing rates of the neurons in a neural group for a semantic pointer, then the brain switches to slow mode. Implementation intentions, construed as semantic pointers that are important enough to become conscious, are one factor that can contribute to the transition from fast to slow and make actions more deliberate.

Alternatively, if you are in slow mode and factors such as fatigue, stress, and cognitive load reduce the activity of conscious semantic pointers below a threshold, then the brain switches back to the fast, automatic mode. Implementation intentions are lost, and involuntary behaviors dominate.

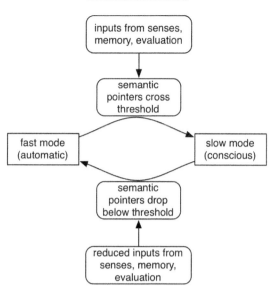

FIGURE 9.3 Transitions between fast and slow modes resulting from semantic pointer mechanisms.

These transitions are illustrated in Figure 9.3. Whether semantic pointers cross the consciousness threshold is determined by inputs from the senses, memory, and evaluation of importance including emotions, as well as by competition among the semantic pointers. Strong inputs lead to transition from the fast mode to the slow mode, but weakening of inputs leads to transition in the opposite direction. These mechanisms show that it is misleading to talk of dual processes and two systems rather than just of two modes, which result from neural firing, semantic pointers, and competition.

The Will

By far the most contentious philosophical issue connected with action and intention concerns the existence of free will, a topic important for ethics because of the common view that moral and legal responsibility require free action. Some neuroscientists and psychologists have argued that empirical findings make it implausible that free will exists. Dualist philosophers reject these claims out of hand, but even some nondualists argue for conceptions of free will that they think are compatible with increased neuropsychological understanding of mental causation. All of these debates have taken place without any specification of the neural mechanisms that plausibly link intention and action.

In a 2014 blog post, I boldly asserted that there is no free will because there is no will, but I later changed my mind. The reason that I had concluded that there is no will is that the model of intention and action in Figure 9.2 does not seem to have any place for will. The interactions of multiple brain areas, such as the prefrontal cortex, the anterior cingulate, and the amygdala, yield actions without any operation that involves will. But combining the neural model of intention and action with neural theories of emotion and consciousness provides a way of understanding what will might be.

On the expanded view, will is the ability to make choices resulting from the interaction of numerous brain areas that perform intention, action, emotion, and consciousness. In accord with the distinction between automatic and deliberate modes of cognition, there are both automatic and deliberate actions. Many of our routine actions are largely unconscious, for example putting on a coat by inserting one arm and then the other.

At the other extreme, consider a decision that I made in 2014 about whether to accept an invitation to speak at a conference in India. On the one hand, I wanted to visit India and see the Taj Mahal in Agra, the site of the conference. On the other hand, the two flights each way would take almost 24 hours and involve substantial amounts of jet lag, severely cutting into my sabbatical plans to work on this book. The decision not to go to India took me several days and was based on extensive conscious deliberation, explainable by combining the neural model of intention in this chapter with the semantic pointer theory of consciousness in chapter 8. Similarly, I had to change my automatic process of putting my coat on with my right arm first, because I had a sore left shoulder. Making this change required consciously reminding myself to insert my left arm before the right one.

In these cases, conscious will operates when semantic pointers such as *India, flights, coat,* and *shoulder* become conscious by outcompeting many other representations in my brain by virtue of their emotional significance and goal relevance. I was conflicted about going to India but needed to decide, and in the other case I wanted to avoid producing pain in my shoulder. The operation of these concepts enables them to become bound into intentions that also achieve consciousness, such as *Don't go to India* and *Put my left arm in the coat first.* The consciousness of these intentions results from neural firings in areas such as the dorsolateral prefrontal cortex, which contribute to actions through the interactive process shown in Figure 9.2. When I emailed to decline the India trip, and when I first started putting my coat on differently, my actions were caused in part by a deliberate process involving conscious goals, emotions, and intentions. In contrast to actions that result automatically from unconscious processing, we could say that the will is the use of conscious deliberate processes resulting from intentions of which we are aware.

If the will exists as this kind of complicated neural process, is it free? Obviously, such will is not free in the way that the actions of a nonmaterial, immortal soul are supposed to be free, operating independently of causal forces. My decision to turn down the trip to India had many causes operating at neural and molecular levels. However, my decision was apparently unaffected by external coercion, internal mental illness, and random quantum fluctuations. More positively, my decision required much conscious deliberation as opposed to routine automatic behaviors. Therefore, I now think that there are at least some cases of human action that result from direction of action by deliberate conscious control.

On the other hand, there are many limitations to will understood as this kind of process. First, it depends on causal processes of neural firing that include potentially nonrational factors, such as the physiological changes that contribute to emotions. Second, as described in chapter 8, people do not have conscious, deliberate control over whether they are in automatic mode or deliberate mode, because they do not have conscious control over which semantic pointers win the competition to become conscious. Conscious deliberate actions are different from automatic ones, but no one gets to choose which mode is operating at a particular moment. Hence I am reluctant to say that will is free, even in cases of conscious deliberation.

Alternatively, I propose to label this kind of will "freeish." Freeish will occurs in deliberate, conscious decisions that are not influenced by external coercion or internal mental illness. This characterization may not be all that one would want from a religious perspective, but it suffices for allowing human actions to be valuable, meaningful, and responsible. In legal and moral contexts, it is socially appropriate to hold people responsible for freeish actions. One of the important roles of socialization and legal systems is to encourage people to have implementation intentions that enable them to operate in deliberate rather than automatic mode in cases where they may cause harm to others. If you want to make your will more freeish, try to use implementation intentions to help accomplish your most important goals. For example, if you have the goal of getting more work done but are easily distracted by the Internet, plan to close your browser and start work at a set time each morning.

Sometimes people have difficulty carrying out actions because they are ambivalent; they just cannot decide whether to do one action, or a different action, or nothing. On the belief-desire-intention model of action, ambivalence occurs because some beliefs and desires support one action, whereas other beliefs and desires support another action, resulting in a tie. Similarly, on the rational expectations view of decision making, ambivalence could result because the expected utility of one action is close or equal to the expected utility of another action, so that there is no basis for choosing between them.

The neural mechanism account of action provides a different explanation of ambivalence that is much more dynamic. On this view, ambivalence does not result from ties but from emotional gestalts. Attention to particular aspects of the situation can lead you to flip back and forth, just as happens in perceptual gestalt switches like the cube in Figure 3.1. If action results from competition among semantic pointers, then what wins the competition can be subject to local influences, such as which aspects of the problem are currently conscious.

For example, if you are trying to decide between two job offers, one of which offers more money while the other has more interesting work, then you may be ambivalent: not in the sense of there being a tie but in the sense that you switch back and forth depending on which goal is more salient at a particular time. If you are short of money because you do not have enough to cover a bill that just arrived, then the goal of making money will be more salient and will tip you toward taking the high-paying job. On the other hand, if you talk to someone who is enjoying the work that goes with the other job, then you may tip toward that choice. From this perspective, ambivalence is not a matter of ties among choices but rather of tipping points between emotional gestalts reflecting the overall desirability of the different choices.

If will is only freeish, what is willpower? Neural explanations of consciousness and intention make it implausible that willpower is a magical property of the soul, and they also undermine the popular metaphor that willpower is like a muscle that can be strengthened by effort and depleted from overuse. A more neutral characterization is that willpower is the ability to resist short-term temptations in order to meet long-term goals. Oscar Wilde said that he could resist anything except temptation, but most people can resist at least some temptations at least some of the time. Such resistance is crucial for avoiding intention-action gaps with respect to eating and other behaviors. From a neural perspective, what gives people the ability to pursue long-term goals without distraction from temptations?

This ability results from many cognitive and emotional processes. To take a concrete example, suppose that your long-term goal is career success, and your temptation is to spend time on Facebook rather than working hard. First, your success in resisting temptation will depend on how much you care about success and how much you enjoy Facebook. Both caring and enjoying are emotional, so the relative intensity depends on the binding of the representations for career and Facebook with semantic pointers for emotions that in turn bind appraisal and physiology.

Resisting temptation is a lot easier if you have a strong emotional pull toward career success and only a weak inclination toward social media.

A second factor in resisting temptation is the mental balance between automatic and deliberative modes of decision and action. If you are in deliberate mode, then you operate more slowly and consciously, allowing you to reflect that you really do care more about success than you do about Facebook. So willpower can partly be a function of the extent to which you are prone to making decisions consciously or unconsciously. Having strong goals such as career success can help to keep you in deliberate mode, because the goals' emotional intensity can help them to break through the consciousness threshold and to outcompete distractions. The result can be actions that are more influenced by the prefrontal cortex than the amygdala or nucleus accumbens.

A third factor in having willpower is learning techniques such as implementation intentions to deal with situations in which intention-action gaps are endemic. I love dark chocolate, but I made a conscious decision not to keep it at home, because I know that when I am tired, hungry, or stressed I am likely to eat too much of it. Conscious planning can thereby contribute to the successful decision making usually attributed to the possession of willpower, which can now be reinterpreted as the advantageous operation of neural mechanisms for emotions, consciousness, and intentions.

SUMMARY AND DISCUSSION

Actions results from the same neural mechanisms used in previous chapters to explain sensation, imagery, concepts, rules, analogies, emotions, and consciousness. Neural representations govern motor operations such as walking and talking. Action selection, however, goes beyond simple associations of perception and motor control, because of deliberations in humans using beliefs, desires, and intentions. These three kinds of mental representation should not be understood as abstract propositional attitudes but rather as semantic pointers that bind multimodal information into rich neural representations that compress sensory, emotional, and verbal information into a form that can be used for directing action. Which actions are selected depends on parallel constraint satisfaction, not on logical inference as in the belief/desire/intention scheme or on simple calculation as in the expected utility model.

The basic neural mechanisms of representation, binding into semantic pointers, and competition among pointers function to produce actions, just as they did with inference, emotion, and consciousness. Intentions are semantic pointers that bind representations of the relevant situation, doing, evaluation, and self. Intentions are embodied in that representing the situation includes perceptions, doing the action includes motor representations, and performing the evaluation is an emotional process that includes physiology.

But intentions can also be transbodied, when representations for the situation, cognitive appraisal, and the self are abstracted by recursive bindings that far surpass sensory-motor inputs. For example, religious persons may mark a situation as the result of divine will, perform appraisals based on goals like getting to heaven, and think of themselves as holy. In nonreligious persons also, intentions can be transbodied when they derive from abstract ideals such as justice and truth and are aimed at nonmotor actions such as solving an intellectual problem.

Consciousness is not a requirement for action but can work to support actions that go against more immediate inclinations based on bodily desires. Intention-action gaps arise because of a mismatch between our conscious goals and biological drives. The ubiquity of weakness of will is not a philosophical puzzle but a psychological commonplace because of this mismatch. Self-control and self-regulation are difficult but can be enhanced by adopting techniques such as implementation intentions and by avoiding factors such as fatigue, hunger, stress, and cognitive overload that contribute to the diminishment of conscious control of action.

Understanding actions as resulting from neural mechanisms makes it tempting to conclude that there is no such thing as will and that the traditional way of explaining actions in terms of conscious intentions needs to be abandoned. Such abandonment would be hasty, however, because there are situations where consciousness plays a part. There are many unconscious actions, but there are also actions where consciousness, resulting from semantic pointer competition, plays a causal role in determining which actions people make. In this sense, will exists, approximately, even though it does not play the noncausal, nonmaterial role assumed by dualist conceptions.

But will is not free absolutely in being immune from causal forces. Rather, it is a neural process connected with external causality via the senses in physical and social environments. For social and political reasons discussed in *Mind–Society*, as well as for ethical reasons considered in *Natural Philosophy*, it is important to retain some notion of freedom or autonomy. One crucial distinction is between (a) actions whose causes are primarily internal through neural processing of beliefs, desires, and intentions and (b) actions whose causes are external as a result of coercion by others against a person's own beliefs, desires, and intentions. Another crucial distinction is between neural mechanisms for normal functioning and ones that are disrupted by diseases such as schizophrenia or by drugs such as alcohol. Actions can be deemed freeish when they result from normal thinking in deliberate mode, without disruption by external coercion or internal defects. Some people will lament the loss of absolute free will and immortality that accompanies the revolutionary view of mind as brain. But we should rejoice over the banishment of noxious ideas like retribution and fear of eternal damnation. Blame and punishment can be justified when they have good social consequences, not because actions are uncaused.

The theory of action has implications for general questions about the nature of the self in chapter 12. Questions about the causes of actions and decisions are also relevant to issues discussed in *Mind–Society*, including economic choices, political decisions, mental illness, and legal responsibility. Issues about responsibility arise in *Natural Philosophy* in connection with ethics and justice.

NOTES

The semantic pointer theory of intention is from Schröder, Stewart, and Thagard 2014, from which extracts here are reprinted by permission of Wiley. This paper includes mathematical analysis, computer simulations, and many more references.

The joke about American and German animals is from Russell 1960 (originally 1927), p. 33. The list of activities is from Heinlein 1974 (p. 248).

On differences in Asian versus Western views of action, see Nisbett 2003 and Heine 2015.

On intention, see Fishbein and Ajzen 1975 for psychology, Bratman 1987 for philosophy, and Wooldridge 2000 for artificial intelligence, where BDI (belief-desire-intention) models are popular. Aflalo et al. 2015 identify neurons in the posterior parietal cortex that represent action planning and that can be used by paralyzed patients to control robotic arms.

According to Glenberg, Witt, and Metcalfe 2013, actions can also influence perceptions, so there should be feedback loops in Figure 9.2 from action back to cognitive processes. Blouw, Eliasmith, and Tripp 2016 describe a spiking neural model of action planning. Floresco 2015 describes the role of the nucleus accumbens (part of the basal ganglia) in action selection.

On decision making as parallel constraint satisfaction, see Thagard and Millgram 1995 and Thagard 2000.

Gollwitzer 1999 provides evidence for the efficacy of implementation intentions.

Arnsten 2009 reviews the effects of stress on prefrontal cortex.

On dual process theories and Systems 1 and 2, see Kahneman 2011 and Evans and Stanovich 2013. Spunt 2015 summarizes the problems with mapping System 1 and System 2 onto brain anatomy.

My view of will is akin to Norman and Shallice 1986 (p. 15), who say that will is "direction of action by deliberate conscious control." My description of willpower is from http://www.apa.org/helpcenter/willpower.aspx. See also Baumeister and Tierney 2011; Job, Walton, Bernecker, and Dweck 2013; Lopez, Hofmann, Wagner, Kelley, and Heatherton 2014; and Sripada, Kessler, and Jonides 2014. Shariff et al. 2014 provide evidence that a mechanistic account of free will reduces retribution.

For philosophical discussions of free will, see Dennett 2003 and Mele 2009. Skeptics about traditional views of will include Greene and Cohen 2006, Harris 2012, Libet 1985, and Wegner 2003. Roskies and Nichols 2008 and Roskies 2006 are skeptical about the skeptics but rely too much on popular opinion concerning the compatibility of neural mechanisms and traditional responsibility. *Natural Philosophy* (chapter 10) has a more thorough discussion of free will. *Mind–Society* (chapter 11) looks at free will in relation to criminal responsibility.

PROJECT

Integrate the intention model in this chapter with the models of consciousness (chapter 8) and emotion (chapter 7) to produce a full computational model of will. Determine its applicability to experiments about free will such as Soon, Brass, Heinze, and Haynes 2008. Use the account of thinking fast and slow in Figure 9.3 to model psychological experiments that have been explained in terms of dual processes.

10

Language

The novelist Virginia Woolf said that language is wine upon the lips. Of course, language is not really wine but nevertheless is *like* wine in being enjoyable and stimulating, even sometimes intoxicating. The metaphorical use of language is one of many linguistic phenomena that need to be explained by cognitive science, along with people's more basic abilities to generate and comprehend utterances. A deep understanding of how the brain works should also explain how human beings in all cultures manage to learn to speak at least one language.

Language and thought in general require an understanding of syntax, semantics, and pragmatics. With respect to language, syntax concerns the grammatical structure of sentences, for example the way in which typical English sentences have the word order subject-verb-object, where the subject and object are nouns. For example, in English one would usually say "The giraffe ate the leaf" rather than "The giraffe the leaf ate," whereas in other languages such as Latin it is standard to place the verb at the end of the sentence.

Semantics concerns the meaning of words and sentences, particularly how the meaning of sentences such as "The giraffe ate the leaf" derives from the meaning of words "giraffe," "ate," and "leaf." Pragmatics concerns the purposes and context of linguistic utterances, for example why it might be appropriate for someone to communicate by using the sentence "The giraffe ate the leaf" in a particular context that makes it clear what "the giraffe" represents. Spoken language also requires attention to phonology, concerning the sounds that are used for conveying words and sentences to other people.

Because of the pioneering work of Noam Chomsky, the dominant approach to language since the 1960s has concentrated on syntax, with semantics, pragmatics, and phonology playing subordinate roles. However, other prominent linguists such as Ray Jackendoff have challenged this syntax-first approach and argued that the study of language needs to integrate syntax with semantics and phonology. The main objective of this chapter is to show how ideas based on semantic pointers can be useful for carrying out this integration. I already suggested in chapter 6 how analogy needs to be appreciated through the integration of syntax, semantics, and pragmatics, and this lesson holds for language and thought in general. Semantic pointers reveal how language, like analogy, can operate in the brain by simultaneously satisfying syntactic, semantic, and pragmatic constraints.

Obviously, language is not just processing in individual brains but also serves to enable people to interact with each other. Language has many social functions, including communication, persuasion, building relationships, and the amusement that comes from telling jokes. Language contributes to all the social phenomena discussed in *Mind–Society* such as economic trading, political argument, social coordination, religious rituals, and legal deliberation. Hence the social sciences and the professions can all benefit from a deep understanding of language deriving from a neural account of how brains work to support social communication. The Semantic Pointer Architecture provides a promising account of syntax, semantics, and pragmatics, with applications to advanced applications such as conceptual blending and metaphor.

By going beyond the syntax-first approach to language, I challenge some widespread assumptions about how the mind works. It is a mistake to say that the mind/brain uses a language of thought, which assumes that mental processes are akin to purely linguistic ones. Without denying that language is an important aspect of human thinking, we can recognize that it is based on a common neural framework that also supports processes such as perception, imagery, and emotion. This appreciation takes us beyond the syntactic dream that has dominated approaches to mind in linguistics and philosophy, toward a full appreciation of how brains operate by integrating syntax with semantics and pragmatics.

SYNTAX FIRST: CHOMSKY

In the 1950s, Noam Chomsky developed a revolutionary approach to linguistics based on mental structures and processes. At the time, linguistics was dominated by behaviorists, who tried to explain language as merely actions resulting from learning by reinforcement. Chomsky presented compelling arguments that the behaviorist approach to language was incapable of explaining the creativity and learnability of language. Language is creative in that people can easily generate new sentences that have never previously been formed. For example, before Virginia Woolf no one had ever uttered the evocative sentence that language is like wine upon the lips. But people have no problem recognizing it as a grammatical sentence in English and attaching some meaning to it. Language is also creative in its capacity to produce complex embeddings, for example by extending Wolfe's remark: if language is like wine upon the lips, then music is like chocolate upon the tongue. Speakers of all languages are capable of generating an unlimited variety of sentences that can be understood by others in a way that cannot be explained by supposing that language is just verbal behavior resulting from simple kinds of association. Rather, according to Chomsky, language needs to be explained by the operation of complex mental structures and processes.

Such hypotheses are also important for explaining the speed with which children in all cultures learn their local language. There are thousands of different languages, but children rarely have difficulty acquiring fluency in the language to which they are first exposed. Chomsky argued that the ease with which children learn a first language requires an innate linguistic ability, which he called a universal grammar. Although the grammars of individual languages differ substantially, for example in word order and the way they make plurals and possessives, all humans are born with the ability to expect particular kinds of linguistic structures, which facilitates their learning of the language used around them. The Chomskyan approach to language differed markedly from behaviorism in two main ways: first in supposing that mental structures and processes are needed to explain how language works, and second in proposing that many of these mental structures and processes are innately built into the human brain.

From the 1950s through the 1990s, Chomsky offered a series of proposals about the nature of universal grammar and the fundamental structures and processes that explain the creative generation and learnability of language. These proposals focused on syntax, leaving phonology and semantics to be worked on independently; and pragmatics was totally ignored. Chomsky's early proposals concerned numerous kinds of transformations that were thought to govern syntax in English and other languages, for example the transformation that can turn a declarative sentence such as "Ottawa is the capital of Canada" into a question "Is Ottawa the capital of Canada?" His latest proposal claims that syntax can be derived from two fundamental transformations, merge and move. Merge builds up syntactic structures by combining lexical items into phrases and by joining phrases with each other, and move serves to transform some syntactic structures into new ones. For example, merge can build "see giraffe" out of "see" and "giraffe," and move can transform the resulting sentence into another sentence such as "The giraffe was seen."

These proposals assumed that the unique human capacity for syntax was central to explaining language use. When critics pointed out that ordinary speech often violates proposals about syntactic structure, Chomsky insisted that he was not interested in performance but rather in competence, the abstract ability to produce grammatical utterances that might not actually be realized under normal circumstances. He was not interested in weird utterances like "This sentence no verb."

Although Chomskyan linguistics remains dominant in the field, substantial alternatives have arisen. Chomsky is often criticized for retreating from the psychological goal of explaining how people actually use language to the much more abstract, nonempirical concern with competence. Alternative approaches have been developed that attempt to overcome these limitations by accommodating semantics, phonology, and sometimes even pragmatics. These alternatives include the cognitive grammar of Ronald Langacker, the parallel architecture of Ray Jackendoff, and the cognitive linguistics of Gilles Fauconnier and George Lakoff. According to Jackendoff, the function of grammar is to mediate between sound and meaning, so syntax cannot be considered as an abstract set of structures and processes independent of phonology and semantics. The Semantic Pointer Architecture is well equipped to develop this approach while illuminating processes of meaning, conceptual blending, and metaphor.

INTEGRATING SYNTAX, SEMANTICS, AND PHONOLOGY

To understand how grammar, meaning, and sound are tied together, we need to consider both words and sentences.

Words

Ray Jackendoff is a distinguished linguist who over several decades has developed a serious alternative to what he calls "syntactocentric" linguistics. Jackendoff does not ignore syntax but argues that a superior approach to it can be developed by appreciating that syntax is not the sole source of generativity, the production of complex linguistic structures from simpler ones. Jackendoff thinks that phonology and semantics are equally generative and need to be treated on an equal footing with syntax. He advocates a parallel architecture in which the mind processes phonological and semantic information at the same time as syntactic information. This architecture enables Jackendoff to explain important phenomena in language, including the role that the lexicon (catalogue of mental words) plays in language processing, and the generation of meanings in increasingly complex words, idioms, and sentences. According to Jackendoff, a theory of syntax should identify the minimum structure needed to mediate between phonology and meaning.

Unfortunately, Jackendoff does not specify neural mechanisms that could carry out the kind of parallel processing required for the integration of phonology, syntax, and semantics. He recognizes the limitations of traditional neural networks for capturing the rich syntactic structure that is needed for an understanding of grammar. He points out serious challenges to providing a neural explanation of the full range of linguistic phenomena. For example, the binding problem is how to keep track of the different parts of a sentence such as "The little star is beside a big star," where the two occurrences of the word "star" play different grammatical roles. Let us now see how the Semantic Pointer Architecture can not only deal with these problems but also more generally handle Jackendoff's agenda of integrating syntax, phonology, and semantics.

To begin, consider a simple word such as "giraffe." Jackendoff claims that words and all other linguistic entities combine sound, meaning, and grammar. Figure 10.1 shows how semantic pointers can carry out this kind of combination using the binding operation described in chapter 2. The word "binding" is often used in linguistics to describe the reference of pronouns and other expressions, for example when "he" refers to Barack Obama. But Jackendoff uses the term, as I do, to describe the function of tying together different features in a representation like

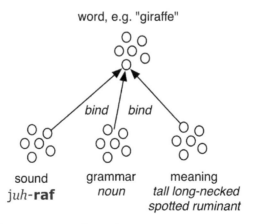

FIGURE 10.1 Mental representation of a word as a semantic pointer integrating phonology, syntax, and semantics.

a perception. Both images and sentences need to distinguish a car being on a road from a road being on a car, which requires binding the representations of car and road to the different roles of being on and being under.

Jackendoff mentions the neural synchrony account of binding, but chapter 2 gave reasons for preferring Eliasmith's account of binding as neural convolution. Here binding is a neural operation that transforms two neural representations into a third one that is also a pattern of firing in a group of neurons serving to integrate the information from the two representations that are bound together.

Figure 10.1 contends that sound, grammar, and meaning are each represented by a neural group that contributes through binding to a new pattern of neural firing. A word is not just a string of letters on a page but a mental representation operating in the brain, combining all the information shown in Figure 10.1. The sound should not be construed as the verbal depiction of the pronunciation of "giraffe" shown on the left of the figure but rather as the usual sound produced when people utter the word. When people say the word "giraffe," they produce sound waves that enter the ears of others, stimulate their sensors, and are encoded by neural populations in their brains.

Grammatically, giraffe is identified as a noun, which allows it to play the syntactic role of the subject or object of a sentence such as "The girl saw the giraffe." Semantically, according to Jackendoff, the meaning of the word "giraffe" is a matter of its relation to other mental representations. But the meaning of concepts is also tied in with perceptual features such as *long neck* and *tall*. Like sounds, these can be encoded nonverbally through visual and other kinds of images. Chapter 4 argued that concepts are not just verbal representations but can also be multimodal, and for the concept *giraffe* visual representations are important for most people. For other people who have had much more personal experience with giraffes, other modalities such as touch, smell, and sound can contribute to the meaning of the word "giraffe." Emotions can also affect the processing of words, because people prefer to attend to ones with positive values.

Sentences

The next linguistic question is how words make up sentences, not only in writing or speech but also with mental representations. Once again, the key is binding by neural convolution, as the words in the mental lexicon encoded as semantic pointers get bound into more complicated representations corresponding to sentences. We have already seen how this works with the construction of beliefs in chapter 4, rules in chapter 5, and desires in chapter 7. The resulting structure for the sentence "The giraffe is beside the tree" is shown in Figure 10.2 as a semantic

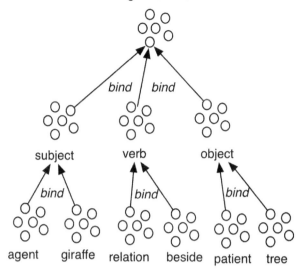

Sentence: The giraffe is beside the tree.

FIGURE 10.2 Mental representation of a sentence as a semantic pointer integrating parts of speech, each of which is a semantic pointer combining sound, grammar, and meaning. The meaning of words like "giraffe," "beside," and "tree" is multimodal, that is, sensory as well as verbal, in accord with the theory of concepts presented in chapter 4 and the theory of meaning.

pointer produced by recursive binding of other semantic pointers. This structure differentiates between the parts of the sentence in the same way that different parts of relations were distinguished for concepts in chapter 4 and analogies in chapter 6.

In Figure 10.2, the word "giraffe" is bound to the grammatical role of agent, while the word "tree" is bound to the grammatical role of patient, that is, what is acted upon. There would be no problem producing a sentence with multiple occurrences of the same word, as in Jackendoff's star example. If the sentence were instead "The little giraffe is beside the big giraffe," its mental representation would include the bindings of *little* and *giraffe* to each other and to *agent*, along with the bindings of *little* and *giraffe* to each other and to *patient*, well within the capabilities of the Semantic Pointer Architecture. Pragmatically, in particular contexts the two giraffes would be also be perceptually distinguishable by appearance and location, so the neural representations for *little giraffe* and *big giraffe* would be different.

The amalgamation of words into sentences by binding operates simultaneously with phonological, syntactic, and semantic information, just as Jackendoff's parallel architecture requires. Binding by neural convolution is equally adept at generating new sounds, grammatical structures, and meaning. Unlike Jackendoff's framework, the Semantic Pointer Architecture describes mathematically specified neural mechanisms to carry out the required operations. The Semantic Pointer Architecture can handle nested representations as recursive bindings of bindings of bindings, making it much more capable than previous neural network models of dealing with the full range of linguistic phenomena identified by Jackendoff and others.

Because of the nested representations that result from recursive binding, semantic pointers can explain the creative, generative aspects of language. This capacity, however, does not provide an infinite or unlimited amount of creativity, because human brains are constrained by the total number, spatial organization, and physically feasible interconnections of neurons available to produce bindings. Hence the Semantic Pointer Architecture approach to language is suitable for explaining performance rather than just abstract competence to produce an unlimited number of sentences of unlimited length. Because of neural limitations arising from the neural cost of binding, relations in spoken language rarely have more than three or four objects tied together, and sentences rarely have more than a few clauses unless they are written down to provide an external memory.

In accord with the standard practice of cognitive science, the adequacy of the Semantic Pointer Architecture for generative syntax and semantics needs to be justified by detailed simulations of complex linguistic phenomena. So far, the Semantic Pointer Architecture has only been applied to simple kinds of syntactic parsing, but it could naturally be extended to include phonology and semantics. Simulations should show how the meaning of a sentence depends not only on the meaning of the words in it but also on the overall context in which the sentence is used, another application of parallel constraint satisfaction.

Jackendoff's integration of syntax with semantics and phonology requires parallel processes rather than step-by-step deductions. We have already seen cases where parallel constraint satisfaction provides a powerful alternative to serial deductions for thinking about how the brain makes inferences: categorization in chapter 4, selection of rules in chapter 5, analogical mapping in chapter 6, cognitive appraisal in chapter 7, competition for consciousness in chapter 8, and decision making in chapter 9. The abandonment of syntax-first approaches to language fits with the general abandonment of sequential and purely verbal approaches to thinking. The alternative encouraged by neural network models is to understand mental processing as parallel constraint satisfaction on multimodal representations. The great advantage of the Semantic Pointer Architecture is that it provides the advantages of multimodal representations and parallel constraint satisfaction with the ability to handle the complexities of syntactic structure.

This section focuses on Jackendoff's parallel architecture, but there are other approaches to linguistics that also challenge the Chomskyan mainstream. Ronald Langacker's cognitive grammar maintains that symbolic structures incorporate semantic and phonological structures, so that syntax is enmeshed with sound and meaning. I discuss ideas about conceptual blending and metaphor that also consider linguistic phenomena in integrated ways that appreciate syntax but notice its connections with meaning.

MEANING

Now we can recognize how linguistic meaning develops for both words and sentences.

Words

Because sentences consist of words, the first question about the meaningfulness of language is: What makes words meaningful? An answer to this question can provide the basis for considering how sentences get their meanings from the meanings of words.

Theories of meaning proposed by philosophers and linguists view it as originating from different directions—upwards, downwards, or sideways. The upwards approach to meaning looks for it in nonworldly realms, as in Plato's theory of forms mentioned in chapter 4. Raphael's painting *The School of Athens* (viewable on Wikipedia) has a famous portrait of Plato and Aristotle that is often interpreted as Plato pointing upward to the heavens as the source of knowledge, whereas the more empirical philosopher Aristotle points outward to the social world around him. For Plato, the sources of the meanings of words are innate concepts, the heavenly forms. Innateness may indeed be a source of some aspects of meaning for some concepts, as we saw in chapter 4. Perhaps some concepts like *object* and *face* are built into our brains through evolutionary history, a nonheavenly source of meaning.

Most theories of meaning today, however, seek meaning downwards or sideways or both. Downwards semantics looks for meaning through the relation of words to the world and sensory experience. Sideway semantics looks for meaning through the relation of words to other words and the corresponding mental representations. The distinction between downwards and sideways semantics is captured in historical distinctions between sense and reference and connotation and denotation. The reference (denotation) of a word is what the word stands for in the world, for example the set of giraffes to which the word "giraffe" refers. In contrast, sense (connotation) concerns how the word relates to other words, for example the connections between "giraffe" and words like "animal" and "mammal."

Jackendoff's conceptual semantics is mainly a sideways theory because he says that the reference of a linguistics expression is just a mental construct. Meanings are mentally encoded by means of principles of combination from a finite, innate stock of primitive concepts. These primitives include basic categories for understanding spatial states and events such as place, path, event, and state. The existence of innate primitive concepts gives Jackendoff's semantics a small upward component, but the origin and meaning for most words is sideways as they relate to other words, especially the primitive concepts.

In contrast, the semantic pointer view of concepts developed in chapter 4 assigns a substantial downwards component to their meaning, resulting from physical interactions with the world. Many concepts such as *dog* have a large sensory-motor component, which can include visual, auditory, tactile, and kinesthetic interactions with dogs. These interactions create causal correlations between dogs in the world and the concept *dog* in our brains. The causal direction is partly from the world to the mind, because that is the causal direction of our sensory mechanisms. Modal retention of sensory information by semantic pointers helps to maintain their causal connection with the world.

For some concepts, we can also go from the mind to the world, when we use our bodies to change the world, for example by patting a dog to make it stay. Patterns of firing correlate with the world as a result of these two kinds of causal interaction, with the world affecting the mind and the mind affecting the world through actions resulting from motor control. Then the downward aspect of meaning results from sensory-motor causal correlations. The meaning of some words can also be indicated partially by gestures, for example when you point to adjacent places to indicate the meaning of "beside" or when you draw two arms away from each other to indicate the meaning "tall."

The semantic pointer view of concepts also allows them to acquire meaning sideways through relations to other concepts, because of their functions in symbolic and imagistic inferences. The semantic pointer for *giraffe* includes connections with other concepts such as *animal* and enables imagistic inferences such as what it would look like if a monkey sat on a giraffe. So semantic pointers corresponding to words can acquire meaning by means of their inferential connections to other semantic pointers for other words. This aspect of semantic pointers fits well with Jackendoff's conceptual semantics.

In sum, the meaning of a word conveyed by semantic pointers comes from all three directions: upwards to a few innate primitives, downwards to the world through causal correlation via sensation and action, and sideways to other conceptual neural processes. Another important source of meaning is social, because individuals do not learn languages on their own but rather through interactions with other people. Both the downwards and sideways aspects of meanings usually derive from forms of social communication. People point out things in the world to other people in order to associate words with the things, and teachers help a child to use language better by corrections, repetitions, and gestures. So meaning results not only from the relationships of words to other words and concepts to other concepts but also through all the social interactions that people have with other people. *Mind–Society* (chapter 3) describes communication as a social mechanism for the approximate transfer of semantic pointers, and *Natural Philosophy* (chapter 8) connects the meaning of language with the meaning of life.

Overall, therefore, the meaning of words is multidimensional, resulting from processes that are downwards, upwards, sideways, and social. Meaning needs to be viewed as a process rather than as a thing. Philosophers often talk of meaning as content, which is something contained, an abstract entity like Plato's forms. Recognizing how the use of words is tied to neural representations shows that meaning depends on several different kinds of causal interactions among neural firing patterns and the world, other firing patterns of firing, and evolutionary history encoded in innate synaptic connections. Hence the term "content" should not be used as a synonym of "meaning," in order to recognize the multidirectional processes that interact to make words and concepts meaningful. Reinterpreting concepts as referring to relational processes rather than objects has often been a mark of scientific progress, for example with *weight, temperature, space, time,* and *life*. The meaning of a word emerges from the interaction of multiple neural and social processes that each can have emergent properties. Like consciousness, meaning results from emergence of emergence.

Sentences

Given this explanation of the meaning of words, the meaning of sentences becomes complicated but comprehensible. We need to avoid several common mistakes, such as supposing that the meaning of a sentence is an abstract entity called a proposition, as ethereal as Plato's forms. Another mistake is to suppose that the meaning of a sentence is captured by its truth conditions based on its logical form, especially when these truth conditions require introducing further abstract entities in the form of possible worlds. Jackendoff's approach to semantics provides a much more psychologically plausible account of how the meanings of sentences can be built up out of the meanings of words, as long as the meanings of words are not construed in the purely mental way that he assumes.

Sentences get their relations to the world indirectly, through the downward connections that many words have through sensory and motor interactions. Some sentences are removed from such interactions, for example ones concerning highly abstract concepts as in "Justice is fairness." The meaning of sentences is mostly a sideways process of relations to the words that compose them but also achieves some downward connections to the world by virtue of the causal correlations with the world possessed by many words and concepts. Similarly, the meaning of larger pieces of language like stories is mostly a sideways process of relations among sentences but also operates downwards thanks to perceptual and emotional images that stories generate in their hearers and readers.

Words and sentences generate new meanings out of old ones, when conceptual combination produces new words such as "caregiver" and speech produces new sentences such as "The caregiver is worried." The generativity of semantics has the same neural basis as the generativity of syntax: binding that produces new neural processes out of old ones. The meaningfulness of sentences tracks the construction of grammatically rich utterances by means of the binding mechanism that builds more and more complicated semantic pointers.

Unlike Chomsky's merge operation, which merely concatenates lexical items, binding by neural convolution ensures that the new semantic pointers carry over some of the connections to the world and other representations. For example, when binding produces the mental representation of the giraffe being beside the tree, then the result carries along with it all the downwards and sideways meaning of the concepts *giraffe, beside,* and *tree.* Similarly, the syntactic processes that produce the sentence "The giraffe is beside the tree" simultaneously generate the sentence's meaning. Meaning in sentences is even messier than it is in words, but can nevertheless be understood by connecting it to neural processes that include interrelations with the world as well as with neural representations, in part mediated by social interactions of a speaker with other people. Meaning emerges from multilevel mechanisms. Molecular mechanisms are also relevant to language, for example through the gene *FOXP2* that is important for language development.

The meanings of sentences can also have a substantial pragmatic component, depending on the context and purpose of their use. For example, Groucho Marx's saying "Hello I must be going" takes on different meanings depending on the person to whom it is said and the reason for him saying it. Extending the Semantic Pointer Architecture account of language to pragmatics is natural for two reasons. First, context is handled because the full set of mental representations used for interpreting linguistic utterances are constructed on the fly, depending on various verbal and sensory inputs. Patterns of firing distributed among various semantic pointers are all operating in response to current contexts. Second, attention to the purposes of utterances is handled by emotional mechanisms of the sort discussed in chapters 7 and 9. Concepts carry with them emotional significance for action. Language is not an abstract entity spinning in the air but rather a tool used by people in real situations for important purposes. Some of these uses can be described as blending.

CONCEPTUAL BLENDING

The linguists Gilles Fauconnier and Mark Turner have developed a theory of conceptual blending relevant to questions about the origins and uses of language. I now show that the semantic pointers provide a neural explanation of how blending works.

To start with a simple example, consider the sentence "Luke is a stockbroker." This utterance requires the blending of two mental spaces, one with representations of Luke and the other with representations of stockbrokers, people who buy and sell securities. This blend produces a new mental space that incorporates aspects of two previously separated mental spaces, both of which belong to a generic space. Much more interesting spaces can be built up by blending multiple spaces, for example by saying "Luke is my brother-in-law and also a stockbroker who plays guitar." This blend brings together mental spaces for family, jobs, and music, weaving them altogether into a mental web.

One cognitive advantage of blends is that they can produce compressed representations that can be used in larger blends. Such small, compressed blends can be unpacked or expanded as needed to connect to what we want to think about. For example, you may develop a new concept of *musical stockbroker* that contributes to understanding of other people besides Luke. Advanced blending (also called "double scope") occurs when two mental spaces have organizing structures that conflict, requiring the development of a new organizing structure as an emergent property. Mental spaces consist primarily of frames, which are representations of familiar elements and relations.

One of Fauconnier and Turner's favorite examples of blending is the riddle of the Buddhist monk who begins at dawn one day to walk up a mountain and then the next day at dawn walks back to the bottom of the mountain. The riddle asks: without making any assumptions about his starting or stopping or his pace, determine whether there is a place on the path that the monk occupies at the same hour of the day on the two trips. You might try to answer this by writing down mathematical equations describing his speed and distance covered for each of the trips, but an answer can be reached more quickly simply by imagining both the ascent and the descent and then blending them into a combined representation. Imagining the monk simultaneously ascending and descending indicates that there must be some spot on the path in the ascent and descent when he meets himself, which will be the same time of day during both of these trips. The blend provides a solution to the riddle.

Fauconnier and Turner have applied the idea of conceptual blending to many important phenomena, including additional forms of creativity. They identify the origin of language with the development of the capability for advanced blending, which enables people to have language, art, religion, culture, science, mathematics, music, and dance. They claim that metaphor and other figures of thought result from the compressions brought about by blending, for example when someone says that stockbrokers are vampires, blending the financial and supernatural mental spaces to generate new inferences.

The blending ideas of Fauconnier and Turner are highly suggestive, but they are also vague. What are frames, and how do they make up mental spaces? What are the mental operations that combine spaces into new ones and reconcile differences in advanced blending? Fauconnier and Turner say that blending is a neural process, with elements in mental spaces corresponding to activated neuronal assembles and linking between elements in different spaces corresponding to neurobiological binding. A much more precise account of blending can be gained by translating ideas about spaces, frames, blends, compression, and emergence into mechanisms of the Semantic Pointer Architecture.

Begin with frames, which are the mental representations corresponding to elements like stockbroker and monk. These are naturally understood as the concepts described in chapter 4 in terms of semantic pointers, a special kind of neural firing pattern. These patterns explain the activated neuronal assemblies mentioned by Fauconnier and Turner, with precise mechanisms for formation by binding, compression, decompression, and contribution to symbolic inference. Semantic pointers are capable of going beyond purely verbal information to include imagistic representations from multiple modalities such as vision. Semantic pointers for concepts like *monk, mountain,* and *walk* include visual and kinesthetic images that are crucial for creating the blended image of the monk walking up and down the mountain. Blending two spaces is just simultaneously activating and binding the semantic pointers from both of them.

Blending also requires neural transformations that operate on these semantic pointers, as when the visual-kinesthetic image of the monk going up the mountain gets combined with the image of the monk going down the mountain. Operation on these images is made possible by their compression into semantic pointers, through the neural mechanisms described in chapter 2. Representations in verbal and nonverbal format can be compressed for the symbol-like functionality of the semantic pointer, and semantic pointers can also be decompressed into their sensory, motor, and other components when required. Hence solutions to problems such as the monk's riddle can rely on the mechanisms of imagery transformation described in chapter 3. Metaphors such as "stockbrokers are vampires" involve conceptual combination by neural binding, including the application of visual images such as a stock seller going for the neck of a purchaser. Binding has to be more than just the simultaneous activation of neuronal assemblies, because it needs to produce representations that can be further bound into combined representations that can be used for other purposes, for example if the concept of *vampire stockbrokers* becomes an ongoing theme in a television show.

Hence blending in mental spaces can be understood in neural terms as operations on semantic pointers. Blending, binding, compression, and decompression are not merely metaphorical, because the theory of semantic pointers shows how they can be described mathematically with sufficient precision to generate computational models of brain mechanisms. It would be a valuable exercise to develop simulations of the full range of blending phenomena described by Fauconnier and Turner. These phenomena should include advanced (double scope) blending when two mental spaces conflict, where resolution of conflicts is achieved by parallel constraint satisfaction as performed by competition among semantic pointers.

Like the parallel architecture of Jackendoff, conceptual blending combines syntax, semantics, and pragmatics. Blending is obviously not a purely syntactic operation, for it assumes that the mental spaces used to generate new spaces are meaningful. Blending sometimes involves analogies, but not the syntax-first kinds of analogy criticized in chapter 6. Fauconnier and Turner contend that blending is a special kind of mental operation, akin to analogy and other basic mental processes, but it is more plausible to describe blending as the result of specific cognitive mechanisms for semantic pointers. Conceptual blending is another valuable departure from the syntactic dream, if it can be rigorously specified by explicit kinds of mental representations and processes. The Semantic Pointer Architecture shows how to carry out this specification.

METAPHOR

Effective language often uses figures of speech such as metaphor and metonymy. Metaphors make comparisons between disparate domains, for example in the song "Love is a rose." Metonymy allows elements associated with each other to substitute for one another, for example in the expression "The pen is mightier than the sword," where "pen" stands in for writing and "sword" stands in for military force. Cognitively, these are not just aspects of speech but are also major determinants of thought and action. Semantic pointers illuminate the cognitive effectiveness of metaphor, not only from discussions of syntax, semantics, and blending in this chapter but also from earlier discussions of imagery, analogy, and emotion.

The cognitive effectiveness of metaphor has been extolled by the linguist George Lakoff and his colleagues Mark Johnson, Mark Turner, and Raphael Nuñez. They convincingly argue that metaphor is not just a literary embellishment but rather a means of grasping much of human experience. For example, time is often understood in terms of space, as in the metaphors "life is a journey" and "time is a river." Emily Dickinson was a master of metaphor, as in the following poem:

> Fame is a fickle food
> Upon a shifting plate
> Whose table once a
> Guest but not
> The second time is set.
> Whose crumbs the crows inspect
> And with ironic caw
> Flap past it to the Farmer's Corn —
> Men eat of it and die.

Literally, fame is not a food, and food is not fickle, but Dickinson (who lived quietly and published little of her poetry during her lifetime) effectively and evocatively conveys the evasiveness and futility of fame by comparing fame to food.

Dickinson's poem uses imagery, including the visual in "shifting plate," the auditory in "caw," and the kinesthetic in "flap past." Chapter 3 describes how semantic pointers explain imagery, because they integrate into a controllable package various kinds of sensory and motor experiences, including shifting, cawing, and flapping. The concept *fame* is too abstract to be much more than verbal, but other concepts in the poem have sensory and motor components. For example, the concept *food* can be understood verbally as a nutritious substance, but people's concepts of it can incorporate aspects of how it looks, how it tastes, and how it feels to be moved into a mouth. Lakoff and his colleagues emphasize the role that the body plays in constructing rich metaphors, and the sensory-motor aspects of semantic pointers show how they can accommodate these embodied aspects of metaphor. But semantic pointers, by virtue of their capacity for recursive binding, can also capture transbodied aspects of more abstract concepts like *fame, guest,* and *die.*

Like all sophisticated metaphors, Dickinson's poem has an underlying analogy, a systematic comparison of the relational structure of human fame and food. Food is fickle because it shifts upon a plate and can cause death, a pattern of relations that the metaphor transfers analogically to fame. This analogy is not merely a syntactic system of isomorphic relations, because the semantic connections are crucial to the mapping. Men do not literally eat the crumbs of fame, but crumbs correspond to the minor features of fame, and eating them corresponds to the pursuit and enjoyment of those features. Without such semantic connections, the analogical metaphor would have no force. We can only guess at Dickinson's purpose in writing this poem, but it clearly accomplishes the goals of both literary creativity and psychological insight. Like the analogies in chapter 6, this metaphor requires interactions of multiple constraints, not just syntax. As with advanced blending, the constraint satisfaction process of mapping does not need to produce a perfectly isomorphic set of correspondences but only semantically insightful matches adequate to accomplish the purposes of the metaphor and its underlying analogy.

The novel *Generosity* by Richard Powers describes a character as running with wolves and scissors, cleverly combining the two metaphors of running with wolves and running with scissors. This mix requires the combination of the concepts of audacity and recklessness, along with the emotional reactions of admiration and reproach. The metaphor *jump the shark* means to introduce a gimmick in a television show to hide a general decline in quality, by analogy to a moment in the comedy *Happy Days* where a character water skis over a shark. This metaphor carries the emotional connotations of embarrassment and scorn from the speaker to the listener.

Dickinson's poem, like all poetic metaphor, also has a substantial emotional component. Emotionally positive words in the poem include "food" and "eat," in contrast to emotionally negative words such as "fickle," "die," "and "caw." The overall accomplishment of the poem is to shift the usual emotionally positive associations of fame toward the emotionally negative associations of fickleness and death. The discussion of emotion in chapter 7 showed how such emotional reactions involve a combination of cognitive appraisal and physiological perception, all bound together via semantic pointers. The emotional impact of poetry requires this kind of cognitive-physiological interaction and integration.

In the terminology of Fauconnier and Turner, we could say that Dickinson's poem requires a blend of mental spaces about fame, food, and fatality. Much of the blending is advanced, in that it requires the reconciliation of what seem to be conflicting concepts, as in "fickle food" and "ironic caw." Such conflicts make the poem all the more interesting and require additional cognitive and emotional work to generate the full impact of the poem. Metaphorical blending in this and other cases depends on the semantic pointer mechanisms of imagery, concepts, analogy, and emotion. All of these rely on representation, binding, transformation, competition, and parallel constraint satisfaction. Hence the important cognitive functions of metaphor are naturally explained by semantic pointer mechanisms.

Like analogies, metaphors can transfer emotions as well as cognitive information. During the 2015 Republican contest for presidential candidate, the front runner Donald Trump was described by his rivals as a rattlesnake with a toothache, a drunken NASCAR driver, a cancer on conservatism, a wrecking ball, a jackass, and nitroglycerine. None of these ascriptions is literally true but serve to transfer negative emotions such as fear and contempt.

INNATENESS AND LANGUAGE LEARNING

Since the 1950s when Chomsky revolutionized linguistics, debate has raged about the extent to which knowledge of language is innate. For the behaviorists, everything about language was learned, but Chomsky argued that the creativity and learnability of language are best explained by the hypothesis that all humans have an innate linguistic ability. His allies have included philosophers such as Jerry Fodor and psychologists such as Stephen Pinker. On the other side, linguists such as Jeff Elman and anthropologists such as Daniel Everett have argued that people have the learning capability and cultural context to learn the huge variety of languages without special innate capacities.

In the abstract, the Semantic Pointer Architecture is neutral on this debate, because it can explain the innateness of some concepts and rules as described in chapters 4 and 5 but it also has the capacity to learn many others. How does the claimed innateness of grammar fare on the five criteria for innateness that I have been using: cultural universality, specific brain areas, animal precursors, adaptiveness during the evolutionary period, and absence of alternative explanations based on learning and culture? The criterion of animal precursors does not apply, because only humans have the full linguistic capability to generate complex sentences. Animals such as chimpanzees and parrots can string sounds and symbols together in small numbers, but they cannot accomplish the kind of recursion of this utterance from the movie *Chinatown*, where Jack Nicholson says to a detective: "You're even dumber than you think I think you are."

Cultural universality of grammar turns out to be tricky, because early claims about language universals were made by generalization from only a few languages, mostly Indo-European. Examination of the approximately 7,000 known languages has brought complications. Everett argues that the Pirahã language of Brazil lacks recursion within sentences, as well as other features of familiar languages such as words for numbers. On the other hand, the language is rich with terms for the jungle environment inhabited by its speakers, and its tonal qualities allow it to be hummed and whistled as well as spoken. Everett contends that language is a cultural tool for communication, satisfying an instinct to be sociable but not requiring a language instinct. If he is right, then cultural learning provides an alternative explanation for the ubiquity of language, undermining claims for innateness.

As for the criterion of adaptiveness during the evolutionary period, too little is known about when language developed in people and the contribution it made at that time to use this as support for the innateness of language. Language does seem to employ important parts of the brain such as Broca's and Wernicke's areas, but these also have nonlinguistic functions, and language requires other areas as well. Hence language is like emotions and consciousness in operating in the brain with a relation between cognitive functions and brain areas that is many-to-many rather than one-to-one.

I suggested that Chomsky's merge operation, fundamental to his latest view of what is universal to language, could be explained by the more general neural operation of binding by convolution. Binding satisfies all the criteria for innateness, as it operates even in the visual systems of newborn chicks and has huge adaptive value for complex perception and cognition. Perhaps the difference between chicks and humans is that we have billions of neurons rather than millions, enabling us to do more repetitions of recursive binding. Moreover, binding in semantic pointers can simultaneously operate with semantic and pragmatic information in addition to syntax. Hence it may be that language results from the combination of neural mechanisms of binding and learning along with social mechanisms of cultural transmission. Then syntax does not need to be innate.

SUMMARY AND DISCUSSION

I have shown the relevance of Eliasmith's Semantic Pointer Architecture for understanding important phenomena about language. Semantic pointers can handle syntactic structure in a way that integrates with other key aspects of language, including semantics, pragmatics, and phonology. Semantic pointers plausibly provide the underlying neural mechanisms for Jackendoff's parallel architecture and for other theories of language that go beyond Chomsky's syntax-first approach. In particular, they show how the mental representation of a word can efficiently combine information about sound, meaning, and grammar to enable the organization of words into sentences. Semantic pointers cast the meanings of words and sentences as multidimensional, relying not just on the relations of words to other words but also on the relation of words to the world through sensory-motor operations, with further contributions from genetic and social processes.

The Semantic Pointer Architecture also provides neural mechanisms for explaining complex linguistic phenomena such as conceptual blending and metaphor. Blending works because mental spaces consist of semantic pointers subject to binding and other transformations that produce useful new representations. Metaphor functions as an important component of thinking as well as language through the operation of images, concepts, analogies, and emotions, all of which work by neural representation, binding, and competition. Semantic pointers include but surpass language, because they can rely on sensory-motor information as well as verbal representations, allowing for the embodiment of metaphorical cognition. At the same time, transbodiment is accomplished by recursive binding of linguistic representations into abstract concepts and utterances. The semantic pointer approach does not rule out the innateness of some aspects of language, but the integration of syntax, semantics, and pragmatics fits well with the view of language as a learned cultural tool.

Because of the pervasive contributions of language to social communication, the linguistic phenomena in this chapter are important for all the topics in *Mind–Society*. Discourse in the social sciences requires attention to the role of metaphors in phenomena such as economic booms and political ideologies. The professions are also replete with complex interactions of syntax, semantics, and pragmatics and with abundant metaphors: some surgeons are gods, some lawyers are sharks, some entrepreneurs are wizards, and so on. Language contributes to the humanities through literary creations, musical lyrics, and the hyperlinguistic endeavors of philosophers (*Natural Philosophy*). Applying the insights of cognitive neuroscience to social processes requires attention to language as a major part of the interfaces connecting minds and environments.

NOTES

On Chomsky's current views, see Chomsky 1995, 2013. Evans 2014 provides a critique.

Cognitive (non-Chomskyan) linguists include Jackendoff 2002, 2010 and Langacker 2013. For an application of semantic pointers to parsing, see Stewart, Choo, and Eliasmith 2014. Blouw and Eliasmith 2017 provide a neural model of inferential role semantics. Frankland and Greene 2015 describe how the brain encodes sentences in left mid-superior temporal cortex.

People prefer to recognize words with positive emotional values: Recio, Conrad, Hansen, and Jacobs 2014. On linguistic comprehension as parallel constraint satisfaction, see Kintsch 1998 and MacDonald and Seidenberg 2006. MacDonald is developing a constraint satisfaction account of language production.

In philosophy, downward approaches to semantics that emphasize the world are called externalist, in opposition to sideways internalist approaches that focus on relations among mental states. Other sideways views of meaning are the procedural semantics of the psychologists George Miller and Philip Johnson-Laird 1976 and the conceptual role semantics of the philosopher Gilbert Harman 1987. For a multidimensional account of the meaning of scientific concepts, see Thagard 2012d. See also the multidirectional neurosemantics of Eliasmith 2005 and the robosemantics of Parisien and Thagard 2008. Advocates of meaning as truth conditions include Davidson 1967. Advocates of meaning as social include Wittgenstein 1968. For more on meaning, including connections between the meaning of language and the meaning of life, see *Natural Philosophy* (chapter 8).

On conceptual blending, see Fauconnier and Turner 2002 and Turner 2014.

On metaphor, see Lakoff 1987, 1994, 1996; Lakoff and Johnson 1980, 1999; Lakoff & Núñez 2000; Lakoff and Turner 1989; Holyoak and Thagard 1995; Bowdle and Gentner 2005. What Lakoff and his collaborators call "image schemas" are, in my terminology, concepts that include imagery.

On the innateness debate, see Chomsky 1980, 2002; Elman et al. 1996; Pinker 1994; Everett 2012. Hauser et al. 2014 (including Chomsky) express skepticism about what can be known about language evolution. Fitch 2011 surveys linguistic universals.

PROJECT

Use semantic pointers to produce computational models of Jackendoff's parallel architecture, of blending in cases such as the monk on the mountain, and of metaphors such as fame is a fickle food.

11

Creativity

According to Apple Computer founder Steve Jobs:

> Creativity is just connecting things. When you ask creative people how they did something, they feel a little guilty because they didn't really *do* it, they just *saw* something. It seemed obvious to them after a while. That's because they were able to connect experiences they've had and synthesize new things.

From the perspective of cognitive science, this quote raises far more questions than it answers. What are the things that get connected? Are they real things in the world, or are they mental representations of things such as images and concepts? Is the connecting done by physical manipulation of the world, as you might connect the hose to a vacuum cleaner? Or is the connecting done by mental operations such as imagery and conceptual combination? Is it enough to connect experiences and synthesize what is already there, or does creativity require going beyond experiences to generate dramatically new mental representations?

Creativity is a major challenge for cognitive science, which aims to explain not only ordinary thinking but also the most impressive mental accomplishments that humans have ever achieved. These accomplishments include Darwin's theory of evolution by natural selection, Gutenberg's printing press, Beethoven's *Ninth Symphony*, and universal healthcare. Each of these was new and surprising in its time and turned out to be valuable with respect to the disparate goals of scientific discovery, technological invention, artistic imagination, and social innovation. This chapter shows how the mental representations and processes described earlier can explain how people make such breakthroughs.

The social impact of creativity has been enormous. Twenty thousand years ago, humans lived in small groups without agriculture, cities, written language, mathematics, science, complex machines, and many other aspects of contemporary life. Human creativity in science, technology, art, and social organization has vastly changed how people interact with each other. These creative accomplishments are not merely the result of individual minds but also of productive social interactions. Creativity helps to explain social change, just as social change helps to explain creativity. This interaction indicates an important feedback loop in human development, not a vicious circularity.

This chapter focuses on the mental mechanisms that produce human creativity, leaving social mechanisms for *Mind–Society* (chapter 13). I describe the ways in which mental representations, including images, concepts, rules, analogies, and emotions, all contribute to human creativity. The transformations of these representations described in previous chapters are capable of producing ideas that are new, surprising, and potentially valuable. The chapter concludes with a cognitive case study of one of the most important advances in recent biology, CRISPR/Cas9.

Most research on creativity in psychology and neuroscience has been correlational, for example finding associations between creative thought and personality or between insight and brain area activation. Instead, this chapter provides a mechanistic theory of creativity, summed up in these hypotheses:

1. Creativity results from combinations and modifications of mental representations to produce ones that are new and valuable.
2. Mental representations and their modifications result from operations on semantic pointers.
3. Emotions foster creativity by providing motivation and evaluation.

WHAT IS CREATIVITY?

By now, readers will know better than to expect a definition of creativity that gives necessary and sufficient conditions for it. Such definitions have major problems, including the difficulty of getting people to agree on a definition, the usual availability of counterexamples to any proposed definition, and the blatant circularity that you often find when you look up a word in dictionary and begin a chain that leads back to the word to be defined. Fortunately, the view of concepts in chapter 4 suggests a much more fruitful way of characterizing creativity using three-analysis. Instead of defining the word "creativity," we need to specify exemplars (standard examples), typical features (prototype), and explanations that indicate both what the concept explains and what explains the concept, as summarized in Table 11.1.

The adjective "creative" applies both to people such as Beethoven and their products such as his symphonies. The creativity of individuals and groups depends on their being able to generate creative products, but what are the products of creativity? Steve Jobs spoke of connecting new things, but did he actually mean ideas about things? Some physical things do get produced through creative thought, such as the first wheel, particular works of art such as the *Mona Lisa*, and specific buildings such as the Taj Mahal. But none of these things could have been produced without new mental representations like images and concepts. The wheel did not come about because of random juxtaposition of pieces of wood or stone, but rather because of conceptual goals such as moving objects easily and images such as how pieces can be shaped and made to fit together. People often describe creative products as ideas, but I prefer to speak more specifically about the production of particular mental representations: images, concepts, rules, and analogies. These are the major products of creative thought, whose operation can lead to the production of solid objects.

Exemplars of creativity are easy to identify in all of the domains so far mentioned: science, technology, art, and society. The following are some of my favorite examples of creative products, not intended to be exclusive or exhaustive. The people who produced them are excellent examples of creative individuals. Other exemplars of creative producers are groups, such as the Wright Brothers, the Beatles, and the huge team of physicists who found evidence for the Higgs boson.

TABLE 11.1

Three-Analysis of *Creativity*

Exemplars	Products such as Beethoven's *Ninth Symphony*, the *Mona Lisa*, the Taj Mahal, the wheel, the theory of relativity, democracy; people such as Beethoven, da Vinci, Edison, Einstein
Typical features	New, valuable, surprising
Explanations	Explains: successes, social changes
	Explained by: neural and social mechanisms

Scientific discovery: Galileo's moons of Jupiter, Hooke's living cells,
Newton's theory of gravity, the wave theories of sound and light,
Einstein's relativity theory, neurons

Technological invention: paper, the telephone, the airplane, the telescope
and microscope, digital computers, electric motors, television, antibiotics

Artistic imagination: da Vinci's *Mona Lisa*, Impressionism, Georgia
O'Keeffe's flower paintings, Vivaldi's *Four Seasons*, the Beatles song
Yesterday, Tchaikovsky's *Nutcracker Suite*, Shakespeare's *Hamlet*, Tolstoy's
War and Peace, Emily Dickinson's poem *The Brain is Wider than the Sky*.

Social innovation: democratic government, public education, old-age pensions, universities, paper currency, hospitals, the United Nations

You might be inclined to challenge some of these examples, but there are many cases that most people would agree are the result of human creativity. Hence even without a strict definition of creativity we can see that there is considerable commonality in the concepts that operate in the minds of different people.

I have already suggested some good candidates for the typical features of creative acts. All of the cases described earlier were new (novel, original) in the contexts in which they arose. The products were also surprising (unexpected, nonobvious), in that they were not simply extensions of things or ideas that were already around. Finally, the products turned out to be valuable (useful, important, appropriate, correct, accurate) for accomplishing the relevant goals such as explanation in science, practical applications in technology, aesthetic enjoyment in art, and improving society in social innovation. The prototype for creativity therefore includes the expectation of products being new, surprising, and valuable.

A product may be new for you but not for society if someone else has already come up with the product. Reinventing the wheel may be a sign that you are clever, but it does not make you creative, because there is little value attached to generating a product that is already available. Surprise is an emotional state that results from the appearance of something unexpected, where expectation comes from coherence with existing beliefs. The emotion of surprise can be either positive or negative, depending on whether the results fits with people's goals. Normally, creative surprises are emotionally positive because they suggest new ways of accomplishing goals, but there are also some creative surprises that are emotionally negative, such as art that is more shocking than beautiful or technology that is potentially powerful but dangerous. Often, the value of a product is not immediately evident but will require ongoing evaluation by other people besides the person who is initially excited about a new and surprising product.

The third aspect of concepts discussed in chapter 4 was explanation, raising two questions. What does creativity explain, and what explains creativity? The creativity of an individual or a group should serve to explain why the individual or group is highly effective at producing results that are new, surprising, and valuable. Such explanations should specify the mental mechanisms that make individuals creative and also the social mechanisms that make groups creative. Then the concept of creativity can play a role in explaining individual and social developments. At the same time, identification of these mechanisms will provide an explanation of creativity, taking it beyond subjectivity and mystery. The result should be a deeply satisfying causal pattern: cognitive and social mechanisms → individual and social creativity → individual and social success.

So we do not need a strict definition to see that progress has been made in understanding creativity through accumulation of exemplars, identification of typical features, and preliminary ideas about mechanisms that explain creativity and then use it to explain individual and social development. Now we can examine in detail the mental mechanisms that underlie creative thinking, focusing on how semantic pointers help to explain creative thought through the power of recursive binding and transformation.

IMAGES

We start with images, which are mental representations based on sensory modalities such as vision, hearing, touch, taste, smell, and pain. Visual images have been strikingly important for creativity in science, technology, and the arts. The following are some scientific examples of discoveries that plausibly involve visual representations, sometimes in the form of physical diagrams or pictures and sometimes in the form of internal mental images: Copernicus's hypothesis that the sun is at the center of the universe, Kepler's view that the orbit of planets is elliptical, Harvey's theory of the circulation of blood pumped by the heart, Hooke's discovery that plants contain cells, Franklin's realization that lightning is like an electric spark, Dalton's ideas about the structure of atoms, Morgan's hypothesis about the existence of genes and chromosomes, Wegener's ideas about continental drift, Hubble's claim about the expanding universe, Fleming's realization that mold can kill bacteria, and Crick and Watson's identification of the helical structure of DNA (chapter 6). All of these are readily visualized. There are also many scientific discoveries that do not rely on visual representations because words and mathematical symbols suffice.

Because creative technology usually produces observable things, visual representations play a large role in invention. Just a few examples of inventions that people can naturally picture are the wheel, light bulbs, gasoline engines, airplanes, the locomotive, electric batteries, stethoscopes, skyscrapers, bicycles, submarines, and windmills. In addition, many creative things also use representations in other modalities such as sounds: radio, telegraph, stethoscope, and phonograph. For creative physical objects, kinesthetic representations can also play a role, for example, with the washing machine, typewriter, hammer, nail, and plow. Visual and kinetic kinesthetic representations can also contribute to artistic products such as paintings and sculptures. Auditory images are obviously useful for creating new songs and dances.

How does creative imagery work? For scientists, inventors, or artists to generate new images in their brains, previous images need to be transformable into novel ones. If an image is formed simply by copying what is already observed in nature, for example the look or the sound of a bird, then the possibility for novelty, surprise, and value are limited. But if the image is not merely a copy of what is observed but rather is compressed into a semantic pointer, then new images can be produced by the operations on imagistic semantic pointers described in chapter 3. Once images are condensed into semantic pointers, they can be juxtaposed, rotated, and combined to produce new images that may turn out to be surprising and valuable. For example, Edison figured out how to juxtapose several elements into an image of a functioning light bulb consisting of a carbonized filament, a wire, and surrounding glass.

Similar transformations can be used to generate novel images in other modalities. For example, a musical composer can take images of sounds and combine them into chords which are then juxtaposed into melodies. A creative chef can take images of taste and smell and combine and juxtapose them to produce dishes that have never previously been produced. A fabric designer can combine materials in novel ways to produce textiles that are pleasant to touch as well as to see. Interrelated systems of perceptual images formed by seeing, hearing, tasting, smelling, or touching can constitute mental models, such as the arrangement of visual and kinesthetic images used by an inventor of a new kind of car.

In these ways, imagery can generate new sensory representations that may turn out to be surprising if they are unlike previous experiences, and may turn out to be valuable if they satisfy the goals of science, technology, arts, or society. Nonhuman animals seem to be capable of creative problem solving using imagery, for example when crows come up with new problem solutions that require sequences of operations such as bending sticks and dropping pebbles into pitchers of water. Crows lack language so these accomplishments are clearly not the result of verbal reasoning.

CONCEPTS

Humans are adept at creative problem solving with imagery, but language gives us an even more powerful tool for generating new representations. Many writers on creativity, going back at least to Dugald Stewart in 1792, have proposed that creativity results from new combinations of ideas, which I construe as either non-verbal images or verbal concepts, which may also have imagistic components as described in chapter 4. Scientific discovery has generated many valuable new concepts such as *gravity, galaxy, virus, photosynthesis, anesthesia, molecule, dinosaur, natural selection, electromagnetism, x-rays, electron, radioactivity, special relativity, isotope, continental drift, insulin, neutron, gene, quark,* and *dark matter.* All of these result from combining previously existing concepts to produce a new one. For example, the word "dinosaur" was formed from combining Greek words for "terrible" and "lizard," when the concept *dinosaur* resulted from conceptual combination of the concepts *reptile, large,* and *powerful.*

Technology also introduces creative new concepts, usually tied to visual and other sensory representations. For every invention, there is a new concept that enables people to think about it, for example *airplane, nuclear reactor, jet engine, thermometer, condom, helicopter,* and *digital video recorder.* Conceptual combination puts together the verbal aspects of two concepts but also carries over the sensory-motor aspects that are also captured by semantic pointers.

Verbal representations of concepts provide new sources of power for creativity. First, word-like concepts make possible representations of things, processes, and relationships that cannot be detected by the senses, such as gravity, atoms, and antimatter. Second, they make it easy to pile creative acts upon creative acts through recursive bindings that are not tied to any sensory modality, for example when the concept *atom* gave way to the surprising concept of *subatomic particle.* Third, they allow concepts to be joined together into expressions of relations among various concepts, for example in scientific laws like Newton's discovery that force equals mass times acceleration. Such creativity is the epitome of transbodiment, taking thought far beyond the bounds of sensation, although some of the contributing concepts may have embodied roots. Newton's gravity is the abstract force between any two bodies that have mass but has a remote connection with bodily experiences of pushes and pulls. Semantic pointers explain both embodied and transbodied creativity, because combining them by binding and transforming them into new images, concepts, and rules generates new representations that can retain sensory origins when they exist.

New concepts are also important for creativity in artistic imagination and social innovation. In some cases, the new concept is formed only after creative projects have begun, as with the concepts *impressionism* in painting, *folk-rock* in music, and *university* in education. But new concepts can also provide creative thinkers with directions and suggestions for how they want their work to develop. For example, the concept *modern dance* directs choreographers in new directions away from classical ballet. By binding verbal concepts together, semantic pointers can go beyond the body to generate new and surprising ways of thinking about the world, such as genetics and relativity theory.

Of course, not all newly generated concepts turn out to be valuable, for in historical development many initially promising concepts are eventually recognized as limited or defective in their explanatory power. Examples of concepts that once played important explanatory roles in science but have been abandoned include *divine creation, bodily humor, luminiferous aether, phlogiston,* and *Oedipus complex.* I once had a dream in which I came up with a new concept so exciting that I woke up to write it down. The concept was *semantic life,* and I still have no clue what it meant or how it could be used. Value in science, technology, art, or social development is not instantly obvious but requires an evaluation that can take years or centuries.

RULES

Concepts are more creatively powerful than images because they allow people to abstract away from sensory-motor inputs. Rules are still more powerful, because they are capable of showing the relations among multiple concepts. For example, Darwin's basic idea about evolution by natural selection can be captured by the rule: *If there is variation in the inheritance of different properties in members of a species, and if there is competition among members for survival and reproduction, then a new species may evolve.* This rule shows relationships among numerous concepts, including *variability, inheritance, competition, survival,* and *reproduction.* No one concept, let alone an image, can capture this kind of cognitive complexity. Hence it is fair to say that rules are the peak of human creativity. Creative rules fall into two main categories: hypotheses that describe the world and methods that specify general ways of doing things. Methods are discussed in the next section on procedural creativity.

Chapter 5 describes mechanisms for generating new rules, some of which may turn out to be new, surprising, and valuable. The easiest but usually least creative way of producing new rules is generalization from examples. Suppose you eat pizza for the first time and it turns out that you like it. You may quickly form the rule: *If something is a pizza then it tastes good.* This rule is multimodal in that both the condition (if part) and action (then part) use concepts that are sensory as well as verbal: *<pizza>* → *<tastes-good>*. Your concept of pizza likely involves representations of what it looks like, what it tastes like, what it smells like, and even what it feels like if it is greasy. The reason that this generalization is not creative is that many other people have previously discovered the appeal of pizza.

More creative generalizations might involve novel combinations of foods, for example pizza made with romanesco, a rare and elegant broccoli-like vegetable that is potentially valuable in providing unexpected tastes and looks to pizza. The rule that romanesco pizza tastes good may result from small-sample generalization, which is more like memory formation than like the gradual processes of Hebbian and reinforcement learning that require many examples.

Chaining of rules into new ones is usually not creative, because the generated rules are just summaries of existing knowledge. For example, I can change the rules *if you want to fly, then buy a ticket* and *if you want to buy a ticket, then go on the Web* into the rule *if you want to fly, then go on the Web*. But there is little about the resulting rule that is new, surprising, or particularly valuable, because I could get the same effect simply by using two steps of rule-based inference to get the same endpoint, although the chained rule may be faster to use.

Abductive generalization is much rarer but potentially much more creative with respect to novelty and value. Whereas generalization from examples sticks with observable features of the world, abductive generalization provides general causal rules involving factors that may not be observable. Scientific theories generally result from abductive generalization into rules that go well beyond what can be observed. From examples, you can generalize the rule *if you drop something, then it falls.* But once the concept of gravity is formed by conceptual combination, then a new causal rule can provide a deeper explanation: *If gravity attracts a dropped object toward a planet, then the object falls.*

Concept formation by conceptual combination and rule formation by abductive generalization are mutually reinforcing. Forming the concept of natural selection makes possible the rule that natural selection and genetic variation cause the evolution of species, while the explanatory power of this rule justifies the value of the concept of natural selection. Natural selection and gravitational attraction cannot be directly observed but must be inferred as part of the best explanation of why things fall. The concepts of gravity and natural selection cannot be abstracted from observed examples, but their value is shown by the explanatory usefulness of associated rules.

Semantic pointers are helpful for understanding the creativity of rules in several ways. First, creative rules such as putting romanesco on pizza often require multimodal concepts, captured by the ability of semantic pointers to combine verbal, sensory, and motor information into a common neural representation. Second, semantic pointers show how such concepts can be combined into rules by binding, as described in chapter 5. Third, allowing the concepts in conditions of rules to be semantic pointers shows how the rules formed by abductive generalization can be meaningful even though they go beyond sensory experience. Chapter 10 describes how meaning results not just from connections to sensory experience but also from conceptual relations in which semantic pointers can participate. The meaning of rules, like other sentences, emerges from the meanings of the concepts they use.

So far, I have been considering rules that describe how the world is. But some of the most valuable rules are not descriptions but rather methods or procedures for doing things. An example is a rule for making pizza: *If you want to make pizza, then put cheese on top of bread and put it in the oven.* Researchers on creativity have surprisingly neglected the importance of procedural creativity that generates new methods expressed as rules.

PROCEDURAL CREATIVITY

Methods are naturally represented by rules about steps that can accomplish a goal, which have the general form: If you want to accomplish the goal, then proceed by using the steps. The following are 50 examples of methods that were new, valuable, and surprising, with approximate dates and creators. I have included recreational improvement as a separate domain of creativity, but all of the examples of it could be moved into technological invention or social innovation.

Scientific Discovery

1. Naturalistic explanation (Thales c. 600 BC): If you want to explain phenomena, look for natural causes rather than theological influences.

2. Experimentation (Ibn al-Haytham c. 1000): If you want to establish scientific truths, use experiments in addition to observations and theory.

3. Mathematical science (Galileo 1590): If you want to describe and explain phenomena, use mathematics in addition to words.

4. Telescope (Galileo 1609): If you want to observe the heavens, use a telescope.

5. Microscope (Malpighi 1660): If you want to study anatomical structure, use a microscope.

6. Calculus (Newton 1666): If you want to describe and explain change mathematically, use the calculus.

7. Statistical inference (Bernoulli 1689): If you want to make inferences about statistics, use probability theory.

8. Taxonomy (Linnaeus 1735): If you want to classify organisms, use the categories of kingdom, class, order, genus, and species.

9. Spectroscopy (Kirchoff and Bunson 1859): If you want to study chemical structure, use a spectroscope.

10. Polymerase chain reaction (PCR; Mullis 1983): If you want to study DNA, use PCR.

Technological Invention

1. Measuring density (Archimedes c. 210 BC): If you want to measure the volume of an object, measure how much water it displaces.

2. Movable type printing (Bi Sheng 1048, Gutenberg 1450): If you want to print books, use movable type and a printing press.

3. Lightning rod (Franklin 1752): If you want to protect a building from lightning, mount a metallic object on it with a wire to the ground.

4. Vaccination (Jenner 1798): If you want to protect people from smallpox, vaccinate them with cowpox.

5. Photography (Daguerre 1839): If you want to take pictures of people, use silver-surfaced plates developed by mercury fumes.

6. Morse code (Morse 1837): If you want to send a message by telegraph, use a code of dots and dashes.

7. Antiseptic surgery (Lister 1866): If you want to perform sterile surgery, use carbolic acid.

8. FORTRAN (Backus 1954): If you want to program a computer efficiently, use a high-level language.

9. Email (van Vleck 1965): If you want to communicate among computers, use electronic mail.

10. World Wide Web (Berners-Lee 1990): If you want to exchange information among computers, use a large hypertext database with links.

Artistic Imagination

1. Perspective drawing and painting (Brunelleschi c. 1400): If you want to make a realistic drawing or painting, use linear perspective.

2. Anatomical painting (da Vinci c. 1510): If you want to make a realistic drawing or painting of people, use detailed knowledge of their anatomy.

3. Opera (Peri 1597): If you want to provide musical entertainment, combine singing, dancing, and speaking.

4. Science fiction (Shelley 1818): If you want to write a novel, use themes drawn from science and technology.

5. Impressionism (Monet 1872): If you want to paint landscapes, use loose brush strokes that create an impression.

6. Jazz (various artists c. 1900): If you want to provide musical entertainment, combine African rhythms, European melodies, and improvisation.

7. Stream of consciousness writing (Richardson 1915): If you want to describe the psychological processes of characters, narrate their streams of conscious experiences.

8. Abstract sculpture (Moore 1922): If you want to make sculptures, use organic abstract forms rather than realistic depictions.

9. Mobile sculpture (Calder 1926): If you want to make sculptures, make them mobile and dynamic.

10. Modern dance (Duncan 1902): If you want to dance, present natural movements rather than ballet.

Social Innovation

1. Teach for America (Kopp 1989): If you want to improve education in low-income communities, get top recent college graduates to teach there.

2. Hospice (Saunders 1989): If you want to care for dying people, establish a hospice.

3. Facebook (Zuckerberg 2004): If you want to make social connections, use a web-based directory.

4. Prison reform (Fry 1817): If you want to improve the condition of prisoners, establish a clothing industry and democratic procedures.

5. Habitat for Humanity (Fuller 1976): If you want to improve housing for the poor and homeless, organize them into partnerships for building their own homes.

6. Microfinance (Yunus 2006): If you want to improve the conditions of poor people, give them small loans to set up businesses.

7. Distance learning (University of London 1858): If you want to educate people who cannot access universities, establish courses that can be taken long distance.

8. Universal healthcare (New Zealand 1941): If you want to ensure public health, provide healthcare and financial protection to all citizens.

9. Affirmative action (United States 1961): If you want to overcome discrimination against some groups, establish policies that benefit members of those groups.

10. Old-age pensions (Bismarck 1889): If you want to ensure an income for retired persons, establish a public pension with regular payments.

Recreational Improvement

1. Snowboarding (Carpenter 1977): If you want to enjoy going down hills, use a flexible wooden board with foot straps.

2. Video games (Douglas 1952): If you want to have fun on a computer, use a video display to play a game.

3. Cruise ship (Ballin 1889): If you want to take a pleasure voyage and return to your destination, take a cruise ship.

4. Airliner (Sikorsky 1913): If you want to fly as a passenger, take a commercial airline.

5. Card games (China c. 900): If you want to have fun, make a game using cards.

6. Mixed martial arts (various c. 1900): If you want a competitive fighting sport, combine different styles of combat.

7. Motion pictures (Armat 1896): If you want to entertain people, show them movies.

8. Cable television (Wilson 1948): If you want to improve television reception, use cables to import the signal from distant stations.

9. E-book (Sony 1992): If you want to read books electronically, use a handheld computer device.

10. Public park (Paxton 1843): If you want to increase enjoyment of the out-
    doors, build parks accessible by the general public.

Many of these rules are not just verbal, because the steps they suggest have a
large sensory-motor component, for example, using a microscope, snowboarding,
and making loose brush strokes: *<paint-impressions>* → *<brush-strokes>*. Hence it
is important that rules have the capacity described in chapter 5 of incorporating
nonverbal, sensory-motor information, which semantic pointers can accomplish.
Procedural knowledge of how to do things does not reduce to verbal knowledge
that propositions are true.

Cognitive Mechanisms for Generating Methods

These 50 examples make it plausible that methods are naturally represented by
rules. Methods do not seem to have been achieved by generalization from multiple
examples, chaining, or abductive generalization. Rather, they result from small-
sample generalization based on special kinds of inputs, outputs, and processes.

The most important kind of procedural creativity is *method generalization,* which
can produce a new rule from only one example:

Input: One or more goals, techniques consisting of one or more steps, and a
    problem solution showing that using the steps leads to accomplishment
    of the goal.
Output: A method with the structure: If you want to accomplish the goals,
    then use the technique consisting of the steps.
Process: Identify the steps that led to the goal and generalize them into the
    method.

The problem solution can be found by any of the techniques described in previous
chapters, including parallel constraint satisfaction (chapter 2), image manipulation (chapter 3), concept application (chapter 4), rule-based inference (chapter 5),
and analogy (chapter 6). No matter how the problem solution has been found,
it can quickly be generalized into a method without considering a host of examples. In contrast, the methods of rule generalization discussed in chapter 5
require multiple examples, because the neural processes of Hebbian and reinforcement learning are slow and incremental. Instant generalization is possible for
methods because of the knowledge-intensive nature of problem solving to which
new methods are useful. One success is enough to suggest a general way of doing

things, although repetition is required to determine whether the new and sur-prising method actually is valuable.

Another way of generating new methods in the form of rules is to use *method analogizing*. The method of snowboarding came about through a mixture of two source analogs, skiing and skateboarding. Sometimes there are methods that work well in one domain, and creators naturally wonder whether there are other similar domains in which an analogous method might work. Mark Zuckerberg did not set out to create Facebook, but he had successful methods for writing programs and developing websites that he was able to adapt for the different purpose of enabling people to interact electronically. The process of using analogy to produce new methods is something like the following:

> Input: A rule (method) that operates in one domain and another similar
>   domain.
> Output: A new rule that provides a method for operating in the new
>   domain.
> Process: Analogically adapt the original rule to provide a method for the
>   new domain.

The snowboarding method illustrates how method analogizing can also work with more than one source.

To my knowledge, no current rule-based or neural network computational models are sufficiently powerful to perform method generalization or adaptation. The Semantic Pointer Architecture can learn rules and has the advantage that its rules can be multimodal, which is valuable because many of the steps to be carried out by methods have sensory-motor aspects. Methods with rules that appear to have sensory and/or motor aspects include ones for the telescope, microscope, measuring density, movable type printing, photography, perspective drawing, impressionism, jazz, mobile sculpture, modern dance, snowboarding, video games, and mixed martial arts. For example, a new procedure introduced in bas-ketball in the 1940s was the jump shot, expressed verbally as *if you want to shoot over a defender then jump and then shoot with one hand* or nonverbally as <shoot-over-defense> → <jump> <one-hand-shot>, where the brackets indicate semantic pointers that incorporate visual and kinesthetic representations.

Another issue that needs to be investigated concerns how procedural rules can be chained together to produce more complicated methods. For example, the overall method of experimental work in psychology and other fields requires chaining methods for designing experiments, running them, analyzing the data, and developing theories to explain the results.

Applications

In science, the historical record is not sufficient to identify the sources of such general methods as naturalistic explanation, experimentation, and use of mathematics; but other examples look like method generalization from problem solving. Newton's calculus, Linnaean taxonomy, spectroscopy, and PCR were all cases where there was an important problem to be solved and the creator came up with a solution that could be generalized into a method. Other examples from the history of science and technology include Archimedes' technique of measuring density, movable type printing, vaccination, photography, Morse code, antiseptic surgery, FORTRAN, email, and the World Wide Web. In contrast, the telescope and microscope were already existing tools developed by Dutch lens grinders that were adapted for new scientific purposes by Galileo and Malpighi. Galileo improved the design of the telescope and then adapted it for astronomical observation, and Malpighi adapted the microscope for anatomical observation.

My 10 examples of artistic imagination are methods, but it is hard to tell from the historical record whether they came about through rule-based reasoning, analogy, or some other more diffuse process. The development of jazz was not the result of invention by any one musician but rather the result of a social process that involved many different musicians from diverse backgrounds, including African rhythms and European marching bands. In most of the other cases, the creator had a primary artistic goal: architecture for Brunelleschi, painting for da Vinci, music for Peri, painting for Monet, writing for Richardson, dance for Duncan, and sculpture for Moore and Calder.

Examples of social innovation more clearly display goal-directed reasoning, as creators identified a large social need and then came up with a novel way of satisfying it. Such needs included teaching in low-income communities, caring for dying people, reforming prisons, housing the homeless, helping the poor, educating people without access, overcoming discrimination, and helping the aged. The major exception is Zuckerberg's creation of Facebook, whose purpose was not initially clear. Zuckerberg was mostly looking for ways to exercise his substantial Web programming skills, and he produced Facebook more as an experiment than as a solution to some problem. Hence it is best described as an instance of a technique in search of a problem rather than vice versa, with analogy more important than method generalization.

Methods for recreational improvement are sometimes clearly goal directed, as with motion pictures, cable television, and e-books. These are cases where a recognized technological need led to a solution. On the other hand, several cases appear to be more analogical, where an existing technique was adapted for a new purpose.

Snowboards were based on skateboards; cruise ships were based on ocean liners; airliners were based on military planes; mixed martial arts were based on existing combat methods; and public parks were based on landscapes in private estates. But in the other cases, recreational enhancements may have come about through non-focused experimentation, which I suspect produced video games and ancient card games.

It is obvious that the five domains of creativity overlap. Some forms of recreational enhancement depended on new technologies (video games, motion pictures, e-books), and others were also social innovations (public parks). Science and technology are often connected, as in the use of the new technologies of the telescope, microscope, and spectroscope for scientific investigation. Reciprocally, some technologies grew out of scientific research, as in the leaps from Franklin's theory of lightning to lightning rods and from Pasteur's germ theory to Lister's antiseptic surgery. The technologies of movable type printing, email, and the World Wide Web also contributed to social innovations. Advantages in artistic imagination also has social effects, as when people gather for opera, jazz, and modern dance. These are all examples of interactions among the creative domains of science, technology, art, society, and recreation.

Creativity sometimes consists not just in figuring out new ways to accomplish goals but in adopting new goals that no one had thought of pursuing. The cognitive, emotional, and social processes of generating creative goals and questions are greatly in need of investigation. Some questions arise as subordinate steps to answer questions already posed, but original questions come from three major sources: surprise, curiosity, and practical need. The first two are emotions arising, respectively, from incoherence with previous beliefs and from personal interests. Practical need generates questions about how to accomplish goals in technology, medicine, and other areas.

ANALOGIES AND METAPHORS

Analogy is often recognized as a major source of creativity in science and other domains. Some scientific examples are shown in Table 11.2, and technological examples are shown in Table 11.3. In all of these cases, thinkers solved a major target problem by finding a source that could be used to generate a solution that turned out to be new, surprising, and valuable. In addition to words, mathematical representations were often useful, along with visual and other sensory modalities.

TABLE 11.2

Some Scientific Discoveries Based on Analogy

Discovery	Target	Source	Modality
living cells	living cells	monk cells	visual
gravity	planetary motion	projectile motion	visual, mathematical, kinesthetic
fossils	shark teeth	stone teeth	visual
life	hierarchy	tree	visual
lightning	lightning	spark	visual, heat
vaccination	smallpox	cowpox	visual
ultraviolet light	ultraviolet	infrared	mathematical
electromagnetism	magnetism	electricity	visual, mathematical
evolution	natural selection	Malthusian competition	mathematical
periodic table	elements	piano scale	visual
relativity	Gravity	elevator	visual, mathematical
fault lines	rock layers	rubber bands	visual
earth mantle	Earth	egg	visual
quantum theory	electrons	crystals	mathematical

Reproduced by permission of Oxford University Press from Thagard 2012b, p. 394.

TABLE 11.3

Analogies in Technological Inventions

Invention	Target	Source	Modality
printing press	printing	olive press	visual, kinesthetic
telephone	telephone	ear	visual, sound
paper	bark paper	hemp paper	visual, touch
airplane	airplane	bird	visual
stethoscope	stethoscope	wood	sound
microscope	microscope	eyeglasses	visual
Braille	Braille	previous dots	touch
incubator	baby incubator	chick hatchery	visual, heat
cotton gin	cotton machine	hand movements	visual, kinesthetic
windmill	windmill	sail	visual
washing machine	machine	hand movements	visual, kinesthetic
oil derrick	oil	gallows	visual

Reproduced by permission of Oxford University Press from Thagard 2012b, p. 397.

Analogies also often contribute to artistic imagination. Novelists such as Tolstoy and James Joyce based much of their writing on episodes in their own lives, with modifications that make it clear that they were writing fiction rather than autobiography. Poets such as Emily Dickinson used poignant metaphors that were based on underlying analogies, for example when she wrote that hope is the thing with feathers. Composers use analogies when they adapt other pieces of music for their own purposes, for example when John Lennon was inspired by Beethoven's *Moonlight Sonata* to produce the Beatles song "Because." Another Beatles song, "Blackbird," has a guitar accompaniment inspired by J.S. Bach's *Bourrée in E minor*.

Going in the other direction, from popular to classical music, we find composers such as Franz Liszt and Aaron Copeland drawing on folk tunes. Painters usually do not exactly reproduce painted objects but instead produce images that are only analogous to what they actually see. Analogies can also contribute to social innovation, for example when Mark Zuckerberg modeled Facebook partly on student directories.

It is important, however, not to exaggerate the contribution of analogy to creativity. First, many episodes of creativity do not require analogy, because they use other cognitive processes such as conceptual combination and abductive generalization. Only if analogy is loosely construed to be identical to categorization, which I criticized in chapter 6, does it become plausible that all creativity involves analogy. Second, many uses of analogy are woefully uncreative: instead of producing results that are new and surprising, they merely rehash previous ideas that are not in fact relevant to the current situation, like the generals and businesses described in chapter 6. Hence analogy can be a conservative force rather than a creative one. Analogies always need to be evaluated to determine whether the solutions they suggest actually are effective at meeting the goals relevant to a target problem. Otherwise, the results may be not very new, surprising, or valuable. A list of the worst analogies ever made includes the following: John and Mary had never met, just like two hummingbirds who had also never met. The paradox of analogy is that it has contributed to some of the most brilliant creations in history but also to some of the most banal repetitions, such as each year's television shows that try to ape the successes of the previous year.

For those cases where creativity is indeed based on analogies, the semantic pointer mechanisms described in chapter 6 can explain the origins of new and surprising products. Semantic pointers can provide the multimodal representations that are important for visual analogies in fields such as science, technology, and painting, as well as for auditory analogies in musical composition. Creative acts are not purely syntactic manipulations but require mechanisms that integrate syntax with semantics and pragmatics to produce analogies that are meaningful and useful. Creativity in science, technology, art, and social change is far from random, driven by goals such as producing an explanation, an instrument, a work of art, or a valuable social enterprise. The Semantic Pointer Architecture shows how to integrate structure with meaning and purpose, which is often directed by emotions.

EMOTIONS

Chapter 7 described how emotion is not simply an addition to or distraction from cognition but rather an integral part of it. Accordingly, it is not surprising that emotion makes important contributions to creativity. Emotions serve as both inputs and outputs of creativity, as well as an accompaniment for all of the cognitive processes needed to generate new images, concepts, rules, and analogies.

Emotions serve as inputs to creative processes by providing motivations that spur people to generate new ideas. Most creative products in science, technology, art, and social change result from conscious, intentional, goal-driven attempts to solve problems. People do not just pick any goal but rather are driven by goals that are emotionally important to them. Chapter 9 described how goals carry emotional significance through binding of semantic pointers. The mental representation of a desired state becomes bound with emotions such as the desire to accomplish it or the fear of failure. The goal can be a fact to be explained, a device to be produced, a work of art to be generated, or a social change to be accomplished. Most creative acts result from substantial periods of intense and prolonged activity, which people would not attempt without the motivation that comes from these emotionally significant goals. You cannot simply will yourself to be creative, because most of the key mechanisms such as binding and combination of representations are not under conscious control. But you can foster emotions that encourage you to engage intensely in the kinds of thinking that sometimes have novel and productive outcomes.

The semantic pointer theory of emotions in chapter 7 showed how mental representations of goals can be bound to emotions construed as bindings of physiological perceptions and cognitive appraisals. Chapter 9 described how emotions attached to goals can generate intentions and courses of action. A diversity of emotion-laden goals, such as curiosity, avoidance of boredom, fame, and fortune motivate the pursuit of lines of thought that can have creative results. Functional magnetic resonance imaging shows that activity in the midbrain and the nucleus accumbens is enhanced during states of high curiosity.

Emotions are also outputs of the creative process, as evident in the inclusion of surprise as one of the typical features of creativity. Much stronger emotions can occur in the creative process as the result of breakthroughs that accomplishes long-pursued goals. The famous story of Archimedes shouting "Eureka" and running naked through the streets of Syracuse (as a result of coming up with a solution to the problem of how to figure out the density of the king's crown) illustrates the excitement and elation that can result from the creative big breakthrough. Other positive emotions that can result from a creative accomplishment include happiness, pride, and satisfaction.

Emotional outputs are central to the evaluation of a product as valuable, useful, important, appropriate, correct, and accurate. As chapter 7 described, emotions result in part from cognitive appraisal of the extent to which a situation accomplishes relevant goals. Hence the reaction to a new product that accomplishes goals will be positive emotions ranging from contentment to elation. On the other hand, a product that fails can result in disappointment, sadness, and even depression. Emotions can spread in groups of collaborators through social mechanisms such as empathy and emotional contagion, so the emotional evaluation of potentially creative products can be a social as well as an individual process. Recognizing the creativity of others can produce a wide range of emotions from pride to envy.

Emotions are not merely inputs and outputs to creativity; rather they pervade the creative process. During the intense work leading up to a creative breakthrough, people may be subject to various emotions, both positive and negative. In addition to the happiness that can go with a feeling that progress is being made toward a challenging goal, there can also be negative emotions such as frustration, disappointment, fear of failure, and possibly even anger at impediments to progress. Emotions can help to steer people away from disappointments and also to encourage them to move in more promising directions as a result of excitement and enthusiasm. In accord with the semantic pointer theory of consciousness in chapter 8, emotions contribute to the ability of some representations to win out in the battle for consciousness over others, ensuring attention to the paths of thought most likely to produce creative outcomes.

Hence the semantic pointer theory of emotion explains how emotions can make major contributions to creativity, as inputs to, outputs from, and constant accompaniments of cognition. Of course, emotions can sometimes be impediments to creativity, if emotional states such as anxiety, resentment, or sadness make it difficult for a thinker to carry out the intense and prolonged effort that is often required to generate products that are new, surprising, and valuable.

CASE STUDY: CRISPR/CAS9

To see how these mental mechanisms interact, consider one of the most important recent advances in biology. Publications in 2012 announced a major breakthrough in both science and technology. The scientific breakthrough was description of a new mechanism by which bacteria protect themselves from viruses. The technological breakthrough was the realization that the same mechanism could be used as a general tool for editing genes, with enormous potential for practical applications ranging from treating genetic diseases and cancer to creating new foods. By 2018, clinical trials for medical uses were underway, and new agricultural products were in advanced development.

The novel biological theory and the novel technology both go by the awkward name "CRISPR/Cas9," whose development provides a fine illustration of my cognitive account of creativity. Innovation required new concepts, images, rules, and analogies, leading to the generation of a new method and attendant emotions. One of the major contributors to these breakthroughs is an American biochemist, Jennifer Doudna, who in 2017 published an engaging account of her lab's work, *A Crack in Creation*.

Concepts and Images

The concepts *CRISPR* and *cas* were introduced in a 2002 article, "Identification of Genes That Are Associated with DNA Repeats". Using computer databases, Ruud Jansen and his collaborators identified a novel family of repetitive DNA sequences they called CRISPR, for "clustered regularly interspaced short palindromic repeats," where "palindromic" means that the sequences read the same backward as forward.

Doudna learned about CRISPR in 2006 from another Berkeley professor, Jillian Banfield, who sought out a collaboration because of Doudna's experience with RNA. Banfield taught Doudna about CRISPR by drawing a diagram:

> First, she drew a large oval to represent a bacterial cell. Then she drew a circle inside the oval, the bacterial chromosome, and added a series of alternating diamonds and squares along one side of the circle to represent a region of DNA. This region, apparently, was CRISPR. Jill shaded in the diamonds and mentioned that they were all identical stretches of the same thirty-ish letters of DNA. Then she numbered the squares sequentially beginning at 1 while explaining that each one constituted a unique sequence of DNA.

Doudna's book and many papers about CRISPR contain similar illustrations. Banfield reported that the function of CRISPR was unknown but that there were hints that it might contribute to a bacterial immune system that helped to protect them against viruses.

The 2002 Jansen paper also reported the occurrence of CRISPR-associated genes, *cas*, located adjacent to occurrences of CRISPR and presumably functionally associated with them. Further studies revealed that a specific gene, *cas9*, produced a protein, Cas9, that was important for providing antiviral immunity to a kind of bacteria used in yogurt production. The concepts *CRISPR* and *Cas9* were partly derived from observations of DNA sequences in computer databases but also required substantial conceptual combinations, as in the binding of the three ingredients that go into "CRISPR-associated genes."

Rules and Procedures

Mental representation of hypotheses about the functions and uses of CRISPR and Cas9 require rules. The key biological claim about CRISPR/Cas9 is captured by this rule: *If the Cas9 protein is guided by RNA from CRISPR, then the protein can destroy DNA from viruses.* This rule summarizes a mechanism in which the interconnected parts (CRISPR, Cas9, and the viral DNA) interact to accomplish the function of protecting bacteria from viruses. Formation of the rules that summarize the mechanisms was by abductive inference, generating an explanation of numerous experiments that explored the functioning of CRISPR and Cas9.

The mechanisms can be captured more vividly and dynamically by visual images that are commonly used in descriptions of CRISPR/Cas9. The diagrams are particularly useful in indicating interactions and causal directions. Figure 11.1 is

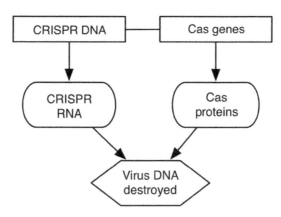

FIGURE 11.1 Sketch of the mechanism by which CRISPR and Cas9 fight viruses.

a simplified depiction of how CRISPR and Cas9 interact to destroy viral DNA and prevent viruses from killing the bacteria they infect.

Doudna and others showed that the mechanism summarized by the rule about Cas9 and RNA can be adapted into a general method of gene editing. This procedural creativity is reflected in a rule: *If you want to edit genes, then use CRISPR RNA and Cas9 to cut and manipulate DNA in the genes.* This rule and similar ones are now the basis for exciting innovations in biotechnology and medicine. The technology and medical treatments are often better represented by pictures that show sequences of DNA in genes being severed and rejoined.

Analogies

Doudna's book uses many educational analogies to make vivid the functions of CRISPR and Cas9. She variously describes their operation as a missile or a weapons system waging warfare in the arms race between bacteria and invading viruses. Cas9 operates like scissors or hedge clippers as part of a Swiss army knife of immune system defenses. This CRISPR-based immune system is analogous to the human immune system, with Cas9 and other proteins protecting bacteria against viruses just as T cells protect humans against viruses, bacteria, and fungi.

Doudna's recounting of the history of ideas about CRISPR shows that her analogies were not just expository. Her thinking about the studies needed to support the procedural rule about using CRISPR and Cas9 to edit genes was guided by her knowledge of other techniques for gene editing, including the recombinant DNA work of the 1970s and subsequent improvements. The analogy with known methods for gene editing suggested how CRISPR might be useful. Filling in the details about the editing mechanisms was a major part of the procedural creativity that led to the new method of gene editing. Method analogizing worked by taking old rules for gene editing procedures and adapting them into new rules for how to use CRISPR and Cas9 to accomplish the same results more efficiently. Development of the new rule exploited previous advances in new biological concepts and hypotheses.

Emotions

The thought processes of Doudna and others exhibit sophisticated cognitive processes using concepts, imagery, rules, and analogy. But Doudna's memoir also exhibits a substantial role for emotions, just as in James Watson's *The Double Helix*, the book that made her want to be a biologist when she was 12 years old. Doudna says that "research scientists are fueled by adventurousness, curiosity, instinct, and grit." She mentions numerous emotional reactions to different stages of work, including exciting and thrilling discoveries, intriguing and alluring hypotheses, amazing and bizarre phenomena, and disappointing experimental results. The following is her description of her reaction on the evening after experiments showed that CRISPR/Cas9 accomplishes gene editing:

> That night, as I stood at my kitchen stove cooking dinner, visions of this tiny machine danced in my head: Cas9 and its guide RNA whizzing around a bacterial cell, hunting for matching DNA sequences. Suddenly, I found myself laughing aloud. How incredible that bacteria had found a way to program a warrior protein to seek and destroy viral DNA! And how miraculous, how fortunate, that we could repurpose this fundamental property for an entirely different use. It was a precious time of pure joy, the joy of discovery.

Scientific creativity clearly interweaves cognition and emotion. Pursuit of challenging questions requires diverse emotions such as interest, doubt, wonder, and enthusiasm.

Collaborations

Doudna's book makes it clear that scientific creativity is a social process. Jillian Banfield spurred Doudna's interest in CRISPR, and her major collaborator on the breakthrough research was the French microbiologist Emmanuelle Charpentier. Their laboratory research depended on the intense efforts of many graduate students and postdoctoral assistants. All of the major papers on CRISPR by Doudna's group and by other laboratories have at least four coauthors. Doudna's interactions with her collaborators required extensive verbal and nonverbal communication. Chapter 12 and *Mind–Society* analyze the social mechanisms responsible for developments in science, technology, and other human activities.

SUMMARY AND DISCUSSION

This neural account of the cognitive and emotional processes sufficient for creativity shows the dispensability of supernatural theories such as divine intervention and Plato's grasping of abstract ideas. Rather, creativity results from neural processes that include binding of representations, generation of new concepts and rules, and the application of analogies. Some of these processes are already well enough understood to be capable of producing simulations using the Semantic Pointer Architecture. For other important phenomena such as the generation of new methods, we can begin to imagine the kinds of computer simulations needed. Like other cognitive processes, creative thinking requires the productive synthesis of syntax, semantics, and pragmatics.

The Semantic Pointer Architecture contributes to the understanding of creativity in several ways. First, it accommodates the full range of multimodal representations needed for creativity in the domains of scientific discovery, technological invention, artistic imagination, and social innovation. Representations may be verbal, mathematical, or tied to sensory and motor processes such as vision and arm movements.

Second, new semantic pointers can be generated by convolution-based bindings in ways that produce new and useful images, concepts, rules, and analogies. Potentially creative products of image manipulation, conceptual combination, rule construction, and analogical inference can all be produced by transformations of semantic pointers. Procedural creativity is the generation of new methods expressed as rules, which can result from generalization and analogy, as illustrated in the case of CRISPR/Cas9.

Third, the pragmatic focus of creative problem solving and the evaluation of the goal relevance of new products can be carried out by emotions, construed as bindings of representations with a combination of appraisal and physiology. Fourth, competition among semantic pointers explains how the delightful realization that you might have done something creative enters consciousness. Fifth, semantic pointers account for the embodied aspects of creativity that require sensory and motor representations but also show how transbodied representations are produced by recursive binding.

Like consciousness, creativity requires emergence of new processes that are themselves emergent, including neural representation, binding into semantic pointers, and evaluation by semantic pointer competition. Molecular, neural, and psychological mechanisms all contribute, along with the social mechanisms described in chapter 12 and *Mind–Society*.

This chapter almost completes the main argument that the Semantic Pointer Architecture is capable of explaining the most challenging aspects of cognition, including problem solving, learning, emotion, consciousness, intentional action, language, and creativity. The remaining chapter considers the last major impediment to a full theory of cognition, the self. Consideration of the self requires attention to social mechanisms, as well as to the cognitive, emotional, and neural mechanisms that have been the main concern of this book. Creativity is not just an individual process but often results from social mechanisms for communication and collaboration. The discussions of professions in *Mind–Society* (chapter 13) and arts in *Natural Philosophy* (chapter 9) describe more ways in which creativity results from the interactions of mental and social mechanisms.

NOTES

The quote from Steve Jobs is at http://archive.wired.com/wired/archive/4.02/jobs_pr.html. For more on Jobs, see *Mind–Society* (chapter 13).

Proponents of the view that creative products are typically new, valuable, and surprising include Boden 2004 and Simonton 2012. On the products of creativity, see, for example, Kaufman and Sternberg 2010; Nersessian 2008; Simonton 1988, 2004; Thagard 1999, 2012d; Thagard and Croft 1999; Ward, Smith, and Vaid 1997; Weisberg 1993.

On surprise as a judgment of emotional coherence, see Thagard 2006.

Where does philosophical creativity fit into my five-fold classification of domains of creativity? I owe to Unnati Patel the observation that some philosophical advances are akin to science (e.g., coherence theories of knowledge), while others are more like social innovation (e.g., theories of justice).

On the contributions of imagery to creativity, see Abraham 2016; Miller 1984; Nersessian 2008; and Finke, Ward, and Smith 1992.

Proponents of the view that creativity requires combination of representations include Stewart 1792, Mednick 1962, Koestler 1967, and Boden 2004. For evidence that all creativity results from combination of representations, see Thagard 2012b (reprinted in Thagard 2012d), Thagard 2014a, Jiang and Thagard 2014, and *Mind–Society* (chapter 13). For advice on how to be more creative, see Thagard 2005a.

Vartanian, Bristol, and Kaufman 2013 discuss the neuroscience of creativity. Kounios and Beeman 2014 review the cognitive neuroscience of insight. Beaty et al. 2018 identify a brain network associated with high creativity. Bayesian models of cognition can simulate some kinds of causal reasoning and learning but have nothing to say about imagery, emotion, analogy, and the generation of new concepts and rules.

On conceptual combination, see Thagard 1988, 2012d; Thagard and Stewart 2011; and Ward, Smith, and Vaid 1997.

On the creative contributions of abduction, see Thagard 1988 and Magnani 2009. Thagard 1999 (pp. 43–44) analyzes how questions are generated. Darden, Pal, Kunda, and Moult 2018 analyze the discovery of disease mechanisms.

I owe to David Park the observation that procedural creativity can sometimes be serendipitous, when people stumble across a new way of doing things that they generalize. According to Sahdra and Thagard 2003, procedural knowledge in molecular biology does not reduce to knowledge-that. *Natural Philosophy* argues that epistemology needs to accommodate verbal knowledge-that, procedural knowledge-how, and perceptual knowledge-of, which each require different kinds of semantic pointers. The nonverbal sorts of knowledge are tacit rather than explicit because they consist of sensory and motor representations that are hard to translate into words. *Mind–Society* argues that the unconscious rules in romantic relationships are tacit for the same reason.

On rule formation, see Anderson 1993; Rosenbloom, Laird, and Newell 1993; Holland, Holyoak, Nisbett, and Thagard 1986; and Thagard 1988. Lenat 1983 describes a computer program that creates new heuristics. According to Greenwald 2012, more Nobel prizes in the sciences have been given for methods rather than theory. Procedural creativity can include new methods for classification, for example of species based on evolutionary descent rather than similarity.

Tables 11.2 and 11.3 are discussed in more detail in Thagard 2012b (reprinted in Thagard 2012d). Many other examples of creative analogies are in Holyoak and Thagard 1995 and in Hofstadter and Sander 2013. For artistic examples, see Thagard 2014a, and for social innovation examples see Jiang and Thagard 2014. For analogy in social contexts, see Dunbar 1997 and Dunbar and Fugelsang 2005. Green 2016 reviews neuroscience research on creativity and analogy.

On the role of emotion in scientific thinking, see Thagard 2006. Activity in the midbrain and the nucleus accumbens is enhanced during states of high curiosity: Gruber, Gelman, and Ranganath 2014. Brain stimulation can boost creativity: Lustenberger et al. 2015. Neurotransmitter-modifying chemicals such as amphetamines and alcohol can also affect creativity. Ritter and Ferguson 2017 report that listening to happy music facilitates creativity. Nested emotions such as fear of embarrassment and desire for pride can also provide motivation for creativity.

Doudna's memoir is Doudna and Sternberg 2017. The quote about drawing CRISPR is from page 41, the quote about what fuels scientists is from page 51, and the quote about the joy of discovery is from pages 83–84. The breakthrough paper by Doudna and her colleagues is Jinek et al. 2012. Other important advances include Gasiunas, Barrangou, Horvath, and Siksnys 2012 and Cong et al. 2013. CRISPR and *cas* were introduced by Jansen, Embden, Gaastra, and Schouls 2002. For images, see Doudna's book and the Wikipedia article https://en.wikipedia.org/wiki/CRISPR. My analysis of the emotions in *The Double Helix* is in Thagard 2002a, reprinted in Thagard 2006.

PROJECT

Develop computational models of method generalization, method analogization, and emotional evaluation of creative products. Apply computational models to the CRISPR/Cas9 case of procedural creativity.

12

The Self

In the play *Hamlet*, Shakespeare has Polonius say: "This above all: to thine own self be true. And it must follow, as the night the day, thou canst not then be false to any man." But what does it mean to be true to yourself? And what is the self to which you are supposed to be true?

The nature of the self is dramatically relevant to all of the aspects of thinking that we have so far examined. Creativity is not an abstract aspect of the universe but rather something that people want to claim for themselves. When Archimedes shouted "Eureka!" after discovering how to measure density, he would not have been so excited if someone else had found it. In language, the word "I" is among the most frequently used in speech and writing. Actions often result from intentions that include the representation of self as having the intent to do something. Consciousness and emotions are not free-floating but rather properties that people naturally apply to themselves: there is a specific person who is aware of pain, happiness, sadness, shame, or pride. Hence, we need to have a good understanding of the self if we want to have a full account of emotions, consciousness, action, language, and creativity.

The role of the self in all these mental phenomena is explicable using semantic pointers, so that many roles of the self in thought and action can be explained in neural-cognitive terms. I argue, however, that there are aspects of the self that require stretching beyond the levels of explanation so far used. Understanding the self requires additional attention to molecular and social mechanisms, because selves depend not just on cognitions and emotions but also on underpinning molecular factors such as genes, neurotransmitters, and hormones. Moreover, a full theory of the self must take into account the social relationships that powerfully influence our feelings, actions, utterances, and even our creativity.

Accordingly, this chapter serves as a bridge between the largely individual psychology discussed in this book and the intensely social phenomena discussed in *Mind–Society*, which applies cognition and emotion to the social sciences and professions. How people think about themselves in relation to their social groups is crucial for understanding economic behavior such as buying and selling, political behavior such as voting, and many other kinds of social behaviors such as practicing religions and waging wars. But understanding of the social self must go hand-in-hand with appreciation of the cognitive and emotional operations that operate in the minds of all participating individuals.

After addressing general questions about the nature of the self, I show the relevance of semantic pointers for crucial characteristics of it. Applications include representational aspects such as self-identity that employ images and concepts, and also dynamic aspects concerning the self's ability or inability to act and its tendency to change. The self is not a supernatural entity like a soul or spirit, but neither is it a mere fiction to be dispensed with in scientific accounts of mind in society. Rather, it is a complex multilevel system that can be understood by bringing to bear the appropriate neural and cognitive mechanisms, supplemented by two additional levels of mechanisms, the molecular and the social.

WHAT IS THE SELF?

My account of the self is radically different from most philosophical approaches, which tend to be either transcendental or deflationary. Transcendental views, held by philosophers such as Plato, Aquinas, Descartes, and Kant, take selves as supernatural entities—souls—that are not open to mechanistic explanation using the methods of natural science. At the other, deflationary extreme, some philosophers have been skeptical of the idea of the self as a determinate kind of thing, proposing instead that the self is just a bundle of perceptions (Hume), a convenient fiction amounting to a "center of narrative gravity" (Dennett), or simply a myth (Metzinger). Similarly, postmodernist sociologists view selves as mere social constructions. In analytical, phenomenological, and Indian traditions, debates continue about whether the self is a substance, non-substance, or nothing at all.

In contrast, social and clinical psychologists make substantial use of the concept of the self in their discussions of a wide range of phenomena. But they have largely shied away from the task of saying what selves are. My multilevel mechanism account is intended to fill this gap while avoiding the metaphysical extravagance of transcendental views and the explanatory impotence of deflationary ones. Figure 12.1 charts more than 80 phenomena about the self that are frequently discussed by psychologists and also sometimes by sociologists and anthropologists. The phenomena are organized into three kinds of self-representing, two kinds of self-effecting, and self-changing. Representing concerns how people portray themselves to themselves and others, effecting concerns how people act to facilitate or

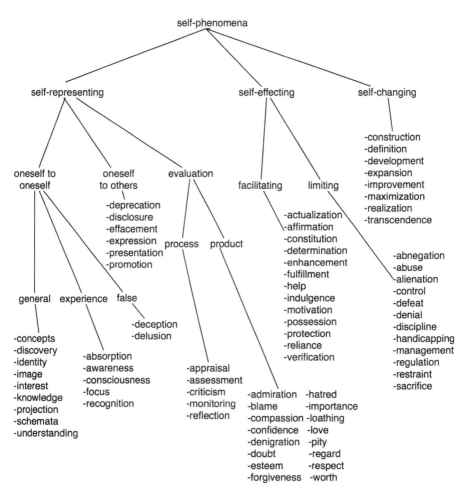

FIGURE 12.1 Grouping of many self-phenomena into six main classes: self-representing (with three subcategories), self-effecting (with two subcategories), and self-changing. Adapted with permission of Routledge from Thagard 2014c.

limit their own behaviors, and changing concerns long-term alterations in representations and behaviors.

The Representing Self

A representation is a structure or activity that stands for something, and many of the self-phenomena listed in Figure 12.1 concern ways in which people represent themselves. The representing self can roughly be divided into three subgroups concerned with (a) depicting oneself to oneself, (b) depicting oneself to others, and (c) evaluating oneself according to one's own standards. For example, you might think of yourself as being anxious but prefer to present yourself to other people as confident because you think being confident is better than being anxious.

The most general terms for depicting oneself to oneself are self-knowledge and self-understanding. Self-concepts and self-schemata are both mental ingredients of self-knowledge, serving as cognitive structures to represent different aspects of the self such as personality traits. Self-interest consists in the collection of your personal goals, both conscious and unconscious. Self-identity and self-image are also ways in which you represent yourself to yourself, although they may also contribute to how you present yourself to others. Self-discovery and self-projection are processes that involve self-representation.

Several aspects of depicting oneself to oneself assume conscious experience, as in self-awareness. Such experience is not purely cognitive, as it can also involve prominent moods and emotions. Another set of phenomena that involve depicting oneself to oneself includes self-deception and self-delusion, in which the representation of self is inaccurate.

The second division within the group of self-representing phenomena involves depicting and communicating oneself to others, which is emotionally positive for self-expression and self-promotion but can be emotionally negative with self-deprecation and self-effacement.

The third subgroup of self-phenomena in the representing category concerns the evaluation of the self, either as an ongoing process or as the product that results from the evaluation. Phenomena concerned with the process of evaluation include self-appraisal, where you decide how well you live up to the standards of yourself and society. There are many products that result from this process, including both general assessments such as self-confidence and particular emotional reactions such as self-admiration and self-pity.

The Effecting Self

The self does more than just represent itself; it also does things to itself, including facilitating its own functioning in desirable ways and limiting its functioning to prevent undesirable consequences. Self-phenomena that have a facilitating effect include self-affirmation and self-protection. Self-evaluation can also produce the self-knowledge that unconstrained actions may have undesirable consequences, as in excessive eating, drinking, drug use, and dangerous liaisons. Accordingly, there is a set of important phenomena concerning limits that people put on their own behavior, including self-control and self-sacrifice. Forms of self-effecting are important for predicting and controlling behavior. For example, self-discipline predicts academic performance better than IQ, and the sum of lovers' self-control predicts relationship quality better than their having different capacities for restraint. All of these results support the need to make sense of the self rather than discarding it.

The self-effecting phenomena involve people encouraging or discouraging their own behaviors, but they do not bring about fundamental, longer lasting changes in the self, which is the third and probably rarest function of the self.

The Changing Self

Over a lifetime, people change as the result of aging and experiences such as major life events. Some self-phenomena such as self-development concern processes of change. The changes can involve alterations in self-representing, when people come to apply different concepts to themselves, and also self-effecting, if people manage to change the degree to which they are capable of either facilitating desired behaviors or limiting undesired ones. Whereas short-term psychotherapy is aimed at dealing with small-scale problems in self-representing and self-efficacy, long-term psychotherapy may aim at larger alterations in the underlying nature of the self. Self-change can build on changes in intentions, emotions, concepts, and rules discussed in previous chapters.

The proposed grouping of self-phenomena summarized in Figure 12.1 is not exhaustive, as there are aspects of self that are described by words without the "self" prefix, such as agency, autonomy, personhood, and resilience, as well as more esoteric terms that do use the prefix. But the diagram serves to provide an idea of the large range of phenomena concerning the self. A theory of the self should explain all of these by specifying causal mechanisms that produce them. The self should not be ignored, as required by deflationary views of the self as non-existing; nor should it be mystified, as required by transcendent views of the self as souls. I show the relevance of semantic pointer accounts of mental representation and inference to the three main aspects of self: representing, effecting, and changing. Then I discuss the relevance of mechanisms at other levels—molecular and social—to understanding these phenomena.

Self-changing and self-effecting depend on self-representing, so the first question to ask is how minds represent themselves. Figure 12.2 displays a semantic pointer for the self that results from binding several other representations, all patterns of neural firing that may in turn be semantic pointers. Your representation of yourself includes your current experiences, for example that you are reading and drinking coffee. But it can also include memories of previous experiences, such as a conversation you had yesterday. Less fleetingly, your self-representation can include concepts that you routinely apply to yourself such as whether you are a man or woman, tall or short, optimistic or pessimistic. Some of these concepts are inherently social in that they describe relationships with other people, such as whether you are a child or parent, student or teacher, and/or employee or boss. The bindings that construct semantic pointers enable your representation of yourself to be complex and dynamic, changing from time to time but with enduring commonalities provided by stable memories and familiar concepts. The self is not a thing but rather a process that emerges from neural mechanisms that also have emergent properties. Again, as with emotions, consciousness, and creativity, the self exemplifies emergence from emergence.

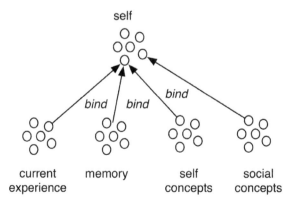

FIGURE 12.2 Semantic pointer for the self, resulting from binding other neural representations.

Images

David Hume argued that philosophers should abandon the concept of self because he could not detect it in any of his sensory experiences. Indeed, our experiences of sights, sounds, pains, and so on do not need to have any explicit representation of ourselves. But Hume did not appreciate how sensations can not only be experienced but can also be bound together into more complicated kinds of images that go well beyond particular sensations. Imagery of all kinds can affect how we represent ourselves, for example as tall or short, heavy or light, strong or weak, fragrant or foul, loud or quiet, happy or sad, confident or afraid, and healthy or in pain. These images need not be as fleeting as sensations, for we can preserve them in memory and retrieve them in appropriate circumstances. Moreover, we can bind them together into packages that provide a coherent depiction of ourselves, for example as someone who is short, strong, and happy.

The semantic pointer account of images in chapter 3 can easily accommodate all of these uses of self-imagery. We saw that sensory images can go beyond sensory experiences by producing new patterns of neural firing that abstract from and synthesize aspects of sensory experience to make images capable of new combinations. You can imagine yourself as having properties that have not in fact been experienced by the senses. You can use images to represent yourself accurately, but you can also imagine yourself as being much taller, thinner, stronger, and happier than you actually are. These operations of self-imagery can all be accomplished by the transformations of images discussed in chapter 3. Self-image can be embodied by virtue of representations of how you see your physical characteristics such as being fit but also transbodied by virtue of abstract concepts that you apply to yourself such as being kind.

Concepts

Social psychologists often discuss self-concepts but rarely take a stand on what concepts are. The semantic pointer theory of concepts in chapter 4 can illuminate the nature of the concepts that we apply to ourselves and that we use to present ourselves to others. Semantic pointers show how to integrate three aspects of concepts that have previously been taken as distinct: exemplars, typical features, and explanations. Consider for example the concepts that personality theorists have found to be most useful for capturing responses to surveys and interviews: openness, conscientiousness, extraversion, agreeableness, and neuroticism. As an illustration, I show how exemplars, features, and explanations all contribute to one of the most familiar of the personality characteristics, extraversion.

Exemplars are standard examples, and the media provide numerous examples of famous people whose behavior marks them as extraverted. Think of movie stars like George Clooney and Jennifer Lawrence, or sports heroes like LeBron James and Venus Williams. More locally, you probably have friends who stand out as being unusually outgoing and gregarious. It also helps to be able to think of counterexemplars who lack the trait of extraversion, such as ordinary people who shun the limelight. Hence the concept of extraversion, which you may or may not apply to yourself, has detectable exemplars associated with it.

It is also easy to identify typical features that belong to most of the exemplars of extraversion. Extraverted people are typically sociable, talkative, confident, and interested in other people. As chapter 4 stresses, these features do not need to be definitional necessary and sufficient conditions, just strongly associated with the concept. You do not need to have a definition of extraversion to apply it to yourself or others, merely an understanding of its typical features. Which concepts you apply to yourself and others may vary with context through the mechanism of parallel constraint satisfaction.

The third feature of concepts accounted for by semantic pointers is the role of explanations. When you apply the concept of extraversion to yourself or others, you often do it for explanatory purposes, in order to account for observed behavior. You might say, for example, that George Clooney had a highly public wedding because he is extraverted, with the assumption that this personality trait is a cause of the behavior. Sometimes, people also know explanations of why they have that trait, for example on the assumption that there is a genetic basis for extraversion that George Clooney inherited from his journalist father. Hence the semantic pointer theory of concepts can readily explain how all three aspects of concepts—exemplars, features, and explanations—can apply to self-representations. Moreover, semantic pointers show how all three aspects can be realized by the same underlying neural processes. The concepts that people apply to themselves constitute their social identities with respect to relationships, occupation, nationality, ethnicity, politics, and religion. For example, I identify as a Canadian retired professor with two sons, mongrel ethnicity, and no religion.

Rules

Rules, which chapter 5 explains as *if–then* structures built of semantic pointers, are also important for understanding self-representations. When you think of yourself as extraverted or introverted, you likely have rules associated with the typical features of the relevant concepts. Pertinent rules in your mind might include: *If a person is extraverted, then he or she wants to meet new people; if a person is introverted then he or she feels uncomfortable at parties.* Typical features naturally translate into rules which can then serve as explanations by immediate causal inference, for example that someone is avoiding a party because of being introverted.

Some of the rules you possess about yourself may be unconscious because they are nonverbal. For instance, I may cringe in gory movies because of the multimodal rule <*see-blood*> → <*recoil*>, where the condition is visual and emotional and the action is motor and emotional. Such unconscious multimodal rules are important for explaining romantic relationships in *Mind–Society*.

Analogies and Metaphors

Analogies are not as central to self-representations as images, concepts, and rules but can contribute to identities. Some people have role models whom they emulate in a way that captures key aspects of themselves. You have a very different way of thinking of yourself if you see your role model as Mother Teresa rather than Gloria Steinem, or Gandhi rather than Bill Gates. Your role models are analogous to you in having relations that connect with actions, not just in having similar features. If your role model is Gandhi, then simple features like height or weight are much less relevant than complex relations that connect goals with actions: his commitment to nonviolence severely constrained the actions he could take in trying to throw off British domination of India. So adopting and presenting Gandhi as your analogical role model will dispose you to nonviolent actions.

Another way in which analogy can affect self-representation is via metaphors, which usually have underlying analogies. The psychotherapist Donald Meichenbaum describes the value of taking into account the metaphors that people apply to themselves, for example when they see themselves as a deer caught in the headlights. These metaphorical representations have underlying analogies that reveal much about how the people think of themselves, for example as someone trapped in a difficult situation. The semantic pointer accounts of analogy and metaphor in chapters 6 and 10 capture this aspect of self-representation.

Emotions

Emotions apply to self-representation in several ways. First, there are the emotion concepts that people self-apply at particular moments when they are not merely experiencing an emotion but are also aware of the emotional experience. For example, you might think of yourself as being happy or worried right now, with awareness that these states apply specifically to you. Second, emotion concepts can be used more enduringly when people apply personality characterizations to themselves, for example when you think of yourself as being agreeable, neurotic, calm, confident, or fun-loving.

The third way in which emotions are relevant to self-representation is more indirect, by virtue of the role that emotions play in all other concepts. A concept such as extraverted is not explicitly emotional, but it likely has emotional associations depending on your appraisal of the value of being extraverted. You may think of being extraverted as positive because of all the fun you have interacting with other people, or you may think of it as negative because it leads you to be distracted from other goals such as work. Similarly, you might view introversion as emotionally positive because it frees you from distractions and disappointments or as emotionally negative if you see it as keeping you from meeting your social needs. Because all concepts have an emotional component, emotion is intrinsic to self-representation.

Emotions operate in all forms of self-evaluation such as admiration, compassion, and denigration. Chapter 7 described how the semantic pointer theory of emotions integrates cognitive appraisal and physiological perception. Physiological variations are most relevant to current emotional states, as when an unsettled stomach contributes to anxiety and self-doubt. But physiological perception can also be relevant to self-representation through the application of dispositional emotional concepts to oneself and the associations of other concepts with emotions. When you think of yourself as being neurotic or confident, you may have an emotional image based on memory of previous cases when you felt worried or secure. Similarly, the emotional associations with concepts like *extraverted* may be tied to images of previous physiological states. All these ways in which emotions are relevant to self-representation are also tied to cognitive appraisal through evaluations of the extent to which the current situation is relevant to your goals and needs. Hence the semantic pointer theory of emotions illuminates the emotional aspects of self-representation by means of the integration of appraisal and physiology.

Consciousness

Other aspects of cognition and emotion discussed in previous chapters are also relevant to self-representation. Chapter 8 discusses self-consciousness as resulting from the same mechanisms as simpler forms: neural representation, binding, and semantic pointer competition. Self-awareness occurs when representations of yourself by images, concepts, rules, or analogies outcompete other representations stimulated by the current situation. Self-consciousness differs from other kinds of consciousness because it requires binding of representations of the situations with aspects of the self. For example, you can drive a car with only basic awareness of features of the road, but you become self-aware if you realize that you are getting sleepy and are in danger of dozing off. Then sensations, images, and concepts applied to the act of driving become bound with the different kinds of representations that refer to you, including images (*you crashing*), concepts (*reckless*), rules (*drive safely*), or analogies (*a reckless celebrity*).

Emotions can also be attached to rules, for example the fear associated with thinking that if you doze off then your car will crash. This fear can help your self-representation to outcompete mere sensations or other distractions, enabling you to focus on avoiding a crash. The Semantic Pointer Architecture illuminates self-representation by explaining how self-concepts can be bound with representations of the situation and by explaining how people become self-conscious when the newly bound self-representation outcompetes other semantic pointers.

The intention-action mechanisms discussed in chapter 9 are also relevant to self-representation. You can think of yourself as having particular intentions, plans, and current or future actions, and you can also use these to present yourself to other people by telling them what you are going to do. Moreover, these self-descriptions may have causal effects on what you actually do. For example, if you think of yourself or present yourself as conscientious, then you may become less likely to perform actions that would betray you as irresponsible. Self-evaluations can be partial causes of actions by leading to new intentions, for example if you judge yourself to be lazy and plan to work harder. These connections between self-representation and action show the relevance of semantic pointers to self-effecting and self-changing as well as self-representing.

SEMANTIC POINTER MECHANISMS FOR SELF-EFFECTING AND SELF-CHANGING

Self-effecting goes beyond representation when the self does things to itself, either facilitating its own functioning to accomplish goals or limiting its functioning to prevent bad consequences. For example, self-help occurs when people consult books or other media to get advice about how to make themselves better at accomplishing their goals, which is self-facilitation. But self-help can also be limiting when it stimulates self-control, as when people try to stop themselves from excessive eating, drinking, gambling, or sex.

Unlike self-representation, self-effecting requires actions that result from intentions. Chapter 9 describes how intentions bind representations of situations, actions, evaluations, and selves into a new neural representation that is intrinsically connected with motor operations. The representation of self that gets bound into an intention can include all of the patterns discussed in the last section, especially a combination of images and concepts. Analogies can also contribute to self-effecting through comparisons to role models that leads people to act in different ways.

Intentions go beyond general representations of self because they include the self as doing something. Accomplishing self-control, for example by stopping yourself from eating unhealthy foods, depends on a combination of self-representation, intention formation, and conscious control of action. Each of these requires semantic pointers of different kinds: self-representations by bindings of images and concepts, intentions by bindings of situations and doings, and consciousness by semantic pointer competition.

When people are limiting or facilitating themselves, their motivations and deliberations are usually emotional, building on the desire and hope that they can make themselves better or at least prevent themselves from becoming worse. For example, substance abusers can be motivated to change both by negative emotions such as fear and disgust and by positive emotions such as pride and hope. Emotions help to connect intentions and actions using both physiological perception and cognitive appraisal. Consciousness resulting from semantic pointer competition also contributes to self-control because self-awareness can help prevent undesired harmful acts such as smoking spurred by stress. For self-control of excessive eating, your ability to limit your consumption will depend partly on how excited you are at the thought of being slim and healthy, and partly on how afraid you are of being overweight and ill. Chapter 9 explains willpower as resulting from emotions, consciousness, and implementation intentions.

Self-changing goes beyond self-effecting in producing results that are longer term than temporary sorts of facilitating and limiting. Self-maximization and self-fulfillment, for example, may require a lifetime. Self-changing depends on prolonged accomplishment of the kinds of facilitating and limiting included under self-effecting. However, it can build on the same semantic pointer mechanisms already discussed: self-representation using images, concepts, rules, analogies, and emotions and control of actions using intentions, emotions, and consciousness. Hence neurocognitive mechanisms are highly relevant to understanding the many self-phenomena involving representation, effecting, and change. But mechanisms at molecular and social levels are also relevant, so it is better to characterize the self as a multilevel system that goes beyond neurons and cognition.

MULTILEVEL SYSTEMS

Recognizing the self as a multilevel system requires identifying the systems, levels, and mechanisms that constitute selves. A system is a structure consisting of Environment, Parts, Interconnections, and Changes (EPIC). Here the parts are the objects (entities) that compose the system. To take a simple example, a bicycle is composed of such parts as the frame, wheels, handlebars, chain, and pedals. The environment is the collection of items that act on the parts, which for a bicycle would include people who push on the pedals, roads that interact with the wheels, and air molecules that provide wind resistance to the handlebars. The interconnections are the relations among the parts, especially the bonds that tie them together. In a bicycle, key relations include the physical connections between the chain and the wheels and between the handlebars and the frame. Finally, the changes are the processes that make the system behave as it does, for example the turning of the bicycle's chain and wheels.

The self cannot be easily decomposed into a single EPIC system. Even a bicycle can be understood at multiple physical levels—for example, with the wheel decomposed into various parts such as the hub, the rim, the tube, and spokes, all consisting of molecules, which consist of atoms, which consist of subatomic particles, which consist of quarks or multidimensional strings. For most purposes, it suffices to consider bicycles at the single level of observable parts such as wheels and pedals in interaction with each other, although an engineer attempting to optimize performance may have reason to work at lower levels, as when nanotechnology is used to design light racing bikes.

To characterize multilevel systems, we can generalize the EPIC idea and think of a multilevel system as consisting of a series of subsystems each with its own relevant environment, parts, interconnections, and changes. The relations among environments, parts, interconnections, and changes at different levels for human selves are shown in Figure 12.3.

MOLECULAR MECHANISMS

In the past two decades, just as cognitive psychology has drawn increasingly on neuroscience, neuroscience has drawn increasingly on molecular biology. Neurons are cells consisting of organelles such as nuclei and mitochondria, and the firing activity of neurons is determined by their chemical inputs and internal chemical reactions. Aspects of the self such as personality are influenced by biochemical factors including genes, neurotransmitters, and hormones and also by factors

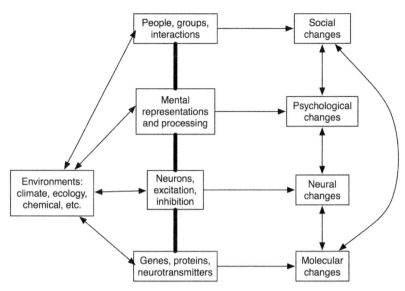

FIGURE 12.3 Diagram of the self as a multilevel system. Lines with arrows indicate causality. Thick lines indicate composition: genes are parts of neurons, which are parts of mental representations, which are parts of people. Reprinted with permission of Routledge from Thagard 2014c.

that modify the expression of genes. Changes in genetic material that affect gene expression independent of differences in the DNA sequence itself are called "epigenetic."

In molecular mechanisms, the parts consist of molecules such as proteins, genes, neurotransmitters, and hormones. The interactions are biochemical reactions involving these molecules, for example the production of proteins by genes, the synthesis of neurotransmitters by enzymes, and the effects of neurotransmitters and hormones on the chemical processes within neurons. There are several ways in which these kinds of interactions can influence processes relevant to the self.

First, personality and other aspects of the self have a genetic component. Characteristics such as intelligence, extraversion, neuroticism, and agreeableness are moderately heritable. Genetic effects on behavior are displayed in studies that find higher correlations between some features in identical twins than in nonidentical ones, for example in tendencies toward mental illnesses such as schizophrenia. Humans have variation in genes that determine the receptors for more than 50 different neurotransmitters that affect neuronal firing. For instance, there are variations in the gene DRD4 that controls the formation of the D_4 receptor for the neurotransmitter dopamine. These variations are associated with behavioral effects such as the personality trait of novelty seeking. It would be naïve, however, to suppose that there are "genes for" particular behaviors, because of evidence showing the importance of multiple genes and of chemical and environmental effects on the operation of genes.

Second, some aspects of the self also have an epigenetic component, which occurs when the operation of genes to produce proteins is affected by the attachment of chemical groups to the genes as the result of environmental conditions. Whether a gene expresses a particular protein depends not only on the gene but also on the attachment of various chemicals such as methyl groups, which are affected by the overall environment of the cells that contain the genes. For example, baby rats that have been nurtured by their mothers have a reduced stress response resulting from repression of the glucocorticoid receptor gene as the result of a chemical attachment.

Third, when aspects of the self such as intelligence and personality are learned, the learning needs to be understood in part as a molecular process. For example, the main neural processes of learning discussed in chapter 2 have a molecular underpinning when synapses are strengthened in Hebbian learning by processes that affect receptors for glutamate, the main excitatory neurotransmitter.

Fourth, neural processes of inference and learning are often influenced by chemical processes more complicated than the ones so far discussed. For maximum simplicity, the brain would need only two neurotransmitters, one to enable one neuron to excite another and another to enable one neuron to inhibit another. But in addition to the neurotransmitters most commonly used for this purpose (glutamate for excitation and GABA for inhibition), there are dozens of additional neurotransmitters that provide various kinds of modulation such as timing.

Moreover, whether a particular neuron builds up enough voltage to fire depends not only on neurotransmitters but also on other chemical processes. Individual neurons can be influenced by hormones such as testosterone, estrogen, cortisol, and oxytocin, which affects peoples' social behaviors such as trust. Some chemical interactions involve not just neurons but also the glia cells that help to keep the neurons alive. The brain contains as many glia cells as neurons, capable of sending and receiving chemical signals that indirectly affect the firing activity of neurons. So it is a mistake to think of the brain as just an electrical computer: it does have digital operations such as firing and resting, but it is also affected by diverse chemical processes as well.

The molecular processes just described can influence all the representations relevant to the self, from images to analogies. This influence is most evident in the role of emotions, which depends on numerous chemicals such as dopamine pathways for positive emotions and the stress hormone cortisol. Molecular processes are involved in both cognitive appraisal, for example when neurotransmitters such as dopamine and serotonin contribute to positive and negative evaluations, and physiological perception, which can be disrupted by drugs such as LSD that dramatically affect serotonin operation.

Molecular processes can also influence self-effecting phenomena such as self-affirmation and self-control. Oxytocin promotes self-regulation with respect to other people, for example leading mothers to tend to their offspring. High cortisol resulting from stress reduces people's working memory and makes it harder for them to resist temptation, contributing to the intention-action gaps discussed in chapter 9. Pleasurable amounts of dopamine help to produce feelings of empathy and self-fulfillment, for example when people take the dopamine-generating drug ecstasy. Serious mental illnesses such as depression that profoundly affect the self are associated with chemical processes like availability of serotonin and cortisol-induced lack of neurogenesis. Hence molecular processes are relevant to all of the kinds of self-phenomena shown in Figure 12.1.

These molecular processes also contribute to all the mental operations discussed in this book, from sensation to creativity. There is no competition between molecular and neural explanations, any more than there is competition between neural and cognitive explanations, which can be synthesized using the Semantic Pointer Architecture. Ongoing progress in understanding the molecular operations of neurons does not produce a simple reduction of the neural to the molecular that would render the neural level irrelevant to further explanations, any more than the semantic pointer account of concepts renders irrelevant psychological explanations in terms of exemplars, typical features, and explanations. My goal is to achieve multilevel explanations, not to reduce one level to a lower one.

SOCIAL MECHANISMS

Accordingly, the self is inherently social as well as mental, neural, and molecular. At the most familiar social level, the set of parts consists of individual persons. Even here, there is a hierarchy of additional sublevels of social organization, such as families, neighborhoods, regions, nations, and states, just as at the neural level there are additional levels of organization such as groups of neurons and brain areas. The social parts are influenced by an environment that includes all the objects that people causally engage, including natural objects such as rocks and lightning bolts, artifacts such as houses and cars, and social organizations such as teams and governments.

The interconnections at the social level consists of the myriad relations among people: mundane perceptual ones such as one person being able to recognize another, deeper bonds such as being in love, and many-person ones such as belonging to the same sports team. The social changes consist of the various processes of human interaction, ranging from talking to playing games to sexual intercourse.

Social mechanisms for the self must be specified precisely by describing their parts, interactions, and changes. The full description of social mechanisms is in *Mind–Society*, but here I sketch the ones most relevant to completing the multilevel account of the self. I focus on interactions that involve various forms of communication, but there are also forms of interaction between people that do not always require communication, such as feeding, fighting, dancing, hugging, having sex, and spreading germs.

In accord with the semantic pointer approach to mental representation, the basic question to be answered is: What are the forms of social interaction that can lead to the approximate transfer of semantic pointers from one person to another? The key word is "approximate," because we should not expect that exactly the same patterns of neural firing would occur in different people. Every individual has a different history of genetics, epigenetics, and learning, so no two individuals will have exactly the same neural patterns. However, given the commonalities in human genetics, physiology, environments, and learning processes, there can be approximate similarity in mental representations such as images, concepts, rules, analogies, and emotions.

For example, even though no two individuals have exactly the same concept of giraffe construed as a pattern of neural firing, there can be substantial similarity in the exemplars, typical features, and explanations that enter into people's concepts, producing similar patterns of firing in brains with similar anatomy and physiology. So it can be reasonable to say that two people have roughly the same concepts and other mental representations. We can therefore describe social mechanisms in terms of the interactions between people that communicate the basic kinds of mental representations, resulting in changes in consciousness, action, language, and creativity.

Communication is not just a verbal process with speech and writing but also a nonverbal process with gestures, body language, and facial expressions. Moreover, communication is not merely a cognitive process with representations such as images and concepts but is also an emotional process with transfer of affective experiences including moods, emotions and motivations, as well as attitudes and values. There are many verbal and nonverbal forms of communication that can produce both cognitive and emotional transfer.

Most obvious are processes of verbal communication in which people use words and sentences to transmit information. Speech has performed this function in the approximately 100,000 years of the existence of our species, *Homo sapiens*. In addition, after humans became literate approximately 6,000 years ago, forms of writing and reading have augmented speech in increasingly diverse ways. Written forms developed as marks on clay tablets but eventually grew into other kinds such as letters, articles, and books. In recent decades, numerous forms of written computer communications have become available, including email, electronic messages, and communications via social media such as Facebook and Twitter. In all these cases, the causal process is the same: the mental representations in one self produce verbal expressions that communicatively cause similar neural firings in another self. Teaching is one of the most productive kinds of social interaction and almost always includes verbal communication.

These verbal connections serve not only to enable one individual to influence the images, concepts, rules, and analogies of another but also indirectly to influence his or her emotional values and attitudes. As chapter 7 notes, words carry with them considerable emotional associations, as in the difference in whether someone is described as a soldier, terrorist, or freedom fighter. Even when verbal communication is not explicitly emotional, it may be implicitly emotional because of the powerful associations of the words that are used by the speaker, helping a self to be emotionally changed by other selves. Empathy is a social interaction that enables one self to understand the emotional state of another by means of analogy and the other modes described in chapter 6. Another kind of emotional communication occurs through reverse empathy, when people attempt to become understood by using analogies to convey to others how they feel. For example, you may tell people you feel like they did when they were in high school in order to get them to empathize with you.

*Non*verbal communication is also important for the interaction of selves, especially for the transfer of largely nonverbal representations such as images and emotions. Chapter 3 mentions the importance of gesture in human communication, and chapter 6 describes how analogies can be enhanced by gestures such as using hand motions to portray rotation in solar systems and atoms. Gestures can also be used for pointing out important aspects of the world that can be encoded nonverbally, for example when you indicate an animal that requires attention. Gestures are most useful for communication of visual images, but they can serve to focus attention on other kinds of images, such as important sounds, smells, body motions, or pains. Gesturing and attention can have strong effects on consciousness, because of the mechanism of semantic pointer competition described in chapter 9.

Other kinds of nonverbal communication involving faces and body language are important for transferring emotions. Mirror neurons enable people and monkeys to emulate the experiences of others observed in motion or in pain. People consciously or unconsciously notice features of others such as faces that are smiling or frowning, arms that are folded or inviting, and stances that are open or closed. Cognitively, this noticing may produce inferences about the mental state of the other person. But people are also susceptible to a more direct form of communication by mimicry, when they unconsciously adopt the same facial or bodily features of the communicator. Then, through the physiological perception aspect of emotion described in chapter 6, people may partially acquire the emotions of others, a process of emotional contagion. This attunement can result not only in the temporary transfer of emotional states but also in the more permanent transfer of attitudes. Electronic communication can also be nonverbal, through the transmission of pictures, diagrams, videos, emoticons, and emojis ☺.

Nonverbal communication of cognitions and emotions can also result from simultaneous interactions among many people, such as group meetings, political demonstrations, military drills, sports practices, dances, and religious rituals. In these situations, people can acquire mental representations from the interactions of the whole group, not just from one individual. Randall Collins describes how joint actions can produce emotional energy in the form of shared enthusiasm, confidence, and initiative. When people interact in groups, they can acquire much more than just the mental representations of the other people with whom they interact; they can also acquire the emotional drives to accomplish collective goals. Such collectivity can sometimes have negative consequences, for example when a charismatic leader like Adolf Hitler leads followers to adopt despicable plans, but group activity can also have benevolent results such as community care. *Mind–Society* says much more about how joint action and communication based on neural mechanisms provide explanations in the social sciences and professions.

My aim in this chapter is merely to illustrate how the social processes of verbal and nonverbal communication shape both cognition and emotion in ways that help to determine the nature of the self. Self-representation, effecting, and changing are not processes that occur merely on one's own but depend very much on the interactions we have with other people. As Hazel Rose Markus says, you can't be a self by yourself. According to the ethical perspective presented in *Natural Philosophy* (chapter 6), you cannot even be a self only for yourself.

Interactions are most obvious with explicitly social processes such as representing oneself to others in self-deprecation, self-disclosure, self-effacement, and self-presentation in general. But even in more apparently individual processes such as self-knowledge and self-appraisal, people rarely ignore the effects of the opinions of others. The goals of different kinds of self-effecting such as self-motivation and self-control are often directly connected to what people are trying to accomplish in their interactions with others. Hence the social self that results from verbal and nonverbal means of communication is just as important as the molecular, neural, and psychological self.

SUMMARY AND DISCUSSION

This chapter has four purposes. First, it fills several gaps from earlier chapters to round out a unified, brain-based account of cognition and emotion. Discussions of imagery, concepts, empathy, consciousness, action, and creativity all alluded to the self. This chapter argues that the self is a complex of mechanisms at multiple levels that include the molecular and the social.

Second, I have described how semantic pointers are crucial to the self with respect to various phenomena, including how you represent yourself to yourself and to others, as well as in how you evaluate yourself. Also explained are operations that the self does to itself in efforts to achieve short-term goals such as self-control and long-term goals such as self-fulfillment. Semantic pointer explanations of images, concepts, and other mental representations are important for understanding how selves accomplish their goals. Representations of the self via semantic pointers can recursively be bound into semantic pointers for beliefs, desires, and intentions.

Third, discussion of the social mechanisms relevant to the self begins to connect neural and mental mechanisms with discussions of social sciences and professions in *Mind–Society*. I emphatically do not attempt to reduce fields such as sociology, economics, politics, anthropology, and history to psychology and neuroscience, even though mechanisms of cognition and emotion contribute mightily to explanations of social phenomena. Rather, an expanded account of the social mechanisms sketched in this chapter meshes with neural and mental mechanisms to explain such social phenomena as environmental ideologies, economic cycles, behavioral norms, religious practices, and wars. The self therefore generates a needed expansion from the largely individual psychological processes discussed in this book to the primarily social ones discussed in the next.

The integration of social and mental mechanisms is also important for answering questions that arise in the professions of medicine, law, education, engineering, and business. Everything about selves applies equally well to persons, providing a bridge to discussions of mental illness and legal responsibility. Just as this book has used semantic pointers to bridge from the neural to the mental, *Mind–Society* uses semantic pointer communication to bridge from the mental to the social. The resulting approach, *social cognitivism*, provides a powerful alternative to rational choice and social construction theories that have dominated the social sciences.

Fourth, the multilevel mechanism account of the self is central for philosophical issues in *Natural Philosophy*. Many questions concerning knowledge, morality, and politics depend on the nature of the self, and I discuss the implications of considering the self as neural and social as well as mental. This integrated account also applies to explaining people's engagement with painting, music, and literature.

How do changes in groups relate to changes to persons, mental representations, neural populations, and molecular configurations? The simplest answer is the reductionist one that property changes at the higher level result just from property changes at the lower level. Such determinations often occur when changes in group interactions derive from changes in mental representations that derive from neural and molecular changes. For example, John approached Mary (social), because she smiled at him (social), because she found him attractive (psychological), because neurons fired in her nucleus accumbens (neural), because dopamine was transmitted (molecular). Often, therefore, the reductionist picture is correct in portraying molecular changes that cause neural changes that cause individual changes that cause social changes.

Frequently, however, causality runs in the opposite direction. When Mary smiles at John, this social interaction is the cause of a course of changes in him that are individual, neural, and molecular. He perceives her smiling and probably infers that she likes him, which are changes in mental representation that are also neural changes. Then social changes cause individual, neural, and molecular changes, as also happens when someone insults you, raising your cortisol, and when someone compliments you, increasing activation of dopamine neurons. Other examples include

- Giving a presentation increases the stress hormone cortisol.
- Men whose favorites sports team have won a game enjoy increased testosterone.
- Male chimpanzees who become dominated have lowered testosterone.
- Women who room together tend to have their menstrual cycles coordinated, altering patterns of estrogen.

Hence social changes cause molecular changes.

Moreover, individual psychological changes can cause neural changes, for example when John's inferring that Mary likes him (a change in mental representation) causes increased neural activity in various brain areas such as the nucleus accumbens. Hence contrary to the reductionist view that causality is always from lower mechanisms to higher ones, my account of the self allows multidirectional causality as in Figure 12.3.

So who are you? My answer is that a self—a person—is a complex system operating at four levels, each of which consists of an EPIC subsystem composed of environment, parts, interconnections, and changes. Each level includes mechanisms consisting of networks of parts whose interactions produce regular changes, as summarized in Figure 12.3. Because the interactions in these subsystems typically involve nonlinear dynamics resulting from feedback loops that magnify effects of small differences in initial conditions, the behaviors of such mechanisms are often hard to predict. In particular, the behavior of the parts at each level is typically difficult to predict from the behavior of parts at lower levels. Forecasting is made even harder by the existence of causal relations among levels, for example social influences on molecular changes and vice versa. Moreover, at all levels the subsystem interacts with environments that include other complex systems such as climate and ecology, each of which can have changes that are difficult to predict.

Earlier discussions from imagery to creativity described the importance of emergent properties, which belong to wholes and result from the interactions of their parts. This basic idea of emergence concerns only the connections of two levels, where the properties of wholes at the higher level (e.g., consciousness) emerge from interactions of parts at the lower levels (e.g., neurons). What I have been calling "emergence from emergence" still only operates at the neural level, through recursive binding producing semantic pointers that integrate other semantic pointers.

Thinking of the self as resulting from multiple interacting mechanisms points to a more complicated kind of emergence that has gone unrecognized. *Multilevel emergence* occurs when the property of a whole such as the self results from interactions in mechanisms at several different levels, in this case molecular and social as well as neural and cognitive. What you are as a self depends on your genes and your social influences as well as on your semantic pointers and mental representations. Major changes in the self such as religious conversions, dramatic career shifts, and recovery from mental illness are critical transitions that result from interactions among multiple levels. For example, recovery from severe depression often requires (a) changes in neurotransmitters through medication operating at the molecular and neural levels and (b) changes in beliefs and goals through psychotherapy operating at the mental and social levels. Multilevel emergence seems dauntingly complex, but *Mind–Society* shows its importance for understanding important phenomena from economic crashes to effective teaching.

The major concern of the present book has been narrower, to provide a unified brain-based account of mental processes of cognition and emotion. I have used Chris Eliasmith's Semantic Pointer Architecture to explain imagery, concepts, rules, analogies, and emotions, with applications to consciousness, action, language, creativity, and the self. Contrary to the syntactic dream of explaining intelligence by formal operations on abstract symbols, semantic pointers show how representation and inference depend on the integration of structure, meaning, and purpose. Because the formation and application of semantic pointers can incorporate sensory and motor information, they can explain the embodied aspects of cognition and the reach of minds into the world. But recursive binding allows representation to surpass bodily limitations and produce transbodiment in the form of abstract self-representations such as *kind, honest,* and *intelligent* that are much more than sensory-motor.

Unification of diverse mental phenomena has been accomplished by showing that they all result from the same mechanisms of semantic pointer construction, modification, and competition. Although some mental processes discussed in this book have been simulated using the Semantic Pointer Architecture (e.g., concepts, rules, emotions, consciousness, and intentions), many other specific models remain to be developed. Moreover, there are currently no neuroscientific methods capable of directly testing semantic pointer hypotheses, but they are falsifiable in the way that scientific theories usually are: by developing new hypotheses that explain more. I have shown that a high standard is set by the theory that the mind operates by semantic pointers, whose explanatory power ranges from imagery to creativity.

The resulting story is utterly scientific, with no room for mystical ideas such as the soul or collective consciousness. But it recognizes the complexity of human mental operations, all the way up to multilevel emergence from mechanisms that are social as well as mental, neural, and molecular. The brain is wider than the sky.

NOTES

This chapter draws on but supersedes Thagard 2014c, with some pages reused by permission of Routledge. It also takes a few paragraphs from Thagard and Wood 2015, for which the authors retain copyright.

The idea of levels of explanation is common in cognitive science, for example in Simon 1962, Newell 1990, Churchland and Sejnowski 1992, Darden 2006, Craver 2007, Wimsatt 2007, and Bechtel 2008. For a comprehensive treatment, see Findlay and Thagard 2012.

Thagard 2014c used the term "multilevelism" as an alternative to reductionism and holism. My approach is similar to the *explanatory pluralism* of McCauley and Bechtel 2001 and to the *systemism* of Bunge 2003.

Skeptics about the self include Hume 1888, Dennett 1991, Metzinger 2009, and Callero 2003. See also Organ 1987; Gallagher 2011; and Siderits, Thompson, and Zahavi 2011.

Psychological discussions of the self include Baumeister 1998; Baumeister, Vohs, and Tice 2007; Leary and Tangney 2003; LeDoux 2002; Markus and Kitayama 1991, Sedikides and Spencer 2007; and hundreds of others: Thagard and Wood 2015 has many references. Yarkoni 2015 reviews the neurobiology of personality.

Examples of the predictive value of self-discipline and self-control include Duckworth and Seligman 2005 and Vohs, Finkenauer, and Baumeister 2011. Inzlicht, Bartholow, and Hirsh 2015 describe the importance of emotions for cognitive control.

Meichenbaum 1994 describes the importance of self metaphors for psychotherapy.

Kunda and Thagard 1996 explain application of social stereotypes in terms of parallel constraint satisfaction.

On epigenetics, see, for example, Weaver et al. 2004. For a neural network model of personality, see Read et al. 2010. Finn et al. 2015 have used functional magnetic resonance imaging to show different patterns of brain connectivity in individuals, for example with respect to intelligence. The self is shaped by social class: Kraus et al. 2012.

On molecular explanations of mind, see Kandel, Schwartz, Jessell, Siegelbaum, and Hudspeth 2012; Thagard 2002a; and Bickle 2003. Philosophical issues about dualism and the "extended mind" are dealt with in *Natural Philosophy* (chapter 2).

Iacoboni 2008 extols mirror neurons, and Hickock 2014 debunks them.

Emotional contagion is discussed by Hatfield, Cacioppo, and Rapson 1994.

Collins 2004 describes how interaction rituals transfer emotional energy.

PROJECT

Model self-representation and self-change using semantic pointers. Use the model of action (chapter 9) to model self-control.

REFERENCES

Abraham, A. (2016). The imaginative mind. *Human Brain Mapping, 37*(11), 4197–4211.

Aflalo, T., Kellis, S., Klaes, C., Lee, B., Shi, Y., Pejsa, K., . . . Heck, C. (2015). Decoding motor imagery from the posterior parietal cortex of a tetraplegic human. *Science, 348*(6237), 906–910.

Akmajian, A., Demers, R. A., Farmer, A. K., & Harnish, R. M. (2010). *Linguistics: An introduction to language and communication* (6th ed.). Cambridge, MA: MIT Press.

Anderson, J. R. (1983). *The architecture of cognition*. Cambridge, MA: Harvard University Press.

Anderson, J. R. (1993). *Rules of the mind*. Hillsdale, NJ: Lawrence Erlbaum.

Anderson, J. R. (2007). *How can the mind occur in the physical universe?* Oxford: Oxford University Press.

Anderson, J. R. (2010). *Cognitive psychology and its implications* (7th ed.). New York: Worth.

Arnsten, A. F. T. (2009). Stress signalling pathways that impair prefrontal cortex structure and function. *Nature Reviews Neuroscience, 10*, 410–422.

Baars, B. J. (1988). *A cognitive theory of consciousness*. Cambridge, UK: Cambridge University Press.

Baars, B. J. (2005). Global workspace theory of consciousness: Toward a cognitive neuroscience of human experience. *Progress in Brain Research, 150*, 45–53.

Baillargeon, R., Kotovsky, L., & Needham, A. (1995). The acquisition of physical knowledge in infancy. In D. Sperber, D. Premack, & A. J. Premack (Eds.), *Causal cognition: A multidisciplinary debate* (pp. 79–116). Oxford: Clarendon Press.

Banich, M. T., & Compton, R. J. (2018). *Cognitive neuroscience* (4th ed.). Cambridge, UK: Cambridge University Press.

Barrett, L. F. (2012). Emotions are real. *Emotion, 12*, 413–429.

Barrett, L. F. (2017). *How emotions are made: The secret life of the brain*. Boston: Houghton Mifflin Harcourt.

Barrett, L. F., Lewis, M., & Haviland-Jones, J. M. (Eds.). (2016). *Handbook of emotions* (4th ed.). New York: Guilford Press.

Barsalou, L. W. (1999). Perceptual symbol systems. *Behavioral and Brain Sciences, 22,* 577–660.

Barsalou, L. W. (2008). Grounded cognition. *Annual Review of Psychology, 59,* 617–645.

Barsalou, L. W. (2009). Simulation, situated conceptualization, and prediction. *Philosophical Transactions of the Royal Society B, 364,* 1218–1289.

Barsalou, L. W. (2016). On staying grounded and avoiding quixotic dead ends. *Psychonomic Bulletin and Review, 23*(4), 1122–1142.

Bartha, P. (2010). *By parallel reasoning: The construction and evaluation of analogical arguments.* Oxford: Oxford University Press.

Baumeister, R. F. (1998). The self. In D. T. Gilbert, S. T. Fiske, & G. Lindzey (Eds.), *The handbook of social psychology,* (4th ed., Vol. 1, pp. 680–740). New York: McGraw-Hill.

Baumeister, R. F., & Tierney, J. (2011). *Willpower: Rediscovering the greatest human strength.* New York: Penguin.

Baumeister, R. F., Vohs, K. D., & Tice, D. M. (2007). The strength model of self-control. *Current Directions in Psychological Science, 16*(6), 351–355.

Bayne, T., Cleeremans, A., & Wilken, P. (Eds.). (2009). *The Oxford companion to consciousness.* Oxford: Oxford University Press.

Beaty, R. E., Kenett, Y. N., Christensen, A. P., Rosenberg, M. D., Benedek, M., Chen, Q., . . . Kane, M. J. (2018). Robust prediction of individual creative ability from brain functional connectivity. *Proceedings of the National Academy of Sciences of the United States of America, 115*(5), 1087–1092.

Bechtel, W. (2008). *Mental mechanisms: Philosophical perspectives on cognitive neuroscience.* New York: Routledge.

Bermudez, J. L. (2014). *Cognitive science: An introduction to the science of the mind* (2nd ed.). Cambridge, UK: Cambridge University Press.

Bernhardt, B. C., & Singer, T. (2012). The neural basis of empathy. *Annual Review of Neuroscience, 35,* 1–23.

Berridge, K. C., Robinson, T. E., & Aldridge, J. W. (2009). Dissecting components of reward: "Liking," "wanting," and learning. *Current Opinion in Pharmacology, 9,* 65–73.

Bickle, J. (2003). *Philosophy and neuroscience: A ruthlessly reductive account.* Dordrecht: Kluwer.

Blackmore, S. (2012). *Consciousness: An introduction* (2nd ed.). Oxford: Oxford University Press.

Blouw, P., & Eliasmith, C. (2017). Inferential role semantics for natural language. In *Proceedings of the 39th Annual Conference of the Cognitive Science Society* (pp. 142–147).

Blouw, P., Eliasmith, C., & Tripp, B. (2016). A scaleable spiking neural model of action planning. In A. Papafragou, D. Grodner, D. Mirman, & J. Trueswell (Eds.), *Proceedings of the 37th Annual Conference of the Cognitive Science Societ* (pp. 1583–1588). Austin, TX: Cognitive Science Society.

Blouw, P., Solodkin, E., Thagard, P., & Eliasmith, C. (2016). Concepts as semantic pointers: A framework and computational model. *Cognitive Science, 40,* 1128–1162.

Boden, M. (2004). *The creative mind: Myths and mechanisms* (2nd ed.). London: Routledge.

Boden, M. (2006). *Mind as machine: A history of cognitive science.* Oxford: Oxford University Press.

Bowdle, B. F., & Gentner, D. (2005). The career of metaphor. *Psychological Review, 112,* 193–216.

Braithwaite, V. (2010). *Do fish feel pain?* Oxford: Oxford University Press.

Bratman, M. E. (1987). *Intention, plans, and practical action.* Cambridge, MA: Harvard University Press.

Broom, D. M., Sena, H., & Moynihan, K. L. (2009). Pigs learn what a mirror image represents and use it to obtain information. *Animal Behavior, 78,* 1037–1041.

Brown, D. E. (1991). *Human universals.* New York: McGraw-Hill.

Bunge, M. (2003). *Emergence and convergence: Qualitative novelty and the unity of knowledge.* Toronto: University of Toronto Press.

Callero, P. L. (2003). The sociology of the self. *Annual Review of Sociology, 29,* 115–133.

Carey, S. (2009). *The origin of concepts.* Oxford: Oxford University Press.

Chalmers, D. (2010). *The character of consciousness.* Oxford: Oxford University Press.

Chalmers, D. J. (1996). *The conscious mind.* Oxford: Oxford University Press.

Chemero, A. (2009). *Radical embodied cognitive science.* Cambridge, MA: MIT Press.

Chi, M. T. H. (2005). Commonsense conceptions of emergent processes: Why some misconceptions are robust. *Journal of the Learning Sciences, 14,* 161–199.

Chi, M. T. H., deLeeuw, N., Chiu, M.-H., & LaVancher, C. (1994). Eliciting self-explanations improves understanding. *Cognitive Science, 18,* 439–477.

Chomsky, N. (1980). *Rules and representations.* New York: Columbia University Press.

Chomsky, N. (1995). *The minimalist program.* Cambridge, MA: MIT Press.

Chomsky, N. (2002). *On nature and language.* Cambridge, UK: Cambridge University Press.

Chomsky, N. (2013). What kind of creatures are we? *Journal of Philosophy, 12,* 645–662.

Churchland, P. S. (2002). *Brain-wise: Studies in neurophilosophy.* Cambridge, MA: MIT Press.

Churchland, P. S. (2011). *Braintrust: What neuroscience tells us about morality.* Princeton, NJ: Princeton University Press.

Churchland, P. S., & Sejnowski, T. (1992). *The computational brain.* Cambridge, MA: MIT Press.

Citron, F. M. M., & Goldberg, A. E. E. (2014). Metaphorical sentences are more emotionally engaging than their literal counterparts. *Journal of Cognitive Neuroscience, 26,* 2585–2595.

Collins, R. (2004). *Interaction ritual chains.* Princeton, NJ: Princeton University Press.

Cong, L., Ran, F. A., Cox, D., Lin, S., Barretto, R., Habib, N., . . . Zhang, F. (2013). Multiplex genome engineering using CRISPR/Cas systems. *Science, 339,* 819–823.

Costa, V. D., Lang, P. J., Sabatinelli, D., Versace, F., & Bradley, M. M. (2010). Emotional imagery: Assessing pleasure and arousal in the brain's reward circuitry. *Human Brain Mapping, 31,* 1446–1457.

Craver, C. F. (2007). *Explaining the brain.* Oxford: Oxford University Press.

Craver, C. F., & Darden, L. (2013). *In search of mechanisms: Discoveries across the life sciences.* Chicago: University of Chicago Press.

Crawford, E., Gingerich, M., & Eliasmith, C. (2016). Biologically plausible, human-scale knowledge representation. *Cognitive Science, 40,* 782–821.

Crick, F. (1994). *The astonishing hypothesis: The scientific search for the soul.* London: Simon & Schuster.

Crick, F., & Koch, C. (2003). A framework for consciousness. *Nature Neuroscience, 6,* 119–126.

Croft, D., & Thagard, P. (2002). Dynamic imagery: A computational model of motion and visual analogy. In L. Magnani (Ed.), *Model-based reasoning: Scientific discovery, technological innovation, values* (pp. 259–274). New York: Kluwer/Plenum.

Csibra, G., & Gergley, G. (2011). Natural pedagogy as evolutionary adaptation. *Philosophical Transactions of the Royal Society of London B: Biological Sciences, 366,* 1149–1157.

Damasio, A. R. (1994). *Descartes' error: Emotion, reason, and the human brain.* New York: Putnam.

Damasio, A. R. (2012). *Self comes to mind: Constructing the conscious brain.* New York: Vintage.

Darden, L. (2006). *Reasoning in biological discoveries.* Cambridge, UK: Cambridge University Press.

Darden, L., Pal, L. R., Kundu, K., & Moult, J. (2018). The product guides the process: Discovering disease mechanisms. In E. Ippoliti & D. Danks (Eds.), *Building theories* (pp. 101–117). Berlin: Springer.

Davidson, D. (1967). Truth and meaning. *Synthese, 17,* 304–323.

Davidson, R. J., & Begley, S. (2012). *The emotional life of your brain: How its unique patterns affect the way you think, feel, and live—and how you can change them.* New York: Penguin.

Dayan, P., & Abbott, L. F. (2001). *Theoretical neuroscience: Computational and mathematical modeling of neural systems.* Cambridge, MA: MIT Press.

de Sousa, R. (2013). Emotion. In E. Zalta (Ed.), *Stanford encyclopedia of philosophy.* https://plato.stanford.edu/entries/emotion/

DeCasien, A. R., Williams, S. A., & Higham, J. P. (2017). Primate brain size is predicted by diet but not sociality. *Nature Ecology and Evolution, 1.* https://www.nature.com/articles/s41559-017-0112

Decety, J. (Ed.). (2014). *Empathy: From bench to bedside.* Cambridge, MA: MIT Press.

Dehaene, S. (2011). *The number sense: How the mind creates mathematics* (2nd ed.). Oxford: Oxford University Press.

Dehaene, S. (2014). *Consciousness and the brain: Deciphering how the brain codes our thoughts.* New York: Viking.

Dennett, D. (1991). *Consciousness explained.* Boston: Little, Brown.

Dennett, D. (2003). *Freedom evolves.* New York: Penguin.

Dennett, D. C. (2017). *From bacteria to Bach and back: The evolution of minds.* New York: W. W. Norton.

Desimone, R., & Duncan, J. (1995). Neural mechanisms of selective visual attention. *Annual Review of Neuroscience, 18,* 193–222.

Doudna, J. A., & Sternberg, S. H. (2017). *A crack in creation: Gene editing and the unthinkable power to control evolution.* New York: Houghton Mifflin Harcourt.

Duckworth, A. L., & Seligman, M. E. P. (2005). Self-discipline outdoes IQ in predicting academic performance in adolescents. *American Psychologist, 16,* 939–944.

Dunbar, K. (1997). How scientists think: On-line creativity and conceptual change in science. In T. B. Ward, S. M. Smith, & J. Vaid (Eds.), *Creative thought: An investigation of conceptual structures and processes* (pp. 461–493). Washington, DC: American Psychological Association.

Dunbar, K., & Fugelsang, J. (2005). Scientific thinking and reasoning. In K. J. Holyoak & R. Morrison (Eds.), *Cambridge handbook of thinking and reasoning* (pp. 705–726). Cambridge, UK: Cambridge University Press.

Dunbar, R. I. (2009). The social brain hypothesis and its implications for social evolution. *Annals of Human Biology, 36,* 562–572.

Dunning, D., & Balcetis, E. (2013). Wishful seeing: How preferences shape perception. *Current Directions in Psychological Science, 22,* 33–37.

Eichenbaum, H. (2014). Time cells in the hippocampus: A new dimension for mapping memories. *Nature Neuroscience, 15,* 732–744.

Einstein, A. (1954). *Ideas and opinions.* New York: Crown.

Ekman, P. (2003). *Emotions revealed: Recognizing faces and feelings to improve communication and emotional life.* New York: Henry Holt.

Ekman, P. (2016). What scientists who study emotion agree about. *Perspectives on Psychological Science, 11*(1), 31–34.

Eliasmith, C. (1996). The third contender: A critical examination of the dynamicist theory of cognition. *Philosophical Psychology, 9,* 441–463.

Eliasmith, C. (2005). Neurosemantics and categories. In H. Cohen & C. Lefebvre (Eds.), *Handbook of categorization in cognitive science* (pp. 1035–1054). Amsterdam: Elsevier.

Eliasmith, C. (2013). *How to build a brain: A neural architecture for biological cognition.* Oxford: Oxford University Press.

Eliasmith, C., & Anderson, C. H. (2003). *Neural engineering: Computation, representation and dynamics in neurobiological systems.* Cambridge, MA: MIT Press.

Eliasmith, C., Stewart, T. C., Choo, X., Bekolay, T., DeWolf, T., Tang, Y., & Rasmussen, D. (2012). A large-scale model of the functioning brain. *Science, 338,* 1202–1205.

Eliasmith, C., & Thagard, P. (2001). Integrating structure and meaning: A distributed model of analogical mapping. *Cognitive Science, 25,* 245–286.

Elman, J. L., Bates, E. A., Johnson, M. H., Karmiloff-Smith, A., Parisi, D., & Plunkett, K. (1996). *Rethinking innateness: A connectionist perspective on development.* Cambridge, MA: MIT Press.

Engel, A. K., Fries, P., König, P., Brecht, M., & Singer, W. (1999). Temporal binding, binocular rivalry, and consciousness. *Consciousness and Cognition, 8,* 128–151.

Evans, J. S. B., & Stanovich, K. E. (2013). Dual-process theories of higher cognition: Advancing the debate. *Perspectives on Psychological Science, 8*(3), 223–241.

Evans, V. (2014). *The language myth: Why language is not an instinct.* Cambridge, UK: Cambridge University Press.

Everett, D. L. (2012). *Language: The cultural tool.* New York: Pantheon.

Falkenhainer, B., Forbus, K. D., & Gentner, D. (1989). The structure-mapping engine: Algorithms and examples. *Artificial Intelligence, 41,* 1–63.

Fauconnier, G., & Turner, M. (2002). *The way we think.* New York: Basic Books.

Fazio, R. H. (2001). On the automatic activation of associated evaluations: An overview. *Cognition and Emotion, 15,* 115–141.

Feinberg, T. E., & Mallatt, J. (2016). *The ancient origins of consciousness: How the brain created experience.* Cambridge, MA: MIT Press.

Findlay, S. D., & Thagard, P. (2012). How parts make up wholes. *Frontiers in Physiology, 3.* doi:10.3389/fphys.2012.00455

Finger, S. (1994). *Origins of neuroscience: A history of explorations into brain function.* New York: Oxford University Press.

Finke, R., Ward, T. B., & Smith, S. M. (1992). *Creative cognition: Theory, research and applications.* Cambridge, MA: MIT Press/Bradford Books.

Finn, E. S., Shen, X., Scheinost, D., Rosenberg, M. D., Huang, J., Chun, M. M., . . . Constable, R. T. (2015). Functional connectome fingerprinting: Identifying individuals using patterns of brain connectivity. *Nature Neuroscience, 18*(11), 1664–1671.

Firestone, C., & Scholl, B. J. (2016). Cognition does not affect perception: Evaluating the evidence for "top-down" effects. *Behavioral and Brain Sciences, 39.* doi:10.1017/S0140525X15000965

Fishbein, M., & Ajzen, I. (1975). *Belief, attitude, intention, and behavior.* Reading, MA: Addison-Wesley.

Fisher, G. A., & Chon, K. K. (1989). Durkheim and the social construction of emotions. *Social Psychology Quarterly, 52,* 1–9.

Fitch, W. T. (2011). Unity and diversity in human language. *Philosophical Transactions of the Royal Society of London B: Biological Sciences, 366,* 376–388.

Floresco, S. B. (2015). The nucleus accumbens: An interface between cognition, emotion, and action. *Annual Review of Psychology, 66,* 25–52.

Fodor, J. (1975). *The language of thought.* New York: Crowell.

Fodor, J. A., & Pylyshyn, Z. W. (1981). How direct is visual perception? Some reflections on Gibson's "Ecological Approach." *Cognition, 9*, 139–196.

Forbus, K. D., Ferguson, R. W., Lovett, A., & Gentner, D. (2017). Extending SME to handle larger-scale cognitive modeling. *Cognitive Science, 41*, 1152–1201.

Frank, M. C., Vul, E., & Johnson, S. P. (2009). Development of infants' attention to faces during the first year. *Cognition, 110*(2), 160–170.

Frankland, S. M., & Greene, J. D. (2015). An architecture for encoding sentence meaning in left mid-superior temporal cortex. *Proceedings of the National Academy of Sciences of the United States of America, 112*(37), 11732–11737.

Friedenberg, J., & Silverman, G. (2011). *Cognitive science: An introduction to the study of mind* (2nd ed.). Thousand Oaks, CA: SAGE.

Gallagher, S. (Ed.). (2011). *The Oxford handbook of the self.* Oxford: Oxford University Press.

Gardner, H. (1985). *The mind's new science.* New York: Basic Books.

Gasiunas, G., Barrangou, R., Horvath, P., & Siksnys, V. (2012). Cas9-crRNA ribonucleoprotein complex mediates specific DNA cleavage for adaptive immunity in bacteria. *Proceedings of the National Academy of Sciences of the United States of America, 109*(39), E2579–E2586.

Gendron, M., Roberson, D., van der Vyver, J. M., & Barrett, L. F. (2014). Perceptions of emotion from facial expressions are not culturally universal: Evidence from a remote culture. *Emotion, 14*, 251–262.

Gentner, D. (1983). Structure mapping: A theoretical framework for analogy. *Cognitive Science, 7*, 155–170.

Gentner, D., Holyoak, K. J., & Kokinov, B. K. (Eds.). (2001). *The analogical mind: Perspectives from cognitive science.* Cambridge, MA: MIT Press.

Gibbs, R. W. (2005). *Embodiment and cognitive science.* Cambridge, UK: Cambridge University Press.

Gibson, J. J. (1979). *The ecological approach to visual perception.* Boston: Houghton-Mifflin.

Gieling, E. T., Mijdam, E., van der Staay, F. J., & Nordquist, R. E. (2014). Lack of mirror use by pigs to locate food. *Applied Animal Behaviour Science, 154*, 22–29.

Glenberg, A. M., Witt, J. K., & Metcalfe, J. (2013). From the revolution to embodiment: 25 years of cognitive psychology. *Perspectives on Psychological Science, 8*, 573–585.

Goldin-Meadow, S. (2003). *Hearing gesture: How our hands help us think.* Cambridge, MA: Harvard University Press.

Gollwitzer, P. (1999). Implementation intentions: Strong effects of simple plans. *American Psychologist, 54*, 493–503.

Green, A. E. (2016). Creativity, within reason: Semantic distance and dynamic state creativity in relational thinking and reasoning. *Current Directions in Psychological Science, 25*(1), 28–35.

Green, A. E., Kraemer, D. J., Fugelsang, J. A., Gray, J. R., & Dunbar, K. N. (2012). Neural correlates of creativity in analogical reasoning. *Journal of Experimental Psychology: Learning, Memory, and Cognition, 38*(2), 264.

Greene, J. D., & Cohen, J. (2006). For the law, neuroscience changes nothing and everything. In S. Zeki & O. Goodenough (Eds.), *Law and the brain* (pp. 207–226). Oxford: Oxford University Press.

Greenwald, A. G. (2012). There is nothing so theoretical as a good method. *Perspectives on Psychological Science, 7*(2), 99–108.

Gregory, R. (1970). *The intelligent eye.* London: Weidenfeld and Nicolson.

Gruber, M. J., Gelman, B. D., & Ranganath, C. (2014). States of curiosity modulate hippocampus-dependent learning via the dopaminergic circuit. *Neuron, 84*(2), 486–496.

Harman, G. (1987). (Nonsolopsistic) conceptual role semantics. In E. LePore (Ed.), *Semantics of natural language* (pp. 55–81). New York: Academic Press.

Harré, R. (Ed.). (1989). *The social construction of emotions*. Oxford: Blackwell.

Harris, S. (2012). *Free will*. New York: Free Press.

Hatfield, E., Cacioppo, J. T., & Rapson, R. L. (1994). *Emotional contagion*. Cambridge, UK: Cambridge University Press.

Hauser, M. D., Yang, C., Berwick, R. C., Tattersall, I., Ryan, M., Watumull, J., . . . Lewontin, R. (2014). The mystery of language evolution. *Frontiers in Psychology, 5*. doi:10.3389/fpsyg.2014.00401

Hebb, D. O. (1949). *The organization of behavior*. New York: Wiley.

Heine, S. J. (2015). *Cultural psychology* (3rd ed.). New York: Norton.

Heinlein, R. A. (1974). *Time enough for love*. New York: Putnam.

Hickock, G. (2014). *The myth of mirror neurons: The real science of communication and cognition*. New York: Norton.

Hofstadter, D., & Sander, E. (2013). *Surfaces and essences: Analogy as the fuel and fire of thinking*. New York: Basic Books.

Holland, J. H., Holyoak, K. J., Nisbett, R. E., & Thagard, P. R. (1986). *Induction: Processes of inference, learning, and discovery*. Cambridge, MA: MIT Press.

Holyoak, K. J. (2012). Analogy and relational reasoning. In K. J. Holyoak & R. G. Morrison (Eds.), *The Oxford handbook of thinking and reasoning* (pp. 234–259). Oxford: Oxford University Press.

Holyoak, K. J., & Morrison, R. G. (Eds.). (2012). *The Oxford handbook of thinking and reasoning*. New York: Oxford University Press.

Holyoak, K. J., & Thagard, P. (1995). *Mental leaps: Analogy in creative thought*. Cambridge, MA: MIT Press/Bradford Books.

Hubbard, T. L. (2010). Auditory imagery: Empirical findings. *Psychological Bulletin, 136*, 302–329.

Hughes, B. L., & Zaki, J. (2015). The neuroscience of motivated cognition. *Trends in Cognitive Sciences, 19*(2), 62–64.

Hume, D. (1888). *A treatise of human nature*. Oxford: Clarendon Press.

Hummel, J. E., & Holyoak, K. J. (1997). Distributed representations of structure: A theory of analogical access and mapping. *Psychological Review, 104*, 427–466.

Hummel, J. E., & Holyoak, K. J. (2003). A symbolic-connectionist theory of relational inference and generalization. *Psychological Review, 110*, 220–264.

Iacoboni, M. (2008). *Mirroring people: The new science of how we connect with others*. New York: Farrar, Straus and Giroux.

Inzlicht, M., Bartholow, B. D., & Hirsh, J. B. (2015). Emotional foundations of cognitive control. *Trends in Cognitive Sciences, 19*(3), 126–132.

Jack, R. E., Oliver, G. B., Yu, H., Caldara, R., & Schyns, P. G. (2012). Facial expressions of emotions are not culturally universal. *Proceedings of the National Academy of Sciences of the United States of America, 109*, 7241–7244.

Jackendoff, R. (2002). *Foundations of language: Brain, meaning, grammar, evolution*. Oxford: Oxford University Press.

Jackendoff, R. (2010). *Meaning and the lexicon: The parallel architecture 1975–2010*. Oxford: Oxford University Press.

James, W. (1884). What is an emotion? *Mind, 9*, 188–205.

Jansen, R., Embden, J., Gaastra, W., & Schouls, L. (2002). Identification of genes that are associated with DNA repeats in prokaryotes. *Molecular Microbiology, 43*(6), 1565–1575.

Jaynes, J. (1976). *The origin of consciousness in the breakdown of the bicameral mind.* Boston: Houghton Mifflin.

Jiang, M., & Thagard, P. (2014). Creative cognition in social innovation. *Creativity Research Journal, 26,* 375–388.

Jinek, M., Chylinski, K., Fonfara, I., Hauer, M., Doudna, J. A., & Charpentier, E. (2012). A programmable dual-RNA–guided DNA endonuclease in adaptive bacterial immunity. *Science, 337,* 816–821.

Job, V., Walton, G. M., Bernecker, K., & Dweck, C. S. (2013). Beliefs about willpower determine the impact of glucose on self-control. *Proceedings of the National Academy of Sciences of the United States of America, 110*(37), 14837–14842.

Johnson, M. (1987). *The body in the mind.* Chicago: University of Chicago Press.

Jones, M., & Love, B. C. (2011). Bayesian fundamentalism or enlightenment: On the explanatory status and theoretical contributions of Bayesian models of cognition. *Behavioral and Brain Sciences, 34,* 169–231.

Kahneman, D. (2011). *Thinking fast and slow.* Toronto: Doubleday.

Kahneman, D., & Tversky, A. (Eds.). (2000). *Choices, values, and frames.* Cambridge, UK: Cambridge University Press.

Kajić, I., Schröder, T., Stewart, T. C., & Thagard, P. (forthcoming). The semantic pointer theory of emotions.

Kandel, E. R., Schwartz, J. H., Jessell, T. M., Siegelbaum, S., & Hudspeth, A. J. (2012). *Principles of neural science* (5th ed.). New York: McGraw-Hill.

Kang, Y. H., Petzschner, F. H., Wolpert, D. M., & Shadlen, M. N. (2017). Piercing of consciousness as a threshold-crossing operation. *Current Biology, 27,* 2285–2295.

Kassam, K. S., Markey, A. R., Cherkassky, V. L., Loewenstein, G., & Just, M. A. (2013). Identifying emotions on the basis of neural activation. *PLOS One, 6,* e66032.

Kaufman, J. C., & Sternberg, R. J. (Eds.). (2010). *The Cambridge handbook of creativity.* Cambridge, UK: Cambridge University Press.

Keltner, D., Oatley, K., & Jenkins, J. M. (2013). *Understanding emotions* (3rd ed.). New York: Wiley.

Kintsch, W. (1998). *Comprehension: A paradigm for cognition.* Cambridge, UK: Cambridge University Press.

Klauer, S. G., Guo, F., Simons-Morton, B. G., Ouimet, M. C., Lee, S. E., & Dingus, T. A. (2014). Distracted driving and risk of road crashes among novice and experienced drivers. *New England Journal of Medicine, 370,* 54–59.

Klein, G. (1998). *Sources of power: How people make decisions.* Cambridge, MA: MIT Press.

Koch, C. (2012). *Consciousness: Confessions of a romantic reductionist.* Cambridge, MA: MIT Press.

Koch, C., Massimini, M., Boly, M., & Tononi, G. (2016). Neural correlates of consciousness: Progress and problems. *Nature Reviews Neuroscience, 17*(5), 307–321.

Koestler, A. (1967). *The act of creation.* New York: Dell.

Kolodner, J. (1993). *Case-based reasoning.* San Mateo, CA: Morgan Kaufmann.

Kosslyn, S. M., Thompson, W. L., & Ganis, G. (2006). *The case for mental imagery.* New York: Oxford University Press.

Kounios, J., & Beeman, M. (2014). The cognitive neuroscience of insight. *Annual Review of Neuroscience, 65,* 71–93.

Kraus, M. W., Piff, P. K., Mendoza-Denton, R., Rheinschmidt, M. L., & Keltner, D. (2012). Social class, solipsism, and contextualism: How the rich are different from the poor. *Psychological Review*, 119(3), 546–572.

Kreibig, S. D. (2010). Autonomic nervous system activity in emotion: A review. *Biological Psychology*, 84, 394–421.

Kriete, T., Noelle, D. C., Cohen, J. D., & O'Reilly, R. C. (2013). Indirection and symbol-like processing in the prefrontal cortex and basal ganglia. *Proceedings of the National Academy of Sciences of the United States of America*, 110, 16390–16395.

Kunda, Z. (1990). The case for motivated reasoning. *Psychological Bulletin*, 108, 480–498.

Kunda, Z. (1999). *Social cognition: Making sense of people*. Cambridge, MA: MIT Press.

Kunda, Z., Miller, D., & Claire, T. (1990). Combining social concepts: The role of causal reasoning. *Cognitive Science*, 14, 551–577.

Kunda, Z., & Thagard, P. (1996). Forming impressions from stereotypes, traits, and behaviors: A parallel-constraint-satisfaction theory. *Psychological Review*, 103, 284–308.

Laird, J. E., Lebiere, C., & Rosenbloom, P. S. (2017). A standard model of the mind: Toward a common computational framework across artificial intelligence, cognitive science, neuroscience, and robotics. *AI Magazine*, 38(4), 13–26.

Lakoff, G. (1987). *Women, fire, and dangerous things*. Chicago: University of Chicago Press.

Lakoff, G. (1994). What is metaphor? In J. A. Barnden & K. J. Holyoak (Eds.), *Advances in connectionist and neural computation theory, Vol. 3: Analogy, metaphor, and reminding* (pp. 203–257). Norwood, NJ: Ablex.

Lakoff, G. (1996). *Moral politics: What conservatives know that liberals don't*. Chicago: University of Chicago Press.

Lakoff, G., & Johnson, M. (1980). *Metaphors we live by*. Chicago: University of Chicago Press.

Lakoff, G., & Johnson, M. (1999). *Philosophy in the flesh: The embodied mind and its challenge to western thought*. New York: Basic Books.

Lakoff, G., & Núñez, R., E. (2000). *Where mathematics comes from: How the embodied mind brings mathematics into being*. New York: Basic Books.

Lakoff, G., & Turner, M. (1989). *More than cool reason: A field guide to poetic metaphor*. Chicago: University of Chicago Press.

Langacker, R. W. (2013). *Essentials of cognitive grammar*. Oxford: Oxford University Press.

Leary, M. R., & Tangney, J. P. (Eds.). (2003). *Handbook of self and identity*. New York Guilford Press.

Lebrecht, S., Bar, M., Barrett, L. F., & J., T. M. (2012). Micro-valences: Perceiving affective valence in everyday objects. *Frontiers in Psychology*, 3.

LeDoux, J. (2002). *The synaptic self*. New York: Viking.

LeDoux, J. E., & Brown, R. (2017). A higher-order theory of emotional consciousness. *Proceedings of the National Academy of Sciences of the United States of America*, 110, E2016–E2025.

Lenat, D. (1983). EURISKO: A program that learns new heuristics and domain concepts. *Artificial Intelligence*, 21, 61–98.

Lerner, J. S., Li, Y., Valdesolo, P., & Kassam, K. S. (2015). Emotion and decision making. *Annual Review of Psychology*, 66, 799–823.

Libet, B. (1985). Unconscious cerebral initiative and the role of conscious will in voluntary action. *Behavioral and Brain Sciences*, 8, 529–566.

Lindquist, K. A., Wager, T. D., Kober, H., Bliss-Moreau, E., & Barrett, L. F. (2012). The basis of emotion: A meta-analytic review. *Behavioral and Brain Sciences*, 35, 121–143.

Lipton, P. (2004). *Inference to the best explanation* (2nd ed.). London: Routledge.

Litt, A., Eliasmith, C., & Thagard, P. (2008). Neural affective decision theory: Choices, brains, and emotions. *Cognitive Systems Research, 9*, 252–273.

LoBue, V., Rakison, D. H., & DeLoache, J. S. (2010). Threat perception across the life span: Evidence for multiple converging pathways. *Current Directions in Psychological Science, 19*, 375–379.

Lomas, T. (2016). Towards a positive cross-cultural lexicography: Enriching our emotional landscape through 216 "untranslatable" words pertaining to well-being. *The Journal of Positive Psychology, 11*(5), 546–558.

Lopez, R. B., Hofmann, W., Wagner, D. B., Kelley, W. M., & Heatherton, T. F. (2014). Neural predictors of giving in to temptation in daily life. *Psychological Science, 10*, 1337–1344.

Lovett, A., Tomai, E., Forbus, K. D., & Usher, J. (2009). Solving geometric analogy problems through two-stage analogical mapping. *Cognitive Science, 33*, 1192–1231.

Lustenberger, C., Boyle, M. R., Foulser, A. A., Mellin, J. M., & Fröhlich, F. (2015). Functional role of frontal alpha oscillations in creativity. *Cortex, 67*, 74–82.

MacDonald, A. A., Naci, L., MacDonald, P. A., & Owen, A. M. (2015). Anesthesia and neuroimaging: Investigating the neural correlates of unconsciousness. *Trends in Cognitive Sciences, 19*(2), 100–107.

MacDonald, M. C., & Seidenberg, M. S. (2006). Constraint satisfaction accounts of lexical and sentence comprehension. In M. Traxler & M. A. Gernsbacher (Eds.), *Handbook of psycholinguistics* (2nd ed., pp. 581–611). San Diego: Academic Press.

Machery, E. (2009). *Doing without concepts.* Oxford: Oxford University Press.

Magnani, L. (2009). *Abductive cognition: The epistemological and eco-cognitive dimensions of hypothetical reasoning.* Berlin: Springer.

Maia, T. V., & Cleeremans, A. (2005). Consciousness: Converging insights from connectionism modeling and neuroscience. *Trends in Cognitive Neuroscience, 9*, 397–404.

Mandik, P. (2013). *This is philosophy of mind: An introduction.* Chichester, UK: Wiley-Blackwell.

Mandler, J. M. (2012). On the spatial foundations of the conceptual system and its enrichment. *Cognitive Science, 36*, 421–451.

Margolis, E., & Laurence, S. (Eds.). (1999). *Concepts: Core readings.* Cambridge, MA: MIT Press.

Margolis, E., & Laurence, S. (Eds.). (2015). *The conceptual mind: New directions in the study of concepts.* Cambridge, MA: MIT Press.

Markus, H. R., & Kitayama, S. (1991). Culture and the self: Implications for cognition, emotion, and motivation. *Psychological Review, 98*(2), 224–253.

Marr, D. (1982). *Vision.* San Francisco: Freeman.

McCauley, R. N. (2007). Reduction: Models of cross-scientific relations and their implications for the psychology-neuroscience interface. In P. Thagard (Ed.), *Philosophy of psychology and cognitive science* (pp. 105–158). Amsterdam: Elsevier.

McCauley, R. N., & Bechtel, W. (2001). Explanatory pluralism and the heuristic identity theory. *Theory & Psychology, 11*, 736–760.

McClelland, J. L., & Patterson, K. (2002). Rules or connections in past-tense inflections: What does the evidence rule out? *Trends in Cognitive Sciences, 6*, 465–472.

McGreggor, K., Kunda, M., & Goel, A. (2014). Fractals and ravens. *Artificial Intelligence, 215*, 1–23.

McNorgan, C. (2012). A meta-analytic review of multisensory imagery identifies the neural correlates of modality-specific and modality-general imagery. *Frontiers in Human Neuroscience, 6.* doi:10.3389/fnhum.2012.00285

Medin, D. L. (1989). Concepts and conceptual structure. *American Psychologist, 44*, 1469–1481.

Mednick, S. A. (1962). The associative basis of the creative process. *Psychological Review, 69,* 220–232.

Meichenbaum, D. (1994). *A clinical handbook/practical therapist manual for assessing and treating adults with post-traumatic stress disorder (PTSD).* Waterloo, Ontario: Institute Press.

Mele, A. R. (2009). *Effective intentions.* Oxford: Oxford University Press.

Metzinger, T. (2009). *The ego tunnel: The science of the mind and the myth of the self.* New York: Basic Books.

Miller, A. I. (1984). *Imagery in scientific thought: Creating twentieth century physics.* Boston: Birkhauser.

Miller, G., & Johnson-Laird, P. (1976). *Language and perception.* Cambridge, MA: Harvard University Press.

Minsky, M. (1975). A framework for representing knowledge. In P. H. Winston (Ed.), *The psychology of computer vision* (pp. 211–277). New York: McGraw-Hill.

Minsky, M. (1986). *The society of mind.* New York: Simon & Schuster.

Mnih, V., Kavukcuoglu, K., Silver, D., Rusu, A. A., Veness, J., Bellemare, M. G., . . . Ostrovski, G. (2015). Human-level control through deep reinforcement learning. *Nature, 518*(7540), 529–533.

Moser, E. I., Kropff, E., & Moser, M. (2008). Place cells, grid cells, and the brain's spatial representation system. *Annual Review of Neuroscience, 31,* 68–89.

Murphy, G. L. (2002). *The big book of concepts.* Cambridge, MA: MIT Press.

Naci, L., Cusack, R., Anello, M., & Owen, A. M. (2014). A common neural code for similar conscious experiences in different individuals. *Proceedings of the National Academy of Sciences of the United States of America, 111*(39), 14277–14282.

Nersessian, N. (2008). *Creating scientific concepts.* Cambridge, MA: MIT Press.

Newell, A. (1990). *Unified theories of cognition.* Cambridge, MA: Harvard University Press.

Newell, A., & Simon, H. A. (1972). *Human problem solving.* Englewood Cliffs, NJ: Prentice-Hall.

Niedenthal, P. M., Barsalou, L. W., Ric, F., & Krauth-Gruber, S. (2005). Embodiment in the acquisition and use of emotion knowledge. In L. Barrett, P. M. Niedenthal, & P. Winkielman (Eds.), *Emotion and consciousness* (pp. 2–50). New York: Guilford Press.

Niedenthal, P. M., & Brauer, M. (2012). Social functionality of human emotion. *Annual Review of Psychology, 63,* 259–285.

Nisbett, R. (2003). *The geography of thought: How Asians and Westerners think differently . . . and why.* New York: Free Press.

Nokes, T. J., Schunn, C. D., & Chi, M. T. (2010). Problem solving and human expertise. In P. Peterson, R. Tierney, E. Baker, & B. McGraw (Eds.), *International encyclopedia of education* (Vol. 5, pp. 265–272). Amsterdam: Elsevier.

Norman, D. A., & Shallice, T. (1986). Attention to action: Willed and automatic control of behavior. In R. J. Davidson, G. E. Schwartz, & D. Shapiro (Eds.), *Consciousness and self-regulation: Advances in research and theory* (Vol. 4, pp. 1–18). New York: Plenum Press.

Nummenmaa, L., Glerean, E., Hari, R., & Hietanen, J. K. (2014). Bodily maps of emotions. *Proceedings of the National Academy of Sciences of the United States of America, 111,* 646–651.

Nummenmaa, L., Glerean, E., Viinikainen, M., Jääskelänen, P., Hari, R., & Sams, M. (2012). Emotions promote social interaction by synchronizing brain activity across individuals. *Proceedings of the National Academy of Sciences of the United States of America, 109,* 9599–9604.

Nussbaum, M. (2001). *Upheavals of thought.* Cambridge, UK: Cambridge University Press.

O'Reilly, R. C., & Munakata, Y. (2000). *Computational explorations in cognitive neuroscience.* Cambridge, MA: MIT Press.

O'Reilly, R. C., Munakata, Y., Frank, M. J., Hazy, T. E., & Contributors. (2012). *Computational cognitive neuroscience*. http://ccnbook.colorado.edu/

Oatley, K. (1992). *Best laid schemes: The psychology of emotions*. Cambridge, UK: Cambridge University Press.

Organ, T. W. (1987). *Philosophy and the self: East and west*. Selinsgrove, PA: Susquehanna University Press.

Palmer, S. E. (1999). *Vision science: Photons to phenomenology*. Cambridge, MA: MIT Press.

Panksepp, J. (1998). *Affective neuroscience: The foundations of human and animal emotions*. Oxford: Oxford University Press.

Parisien, C., & Thagard, P. (2008). Robosemantics: How Stanley the Volkswagen represents the world. *Minds and Machines, 18*, 169–178.

Pessoa, L. (2013). *The cognitive-emotional brain: From interactions to integration*. Cambridge, MA: MIT Press.

Pinker, S. (1991). Rules of language. *Science, 253*, 530–535.

Pinker, S. (1994). *The language instinct: How the mind creates language*. New York: William Morrow.

Pinker, S. (1999). *Words and rules: The ingredients of language*. New York: HarperCollins.

Plate, T. (2003). *Holographic reduced representations*. Stanford, CA: CSLI.

Poldrack, R. A., & Yarkoni, T. (2016). From brain maps to cognitive ontologies: Informatics and the search for mental structure. *Annual Review of Psychology, 67*, 587–612.

Prentice, D. A., & Miller, D. T. (2007). Psychological essentialism of human categories. *Current Directions in Psychological Science, 16*, 202–206.

Prinz, J. (2004). *Gut reactions: A perceptual theory of emotion*. Oxford: Oxford University Press.

Prinz, J. (2012). *The conscious brain: How attention engenders experience*. Oxford: Oxford University Press.

Prior, H., Schwarz, A., & Güntürkün, O. (2008). Mirror-induced representation in magpies: Evidence of self-recognition. *PLoS Biology, 6*(8), e202.

Putnam, H. (1975). *Mind, language, and reality*. Cambridge, UK: Cambridge University Press.

Quiroga, R. Q. (2012). Concept cells: The building blocks of declarative memory functions. *Nature Reviews Neuroscience, 13*, 589–597.

Quiroga, R. Q., Reddy, L., Kreiman, G., Koch, C., & Fried, I. (2005). Invariant visual representation by single neurons in the human brain. *Nature, 435*(7045), 1102–1107.

Rasmussen, D., & Eliasmith, C. (2014). A spiking neural model applied to the study of human performance and cognitive decline on Raven's Advanced Progressive Matrices. *Intelligence, 42*, 53–82.

Read, S. J., Monroe, B. M., Brownstein, A. L., Yang, Y., Chopra, G., & Miller, L. C. (2010). A neural network model of the structure and dynamics of human personality. *Psychological Review, 117*(1), 61.

Read, S. J., Vanman, E. J., & Miller, L. C. (1997). Connectionist, parallel constraint satisfaction, and Gestalt principles: (Re)Introducing cognitive dynamics to social psychology. *Personality and Social Psychology Review, 1*, 26–53.

Recio, G., Conrad, M., Hansen, L. B., & Jacobs, A. M. (2014). On pleasure and thrill: The interplay between arousal and valence during visual word recognition. *Brain and Language, 134*, 34–43.

Rips, L. J., Smith, E. E., & Medin, D. L. (2012). Concepts and categories: Memory, meaning, and metaphysics. In K. J. Holyoak & R. G. Morrison (Eds.), *Oxford handbook of thinking and reasoning* (pp. 177–209). Oxford: Oxford University Press.

Ritter, S. M., & Ferguson, S. (2017). Happy creativity: Listening to happy music facilitates divergent thinking. *PLOS One, 12*(9), e0182210.

Rogers, T. T., & McClelland, J. L. (2004). *Semantic cognition: A parallel distributed processing approach*. Cambridge, MA: MIT Press.

Rosch, E. B., & Mervis, C. B. (1975). Family resemblances: Studies in the internal structure of categories. *Cognitive Psychology, 7*, 573–605.

Rose, J. D., Arlinghaus, R., Cooke, S. J., Diggles, B. K., Sawynok, W., Stevens, E. D., & Wynne, C. D. L. (2012). Can fish really feel pain? *Fish and Fisheries, 15*, 97–133.

Rosenbloom, P. S., Laird, J. E., & Newell, A. (Eds.). (1993). *The Soar papers: Research on integrated intelligence*. Cambridge, MA: MIT Press.

Roskies, A. (2006). Neuroscientific challenges to free will and responsibility. *Trends in Cognitive Sciences, 10*, 419–423.

Roskies, A. L., & Nichols, S. (2008). Bringing moral responsibility down to earth. *Journal of Philosophy, 105*, 371–388.

Rumelhart, D. E., & McClelland, J. L. (Eds.). (1986). *Parallel distributed processing: Explorations in the microstructure of cognition*. Cambridge, MA: MIT Press/Bradford Books.

Russell, B. (1960). *An outline of philosophy*. Cleveland: World Publishing.

Russell, S., & Norvig, P. (2009). *Artificial intelligence: A modern approach* (3rd ed.). Upper Saddle River, NJ: Prentice-Hall.

Safina, C. (2015). *Beyond words: What animals think and feel*. New York: Macmillan.

Sahdra, B., & Thagard, P. (2003). Procedural knowledge in molecular biology. *Philosophical Psychology, 16*, 477–498.

Schacter, S., & Singer, J. (1962). Cognitive, social, and physiological determinants of emotional state. *Psychological Review, 69*, 379–399.

Scherer, K. R., Schorr, A., & Johnstone, T. (2001). *Appraisal processes in emotion*. New York: Oxford University Press.

Schlegel, A., Kohler, P. J., Fogelson, S. V., Alexander, P., Konuthula, D., & Tse, P. U. (2013). Network structure and dynamics of the visual workspace. *Proceedings of the National Academy of Sciences of the United States of America, 110*, 16277–16282.

Schröder, T., Stewart, T. C., & Thagard, P. (2014). Intention, emotion, and action: A neural theory based on semantic pointers. *Cognitive Science, 38*, 851–880.

Schröder, T., & Thagard, P. (2013). The affective meanings of automatic social behaviors: Three mechanisms that explain priming. *Psychological Review, 120*, 255–280.

Schutt, R. K., Keshavan, M., & Seidman, L. J. (2015). *Social neuroscience: Brain, mind, and society*. Cambridge, MA: Harvard University Press.

Sedikides, C., & Spencer, S. J. (2007). *The self*. New York: Psychology Press.

Shallice, T., & Cooper, R. P. (2011). *The organisation of mind*. Oxford: Oxford University Press.

Shariff, A. F., Greene, J. D., Karremans, J. C., Luguri, J. B., Clark, C. J., Schooler, J. W., . . . Vohs, K. D. (2014). Free will and punishment: A mechanistic view of human nature reduces retribution. *Psychological Science, 25*, 1563–1570.

Shastri, L., & Ajjanagadde, V. (1993). From simple associations to systematic reasoning: A connectionist representation of rules, variables, and dynamic bindings. *Behavioral and Brain Sciences, 16*, 417–494.

Shelley, C. (2003). *Multiple analogies in science and philosophy*. Amsterdam: John Benjamins.

Shelley, C. P. (1996). Visual abductive reasoning in archaeology. *Philosophy of Science, 63*, 278–301.

Siderits, M., Thompson, E., & Zahavi, D. (2011). *Self, no self?* Oxford: Oxford University Press.

Simon, D., Stenstrom, D., & Read, S. J. (2015). The coherence effect: Blending cold and hot cognitions. *Journal of Personality and Social Psychology, 109*, 369–394.

Simon, H. (1962). The architecture of complexity. *Proceedings of the American Philosophical Society, 106*, 467–482.

Simonton, D. (2012). Taking the US Patent Office creativity criteria seriously: A quantitative three-criterion definition and its implications. *Creativity Research Journal, 24*, 97–106.

Simonton, D. K. (1988). *Scientific genius: A psychology of science*. Cambridge, UK: Cambridge University Press.

Simonton, D. K. (2004). *Creativity in science: Chance, logic, genius, and zeitgeist*. Cambridge, UK: Cambridge University Press.

Skinner, B. F. (1976). *About behaviorism*. New York: Vintage.

Slagter, H. A., Johnstone, T., Beets, I. A. M., & Davidson, R. J. (2010). Neural competition for conscious representation across time: An fMRI study. *PLOS One, 5*, e10556. doi:10.1371/journal.pone.0010556

Smith, E., & Medin, D. (1981). *Categories and concepts*. Cambridge, MA: Harvard University Press.

Smith, E. E., & Kosslyn, S. M. (2007). *Cognitive psychology: Mind and brain*. Upper Saddle River, NJ: Pearson Prentice Hall.

Smith, T. W. (2015). *The book of human emotions: An encyclopedia of feeling from anger to wanderlust*. New York: Little, Brown.

Smolensky, P. (1990). Tensor product variable binding and the representation of symbolic structures in connectionist systems. *Artificial Intelligence, 46*, 159–217.

Smolensky, P., & Legendre, G. (2006). *The harmonic mind*. Cambridge, MA: MIT Press.

Soon, C. S., Brass, M., Heinze, H. J., & Haynes, J. D. (2008). Unconscious determinants of free decisions in the human brain. *Nature Neuroscience, 11*(5), 543–545.

Spering, M., Wagener, D., & Funke, J. (2005). The role of emotions in complex problem-solving. *Cognition and Emotion, 19*, 1252–1261.

Spunt, R. P. (2015). Dual-process theories in social cognitive neuroscience. In A. Toga & M. D. Lieberman (Eds.), *Brain mapping: An encyclopedic reference* (pp. 211–215). Amsterdam: Elsevier.

Sripada, C., Kessler, D., & Jonides, J. (2014). Methylphenidate blocks effort-induced depletion of regulatory control in healthy volunteers. *Psychological Science, 25*, 1227–1234.

Stewart, D. (1792). *Elements of the philosophy of the human mind*. London: Strahan, Cadell, and Creech.

Stewart, T. C., Choo, X., & Eliasmith, C. (2014). Sentence processing in spiking neurons: A biologically plausible left-corner parser. In *Proceedings of the 36th Annual Conference of the Cognitive Science Society* (pp. 1533–1538). Quebec City: Cognitive Science Society.

Stewart, T. C., & Eliasmith, C. (2012). Compositionality and biologically plausible models. In W. Hinzen, E. Machery, & M. Werning (Eds.), *Oxford handbook of compositionality* (pp. 596–615). Oxford: Oxford University Press.

Stiles, J. (2008). *The fundamentals of brain development*. Cambridge, MA: Harvard University Press.

Sun, R. (2014). *Anatomy of the mind*. New York: Oxford University Press.

Sutherland, N. S. (1989). *International dictionary of psychology*. New York: Continuum.

Thagard, P. (1988). *Computational philosophy of science*. Cambridge, MA: MIT Press.

Thagard, P. (1992). *Conceptual revolutions*. Princeton, NJ: Princeton University Press.

Thagard, P. (1999). *How scientists explain disease*. Princeton, NJ: Princeton University Press.

Thagard, P. (2000). *Coherence in thought and action*. Cambridge, MA: MIT Press.

Thagard, P. (2002a). How molecules matter to mental computation. *Philosophy of Science, 69,* 429–446.

Thagard, P. (2002b). The passionate scientist: Emotion in scientific cognition. In P. Carruthers, S. Stich, & M. Siegal (Eds.), *The cognitive basis of science* (pp. 235–250). Cambridge, UK: Cambridge University Press.

Thagard, P. (2004). Causal inference in legal decision making: Explanatory coherence vs. Bayesian networks. *Applied Artificial Intelligence, 18,* 231–249.

Thagard, P. (2005a). How to be a successful scientist. In M. E. Gorman, R. D. Tweney, D. C. Gooding, & A. P. Kincannon (Eds.), *Scientific and technological thinking* (pp. 159–171). Mahwah, NJ: Lawrence Erlbaum.

Thagard, P. (2005b). *Mind: Introduction to cognitive science* (2nd ed.). Cambridge, MA: MIT Press.

Thagard, P. (2006). *Hot thought: Mechanisms and applications of emotional cognition.* Cambridge, MA: MIT Press.

Thagard, P. (2009). Why cognitive science needs philosophy and vice versa. *Topics in Cognitive Science, 1,* 237–254.

Thagard, P. (2010). *The brain and the meaning of life.* Princeton, NJ: Princeton University Press.

Thagard, P. (2011). The brain is wider than the sky: Analogy, emotion, and allegory. *Metaphor and Symbol, 26*(2), 131–142.

Thagard, P. (2012a). Cognitive architectures. In K. Frankish & W. Ramsay (Eds.), *The Cambridge handbook of cognitive science* (pp. 50–70). Cambridge, UK: Cambridge University Press.

Thagard, P. (2012b). Creative combination of representations: Scientific discovery and technological invention. In R. Proctor & E. J. Capaldi (Eds.), *Psychology of science: Implicit and explicit processes* (pp. 389–405). Oxford: Oxford University Press.

Thagard, P. (2012c). Mapping minds across cultures. In R. Sun (Ed.), *Grounding social sciences in cognitive sciences* (pp. 35–62). Cambridge, MA: MIT Press.

Thagard, P. (2012d). *The cognitive science of science: Explanation, discovery, and conceptual change.* Cambridge, MA: MIT Press.

Thagard, P. (2014a). Artistic genius and creative cognition. In D. K. Simonton (Ed.), *Wiley handbook of genius* (pp. 120–138). Oxford: Wiley-Blackwell.

Thagard, P. (2014b). Explanatory identities and conceptual change. *Science & Education, 23,* 1531–1548.

Thagard, P. (2014c). The self as a system of multilevel interacting mechanisms. *Philosophical Psychology, 27,* 145–163.

Thagard, P. (2014d). Thought experiments considered harmful. *Perspectives on Science, 22,* 288–305.

Thagard, P. (2019a). *Mind–Society: From Brains to Social Sciences and Professions.* Oxford: Oxford University Press.

Thagard, P. (2019b). *Natural Philosophy: From Social Brains to Knowledge, Reality, Morality, and Beauty.* Oxford: Oxford University Press.

Thagard, P., & Aubie, B. (2008). Emotional consciousness: A neural model of how cognitive appraisal and somatic perception interact to produce qualitative experience. *Consciousness and Cognition, 17,* 811–834.

Thagard, P., & Croft, D. (1999). Scientific discovery and technological innovation: Ulcers, dinosaur extinction, and the programming language Java. In L. Magnani, P. Nersessian, & P. Thagard (Eds.), *Model-based reasoning in scientific discovery* (pp. 125–137). New York: Plenum.

Thagard, P., & Findlay, S. D. (2011). Changing minds about climate change: Belief revision, coherence, and emotion. In E. J. Olsson & S. Enqvist (Eds.), *Belief revision meets philosophy of science* (pp. 329–345). Berlin: Springer.

Thagard, P., & Litt, A. (2008). Models of scientific explanation. In R. Sun (Ed.), *The Cambridge handbook of computational psychology* (pp. 549–564). Cambridge, UK: Cambridge University Press.

Thagard, P., & Millgram, E. (1995). Inference to the best plan: A coherence theory of decision. In A. Ram & D. B. Leake (Eds.), *Goal-driven learning* (pp. 439–454). Cambridge, MA: MIT Press.

Thagard, P., & Nussbaum, A. D. (2014). Fear-driven inference: Mechanisms of gut overreaction. In L. Magnani (Ed.), *Model-based reasoning in science and technology* (pp. 43–53). Berlin: Springer.

Thagard, P., & Schröder, T. (2014). Emotions as semantic pointers: Constructive neural mechanisms. In L. F. Barrett & J. A. Russell (Eds.), *The psychological construction of emotions* (pp. 144–167). New York: Guilford Press.

Thagard, P., & Shelley, C. P. (2001). Emotional analogies and analogical inference. In D. Gentner, K. J. Holyoak, & B. K. Kokinov (Eds.), *The analogical mind: Perspectives from cognitive science* (pp. 335–362). Cambridge, MA: MIT Press.

Thagard, P., & Stewart, T. C. (2011). The AHA! experience: Creativity through emergent binding in neural networks. *Cognitive Science*, *35*, 1–33.

Thagard, P., & Stewart, T. C. (2014). Two theories of consciousness: Semantic pointer competition vs. information integration. *Consciousness and Cognition*, *30*, 73–90.

Thagard, P., & Wood, J. V. (2015). Eighty phenomena about the self: Representation, evaluation, regulation, and change. *Frontiers in Psychology*, *6*. doi:10.3389/fpsyg.2015.00334

Thorstenson, C. A., Pazda, A. D., & Elliot, A. J. (2015). Sadness impairs color perception. *Psychological Science*. doi:10.1177/0956797615597672

Tononi, G. (2012). *PHI: A voyage from the brain to the soul*. New York: Pantheon.

Turner, M. (2014). *The origin of ideas: Blending, creativity, and the human spark*. Oxford: Oxford University Press.

Tversky, B. (2011). Visualizing thought. *Topics in Cognitive Science*, *3*, 499–535.

Ullman, S. (1980). Against direct perception. *Behavioral and Brain Sciences*, *3*, 331–381.

Vartanian, O., Bristol, A. S., & Kaufman, J. C. (2013). *Neuroscience of creativity*. Cambridge, MA: MIT Press.

Vohs, K. D., Finkenauer, C., & Baumeister, R. F. (2011). The sum of friends' and lovers' self-control scores predicts relationship quality. *Social Psychological and Personality Science*, *2*, 138–145.

Vuilleumier, P., & Huang, Y. (2009). Emotional attention: Uncovering the mechanisms of affective bias in perception. *Current Directions in Psychological Science*, *18*, 148–152.

Wagar, B. M., & Thagard, P. (2004). Spiking Phineas Gage: A neurocomputational theory of cognitive-affective integration in decision making. *Psychological Review*, *111*, 67–79.

Wang, H., & Fan, J. (2007). Human attentional networks: A connectionist model. *Journal of Cognitive Neuroscience*, *19*(10), 1678–1689.

Ward, T. B., Smith, S. M., & Vaid, J. (Eds.). (1997). *Creative thought: An investigation of conceptual structures and processes*. Washington, DC: American Psychological Association.

Weaver, I. C., Cervoni, N., Champagne, F. A., D'Alessio, A. C., Sharma, S., Seckl, J. R., . . . Meaney, M. J. (2004). Epigenetic programming by maternal behavior. *Nature Neuroscience*, *7*, 847–854.

Wegner, D. M. (2003). *The illusion of conscious will*. Cambridge, MA: MIT Press.

Weisberg, R. W. (1993). *Creativity: Beyond the myth of genius*. New York: W. H. Freeman.

Wierzbicka, A. (1999). *Emotions across languages and cultures: Diversity and universals*. Cambridge: Cambridge University Press.

Wimsatt, W. C. (2007). *Re-engineering philosophy for limited beings*. Cambridge, MA: Harvard University Press.

Winer, G. A., Cottrell, J. E., Gregg, V., Fournier, J. S., & Bica, L. A. (2002). Fundamentally misunderstanding visual perception: Adults' belief in visual emissions. *American Psychologist*, 57, 417–424.

Wittgenstein, L. (1968). *Philosophical investigations* (G. E. M. Anscombe, Trans. 2nd ed.). Oxford: Blackwell.

Wood, J. N. (2014). Newly hatched chicks solve the visual binding problem. *Psychological Science*, 25, 1475–1481.

Wooldridge, M. (2000). *Reasoning about intelligent agents*. Cambridge, MA: MIT Press.

Yarkoni, T. (2015). Neurobiological substrates of personality: a critical overview. In M. Mikulincer & P. R. Shaver (Eds.), *APA handbook of personality and social psychology* (Vol. 4, pp. 61–83). Washington, DC: American Psychological Association.

Tables and figures are indicated by an italic *t* and *f* following the paragraph number